Concepts and Activities

Maternal-Neonatal Nursing

Concepts and Activities

Maternal-Neonatal Nursing

Aileen MacLaren, CNM, MSN
Instructor of Gynecology and Obstetrics,
Research Associate and Partner of The Johns Hopkins Nurse-Midwives
Johns Hopkins University School of Medicine
Division of Maternal-Fetal Medicine
Baltimore, Maryland

Springhouse Corporation
Springhouse, Pennsylvania

Staff

Executive Director, Editorial
Stanley Loeb

Senior Publisher, Trade and Textbooks
Minnie B. Rose, RN,BSN,MEd

Art Director
John Hubbard

Editors
Diane Labus, David Moreau, Janice Fisher

Copy Editors
Diane M. Armento, Pamela Wingrod

Designers
Stephanie Peters (associate art director), Mary Stangl (book designer), Susan Hopkins, Donald G. Knauss, Laurie Mirijanian, Janice Nawn, Anita Curry (cover design)

Typography
Diane Paluba (manager), Elizabeth Bergman, Joyce Rossi Biletz, Phyllis Marron, Robin Mayer, Valerie L. Rosenberger

Manufacturing
Deborah Meiris (director), Anna Brindisi, Kate Davis, T.A. Landis

Editorial Assistants
Caroline Lemoine, Louise Quinn, Betsy K. Snyder

Library of Congress Cataloging-in-Publication Data

MacLaren, Aileen.
  Maternal-neonatal nursing / Aileen MacLaren.
    p. cm. — (Concepts and activities)
  Includes bibliographical references and index.
  1. Maternity nursing. 2. Infants (Newborn)—Care. I.
Title. II. Series.
  [DNLM: 1. Maternal-Child Nursing. 2. Obstetrical Nursing.   WY157.3 M161m 1994]
RG951.M24 1994
610.73'678—dc20
DNLM/DLC   93-37753
ISBN 0-87434--576-6   CIP

Contents

Acknowledgments

During the early stages of the development of this text, I received helpful guidance from Georgie Labadie, RN, EdD, Professor, University of Miami; Patricia Moccia, RN, PhD, FAAN, Executive Vice President, NLN Competencies Committee, New York; and Susan Sherman, RN, MA, Head Director of Nursing, Community College of Philadelphia. Lorraine Harbold, RN,C, MSEd, NICU Education Coordinator, Johns Hopkins Hospital, Baltimore, also graciously spent several hours lending her expertise to this project.

I especially wish to thank those whose constant friendship and unyielding support sustained me through the trials of writing while doing full-time doctoral studies. I am deeply grateful to my mentor and friend, Terry Gesse, CNM, PhD, for her unfailing belief in my capabilities. Survival would not be possible without the steadfast friendship of Sandy Williamson, CNM, MSN, who braved her own trials during the course of this book. Janice Bowie and Rick, Caroline, and Patrick Driscoll became my invaluable family-away-from-home while at school. My family in Seattle provided love, financial assistance, and a willingness to travel east so that I could continue writing. Bonnie and Ernie also have been faithful companions.

Finally, Pennie Sessler-Branden, CNM, MSN, truly made *all* the difference by contributing her clinical and editorial expertise to the chapter on Antepartal Complications and by kindly bolstering me up to complete the task at hand. Thank you, all, for our unspoken yet integral partnerships.

Dedication
To all my babies, who have shared with me their individual journeys through pregnancy, birth, and their family's unfoldings, so that I may continue to learn what is essential to teach other students of maternal-neonatal nursing.

Preface

Trends in the social structure, economic outlook, and evolving roles within contemporary nursing have shaped the present delivery of nursing care to the childbearing family. Nursing has become increasingly involved in broader aspects of maternal, neonatal, and women's health care; nurses now have specific generalist and specialist roles with different levels of clinical responsibility.

Maternity nurses, integral members of the specialized health care team, are constantly challenged to achieve better maternal-neonatal outcomes. Students of this discipline must become familiar with the expectations involved in providing comprehensive family and maternity care. Students also need to develop an understanding of the basic concepts of nursing care of the childbearing family and be able to apply these in the clinical setting. Further, they must enhance their problem-solving and communication skills within this speciality to be prepared as entry-level providers as well as managers of nursing care for the childbearing family.

This fundamental textbook has been written on the premise that the nursing student will have previously learned basic concepts in anatomy and physiology, particularly of the reproductive system; family dynamics and the relevance of a family-centered approach to nursing care; and the intricacies of using the comprehensive nursing process and its SOAP format. The text highlights the essential content areas in maternal-neonatal nursing and supplies learning objectives to guide the student through each chapter. Each chapter concludes with a wide assortment of study activities designed to assist the student in applying the concepts to clinical situations and to recall important clinical or theorectical information in maternal-neonatal nursing.

Unit One provides the student with an overview of the key areas of conception and fetal development. It begins with a review of all aspects of a healthy pregnancy, including physiological changes, psychosocial concerns, and nutrition, then progresses to more complex issues surrounding antepartal complications.

Unit Two explores nursing care during the intrapartal period, addressing the physiology of labor and childbirth, fetal assessment, stages of labor and delivery, and comfort promotion.

Unit Three discusses the postpartal period, including normal physiology, maternal adaptation, and unexpected complications encountered during this recovery phase of childbirth.

Unit Four offers a review of the physiology of neonatal adaptation, neonatal assessment, care of the healthy neonate, and health concerns of the high-risk neonate.

It is anticipated that the greatest learning and comprehension regarding entry level maternal-neonatal nursing will take place in the dialogue between the nursing instructors and students as they work together to explore each of these content areas. This text is intended to provide a springboard for discussion and a catalyst for a deeper level of investigation, as each student recognizes which areas present the greatest individual challenges to learning. Above all, it is hoped that this text will stimulate an appreciation for this specialized area of clinical practice.

CHAPTER 1

Conception and fetal development

OBJECTIVES After studying this chapter, the reader should be able to:
1. Describe fertilization.
2. Discuss the developmental implications of the embryonic period.
3. Describe the major developmental events of the fetal period.
4. Briefly discuss the functions of the placenta.
5. Identify the special characteristics of fetal circulation.

OVERVIEW OF CONCEPTS Development of a functioning human being from a fertilized ovum involves a complex process of cell division, differentiation, and organization. Development begins with the union of a spermatozoon and an ovum to form a composite cell containing chromosomes from both parents. This composite cell divides repeatedly; individual cells increase in size. Beginning approximately 4 weeks after fertilization, groups of differentiated cells begin to organize into complex structures, such as the brain and spinal cord, liver, kidneys, and other organs that function as integrated units.

A precise timetable governs each developmental step. During this time, the fetus and mother form a relationship via the placenta that provides an environment conducive to fetal growth and well-being.

The time from fertilization to birth is the gestational period. Because few patients know when ovulation occurs, a method using menstrual flow (called "menstrual age") typically is used to estimate the gestational period, from the first day of the last normal menstrual period. Thus, the length of gestation approximates 40 weeks.

Pre-embryonic period Beginning with fertilization, the pre-embryonic period lasts for 3 weeks. Also during this crucial developmental stage, implantation occurs, cells divide rapidly and begin to differentiate, and the placenta and embryo begin to form.

Penetration of an ovum by a spermatozoon marks the beginning of conception. Called fertilization, this event requires coordination of a complex array of physical and chemical factors. (For more information, see *Events leading to conception.*)

When a spermatozoon penetrates an ovum during fertilization, the spermatozoon's tail degenerates and its head enlarges and fuses with the nucleus of the ovum. This restores the cell's genetic component to 46 chromosomes—23 from the spermatozoon and 23 from the ovum.

Successful transfer of genetic information from parents to offspring is a crucial step in normal human development. Genetic disorders may result from monogenic (single gene) factors; chromosomal abnormalities, such as changes in the number or structure of chromosomes; or interactions between genetic alterations and the environment. If a parent's genetic material contains an error or defect, or if an error arises during cell division, offspring may suffer profound deleterious effects.

The fertilized ovum, known as a zygote at the one-cell stage, undergoes a series of mitotic divisions as it continues to travel down the fallopian tube toward the uterus. By the end of the first week after fertilization, the morula (small mass of cells) has begun to implant in the uterine wall.

During the second week of development, the blastocyst cavity develops into two cavities, and the trophoblast differentiates into two cell layers.

During the third week of development, the embryonic disk evolves into three layers,and three new structures are formed: the primitive streak, the notochord, and the allantois. The chorionic villi acquire central cores of mesoderm and now also consist of three layers.

Embryonic period   Early in the fourth week, the flat, pre-embryonic structure becomes a cylindrical embryo that, over the following 4 weeks, nearly triples in size. Embryonic cells undergo complex differentiation and develop into primitive organ systems. (For more information, see *Embryonic development,* page 4.)

Two major events occur during this period: cell differentiation begins and cell organization is initiated.

Especially during this period, drugs ingested by the mother, some viral infections, radiation, and other environmental factors can seriously disturb embryonic development, possibly leading to congenital abnormalities.

In addition, specialized structures that protect and nurture the embryo—including the maternal decidua and fetal membranes—become fully functional during this period.

Each of the germ layers derived from the inner cell mass (ectoderm, mesoderm, and endoderm) will form specific tissues and organs within the developing embryo.

Events leading to conception

A complex process, conception requires the exact coordination of several steps, including gametogenesis, fertilization, and implantation.

The woman's ovaries must produce an ovum, and her body must produce sufficient gonadotropic hormones to allow ovum maturation and release. Her partner's testes must produce sufficient mature, motile spermatozoa (sperm), which must travel through his reproductive system and be ejaculated into her vagina. His reproductive system must produce secretions that permit sperm motility; her vaginal and cervical secretions must allow sperm survival. The ovum must enter a patent fallopian tube at the same time that sperm are present in the tube's distal end. The sperm must penetrate the ovum, and then the fertilized ovum must move through the fallopian tube to the uterus.

The woman's endometrium must have had sufficient hormonal stimulation to allow implantation of the embryo. Her body must maintain appropriate hormone levels to create a uterine environment that allows the embryo to develop and the pregnancy to continue.

If any of these events is interrupted or abnormal, fertilization will not occur or the pregnancy will not be sustained.

Fetal period

Lasting from weeks 8 to 40, the fetal period involves further growth and development of organ systems established in the embryonic period. When fully developed, fetal organs begin to function and supply part of the fetus's metabolic needs. (See *Fetal development,* pages 5 to 7, for illustrations and characteristics of this period.)

Placental development and functions

A flattened, disk-shaped organ of pregnancy that weighs about 500 g, the placenta is derived from the trophoblast and from maternal tissues. The chorion and the villi are formed from the trophoblast and the decidua basalis. The fused amnion and chorion extend from the margins of the placenta to form the fluid-filled sac enclosing the fetus, which ruptures at birth.

The placenta circulates blood between the mother and fetus so that fetal oxygen and nutrients may be provided; in addition, waste products are transferred away from the fetus. This is accomplished through a specialized circulation system in which fetal and maternal blood do not mix. (For more information, see *Placental transfer,* page 8.)

The fetus is connected to the placenta by the umbilical cord, which contains two arteries and a single vein. The arteries follow a spiral course in the cord, divide on the surface of the placenta, and branch to the chorionic villi. Oxygenated arterial blood from the mother is delivered into large spaces between the villi (intervillous spaces) and transferred to the fetus through the single umbilical vein. Oxygen-depleted blood travels from the fetus into the chorionic villi through the two umbilical arteries. This blood leaves the intervillous spaces and flows back into the maternal circulation through maternal veins in the basal part of the placenta.

Embryonic development

During this period, the embryo undergoes rapid growth and differentiation. It develops organ systems, limbs, eyes, and ears; the amnion, yolk sac, and connecting stalk unite to form an umbilical cord with two arteries and one vein.

WEEKS	CHARACTERISTICS
4 weeks	Center of embryonic disk grows more rapidly than periphery as nervous system begins to form; amniotic sac, attached to lateral margins of embryonic disk, follows changing contour of embryo and bends around it; part of yolk sac also becomes enfolded within embryo, and later will form intestinal tract and other important structures; lateral margins of embryonic disk fuse at midline to form ventral (anterior) body wall; fusion is incomplete in middle of body wall where umbilical cord is attached; portion of yolk sac not enfolded within embryo protrudes, still connected to embryo by a narrow duct that eventually degenerates
5 weeks	Head and heart grow rapidly; amnion, yolk sac, and connecting stalk unite to form umbilical cord containing two arteries and one vein; at this time, embryo's four limb buds are most vulnerable to injury by teratogens (such as drugs or radiation)
6 weeks	Head grows larger than trunk and appears to be bent over heart area; eyes, nose, and mouth are more evident; upper limbs have elbows and wrists; hand plates develop ridges called finger rays
7 weeks	Head continues to enlarge and cerebral hemispheres appear; face elongates, placing eyes in a more frontal position; areas over heart and liver are prominent because these organs form earlier than others; limbs continue to develop, especially fingers
8 weeks	Head makes up half of total embryonic mass; a face occupies its lower half, with a flat nose and recognizable mouth; eyelid folds have developed and eyes are far apart; external ears look similar to their final shape; arms, legs, fingers, and toes are distinct; sexual differences may be observed

The fetal-placental unit (umbilical cord, placental layers, and chorionic villi) must have developed properly and be functioning for placental transfer to occur.

In addition to providing the means by which the mother nourishes the developing fetus, the placenta also functions as an endocrine organ; it produces various hormones, including human chorionic gonadotropin (hCG), human placental lactogen (hPL), and the steroid hormones estrogen and progesterone.

HCG can be detected in the mother's serum as early as 8 days after conception, which corresponds to the time the blastocyst is burrowing into the endometrium. For the first 8 weeks of pregnancy, hCG maintains the corpus luteum, which provides the progesterone essential

(Text continues on page 8.)

Fetal development

System development: weeks 8 to 40

The following chart highlights significant events during fetal development and the times they occur.

SYSTEM	WEEKS	CHARACTERISTICS
Nervous	12 to 16 weeks	Structural configuration of brain roughly completed; cerebral lobes delineated; cerebellum assumes prominence
	20 to 24 weeks	Brain grossly formed; myelination of spinal cord begins; spinal cord ends at S-1
	28 to 36 weeks	Cerebral fissures appear; convolutions appear; spinal cord ends at L-3
	40 weeks	Myelination of brain begins
Musculoskeletal	12 weeks	Some bones well outlined; ossification continues
	16 weeks	Joint cavities present; muscular movements detectable
	20 weeks	Ossification of sternum; mother can detect fetal movements (quickening)
	28 to 32 weeks	Ossification continues; fetus can turn head to side
	36 weeks	Muscle tone developed; fetus can turn and elevate head
Cardiovascular	16 to 20 weeks	Fetal heart tone audible with fetoscope
Gastrointestinal	8 to 11 weeks	Intestinal villi form; small intestine coils in umbilical cord
	12 to 16 weeks	Bile is secreted; intestine withdraws from umbilical cord to normal position; meconium present in bowel; anus open
	20 weeks	Enamel and dentin are deposited; ascending colon appears; fetus can suck and swallow; peristaltic movements begin
Genitourinary	8 to 12 weeks	Bladder and urethra separate from rectum; bladder expands as a sac; kidneys secrete urine
	13 to 20 weeks	Kidneys in proper position with definitive shape
	36 weeks	Formation of new nephrons ceases
Respiratory	8 to 12 weeks	Bronchioles branch; pleural and pericardial cavities appear; lungs assume definitive shape
	13 to 20 weeks	Terminal and respiratory bronchioles appear
	21 to 28 weeks	Nostrils open; surfactant production begins; respiratory movements possible; alveolar ducts and sacs appear
	38 to 40 weeks	Pulmonary branching two-thirds complete; lecithin-sphingomyelin (L-S) ratio 2:1
Reproductive	12 to 24 weeks	Testes descend into inguinal canal; external genitalia distinguishable
Endocrine	10 weeks	Islets of Langerhans differentiated
	12 weeks	Thyroid secretes hormones; insulin present in pancreas

(continued)

Fetal development *(continued)*

Physical development: weeks 9 to 40

By the ninth week, the eyelids fuse together, remaining so until the seventh month. The fetus's head remains disproportionately large. Limbs are disproportionately small at week 9, but by week 12 the arms have reached normal proportions. Legs and thighs remain small. The liver begins to produce red blood cells, a function taken over by the spleen at about 12 weeks. At 12 weeks, the placenta is complete and fetal circulation has developed. The skin is pink and delicate. Lacrimal ducts are forming.

By the end of week 16, the head makes up one-third of the total size of the fetus, and the brain is roughly delineated. The forehead is prominent, with lanugo (fine hair) growing on it. The chin is apparent, and the ears are placed higher on the head than previously. Fingernails begin to form. The kidneys function, secreting urine, and the fetus begins to swallow amniotic fluid. Sweat glands form. The lower limbs lengthen and the skeleton ossifies. The intestines withdraw from the umbilical cord to their normal position in the abdomen.

By week 17, the fetus's body is covered with lanugo, and sebaceous glands secrete sebum. This forms the vernix caseosa, a cheeselike material that covers the skin, protecting it from the drying action of the amniotic fluid. Many women feel movement, or quickening, between 16 and 20 weeks. Heart tones may be heard with a fetoscope placed over the symphysis pubis. By 20 weeks, the lower limbs are fully formed.

Although gaining weight steadily, the fetus between weeks 21 and 24 appears lean in comparison with a fetus at term. The wrinkled skin is covered with vernix caseosa. The lungs produce surfactant (a respiratory by-product); meconium (fetal excrement) is present in the rectum. The eyes are structurally complete.

The face matures between 25 and 28 weeks; eyelashes and eyebrows form. Eyelids open and close. Skin is red. Most fetuses are considered viable by week 27 if given highly specialized care.

Between 28 and 32 weeks, subcutaneous fat causes the fetus to grow more rounded. Vernix caseosa forms a thick coat over pink skin. Cerebral fissures and convolutions appear. Born at the end of this period, the neonate has a good chance of survival if adequate care is provided.

Subcutaneous fat increases further during weeks 33 through 38. The fetus has hair and fully formed limbs with fingernails and toenails. Earlobes are soft with little cartilage, but stiffen by week 40. Lanugo disappears from the face but remains on the head. Skin on the fetus's face and body becomes smooth. Amniotic fluid volume declines. The skull continues to be the largest body part. All organ systems are developed and can support extrauterine life. In males, the left testicle descends into the scrotum between 37 and 39 weeks. Both testicles are fully descended by 38 weeks. At week 40 lanugo appears on the upper body.

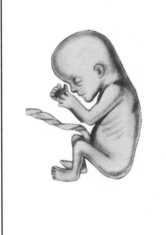

WEEK 12
Approximate length: 70 mm
Approximate weight: 28 g

WEEK 16
Length: 100 to 170 mm
Weight: 55 to 120 g

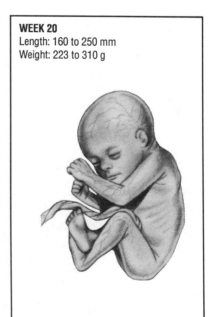

WEEK 20
Length: 160 to 250 mm
Weight: 223 to 310 g

Fetal development *(continued)*

WEEK 24
Length: 240 to 280 mm
Weight: 680 to 1,000 g

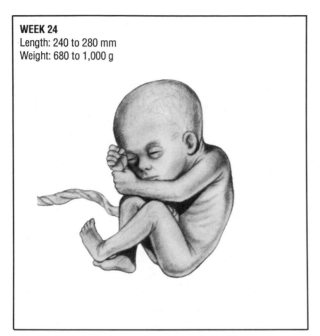

WEEK 28
Length: 350 to 380 mm
Approximate weight: 1,200 g

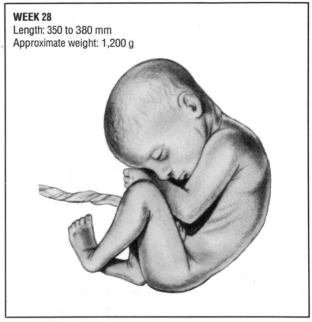

WEEK 32
Length: 380 to 430 mm
Weight: 1,700 to 2,400 g

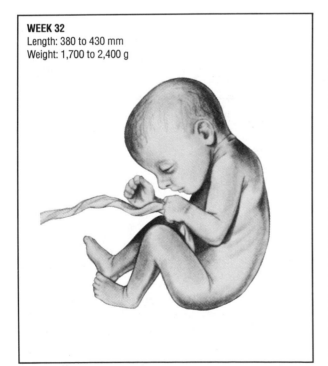

WEEK 38
Length: 480 to 520 mm
Weight: 2,800 to 3,200 g

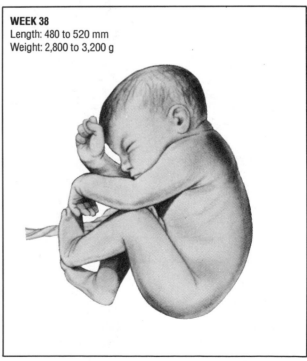

Placental transfer

Many substances can be transported from mother to fetus and back through the placenta. The fetal-placental unit must have developed properly and be functioning for placental transfer to occur.

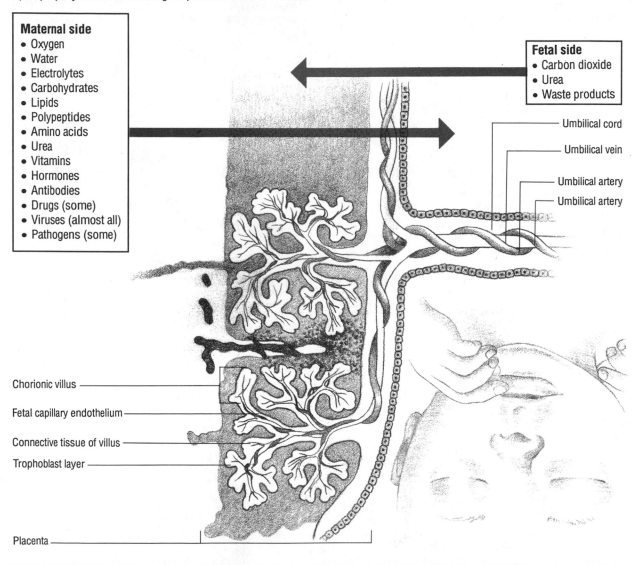

Maternal side
- Oxygen
- Water
- Electrolytes
- Carbohydrates
- Lipids
- Polypeptides
- Amino acids
- Urea
- Vitamins
- Hormones
- Antibodies
- Drugs (some)
- Viruses (almost all)
- Pathogens (some)

Fetal side
- Carbon dioxide
- Urea
- Waste products

Umbilical cord

Umbilical vein

Umbilical artery

Umbilical artery

Chorionic villus

Fetal capillary endothelium

Connective tissue of villus

Trophoblast layer

Placenta

to the pregnancy until the placenta takes over hormone production. This hormone also may regulate maternal and fetal synthesis of steroid hormones, and it stimulates testosterone production by the testes of a male fetus.

The detection of hCG in the blood and urine by immunologic tests is the basis of widely used pregnancy tests. Highly sensitive and specific pregnancy tests can detect hCG in blood and urine even before the first missed menstrual period, and sensitive tests almost invariably are positive if pregnancy causes one missed menstrual period.

HPL stimulates the maternal metabolism of protein and fat to ensure adequate amino and fatty acids for the mother and fetus. It may antagonize the action of insulin in the mother, decreasing maternal glucose use and making it available to the fetus. The hormone also stimulates the growth of the breasts in preparation for lactation. HPL levels rise progressively throughout pregnancy.

Three types of estrogen are produced by the placenta: estrone (E_1), estradiol (E_2), and estriol (E_3). Estrogen production (primarily estriol) and estrogen urinary output increase throughout pregnancy. Progesterone production also increases.

Fetal circulation

Because lungs do not function in a fetus, blood is oxygenated by the placenta. Fetal circulation differs from neonatal circulation in that three shunts bypass the liver and lungs and separate the systemic and pulmonary circulations of the fetus. Because of the shunts, the umbilical vein carries oxygenated blood and the umbilical arteries carry unoxygenated blood. The shunts are:
- the ductus venosus (circulatory pathway that allows blood to bypass the liver)
- the foramen ovale (opening in the interstitial septum that directs blood from the right atrium to the left one)
- the ductus arteriosus (tubular connection that shunts blood away from the pulmonary circulation).

Oxygenated blood returns from the placenta through the umbilical vein. A small amount of this blood passes through the sinusoids of the liver; most is shunted through the ductus venosus into the inferior vena cava. Most of the blood flowing into the right atrium passes through the foramen ovale into the left atrium, bypassing the lungs. Thus, oxygenated blood from the placenta enters the left side of the heart; it is then pumped by the left ventricle into the aorta and then mainly into the vessels of the head and forelimbs.

Unoxygenated blood returns to the right atrium through the superior vena cava and flows downward through the tricuspid valve into the right ventricle. It then is pumped into the pulmonary arteries. Because the lungs are deflated, the blood encounters resistance. Consequently, most of the blood entering the main pulmonary artery bypasses the lungs and flows directly into the aorta through the ductus arteriosus and into the descending aorta. From there, it passes through the two umbilical arteries into the placenta, where the unoxygenated blood can become oxygenated. (See *Fetal circulation*, page 10, for an illustration and description of this specialized process.)

Fetal circulation

This schematic representation of blood flow from the placenta through the fetus and back to the placenta shows the path of oxygenated blood (in white) and unoxygenated blood (in gray) during fetal circulation.

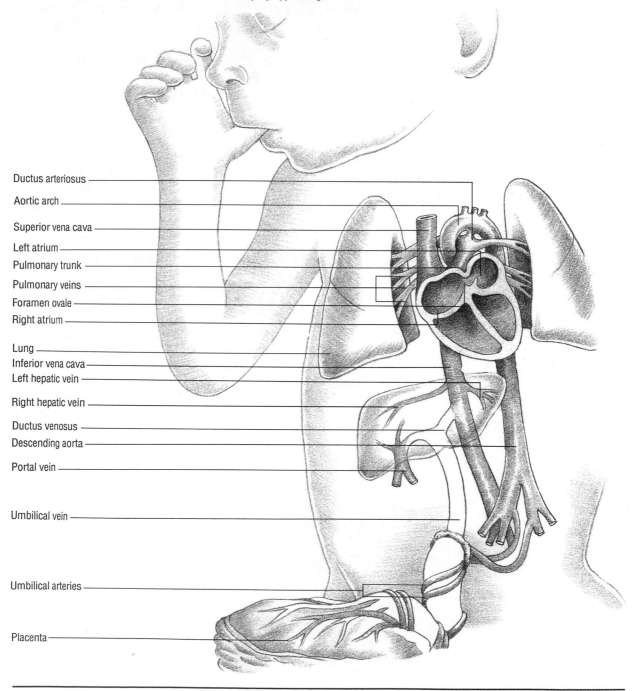

Ductus arteriosus

Aortic arch

Superior vena cava

Left atrium

Pulmonary trunk

Pulmonary veins

Foramen ovale

Right atrium

Lung

Inferior vena cava

Left hepatic vein

Right hepatic vein

Ductus venosus

Descending aorta

Portal vein

Umbilical vein

Umbilical arteries

Placenta

STUDY ACTIVITIES

Short answer

1. Susan and Ernest Delray have been attempting to conceive. Susan asks the nurse how early a pregnancy can be detected. What should the nurse tell her?

_____

2. During a childbirth education class on fetal growth and development, the nurse educator is asked if the mother's blood actually mixes with the fetus's blood. How should the nurse describe the interaction between maternal and fetal circulation?

_____

_____

_____

3. Identify the major functions of the placenta in maintaining maternal-fetal health.

_____

4. How does fetal circulation differ from neonatal circulation?

_____

Fill in the blank

5. The small mass of cells that implants into the uterine wall is known as the _____.

6. _____ occurs when a spermatozoon penetrates the ovum.

7. The prenatal organ derived from the trophoblast and from maternal tissues is called the _____.

8. The _____ is a single cell resulting from the union of female and male gametes.

9. The fused _____ and _____ form the fluid-filled sac enclosing the fetus.

Multiple choice

10. During which gestational period are exposure to drugs, viral infections, radiation, and other environmental factors especially likely to disturb development and lead to congenital anomalies?

    A. Conception
    B. Pre-embryonic
    C. Embryonic
    D. Fetal

11. When fertilization occurs, the genetic component of the newly formed cell is:
   A. 23 chromosomes
   B. 46 chromosomes
   C. 32 chromosomes
   D. 64 chromosomes

12. Certain sensitive pregnancy tests are based on the detection of which hormone?
   A. HCG
   B. Progesterone
   C. HPL
   D. Estradiol

13. Which hormone is responsible for stimulating the maternal metabolism of protein and fat to ensure adequate amino and fatty acids for the mother and fetus?
   A. HPL
   B. Estriol
   C. HCG
   D. Progesterone

True or false

14. Cell differentiation and organization begin during the embryonic period.
   ☐ True   ☐ False

15. The blastocyst burrows into the endometrium as early as 12 days after conception.
   ☐ True   ☐ False

16. At 8 weeks' gestation, the placenta is complete and fetal circulation has developed.
   ☐ True   ☐ False

17. The umbilical cord contains two veins and an artery.
   ☐ True   ☐ False

18. Because lungs do not function in a fetus, fetal blood is oxygenated through the placenta.
   ☐ True   ☐ False

19. Most women feel fetal movement, or quickening, between 13 and 15 weeks' gestation.
   ☐ True   ☐ False

20. Many fetuses are considered viable by week 27 if given highly specialized care.
   ☐ True   ☐ False

21. A neonate born after 32 weeks' gestation has a good chance of survival if adequate care is provided.
   ☐ True   ☐ False

ANSWERS **Short answer**

1. The nurse should tell the patient that certain tests do detect the hormone hCG in the mother's serum as early as 8 days after conception, indicating pregnancy even before the first missed menstrual period. Most commonly, sensitive tests are positive after pregnancy causes one missed period.

2. The placenta circulates blood between the mother and fetus so that fetal oxygen and nutrients may be provided. This is accomplished through a specialized circulation system in which fetal and maternal blood do *not* mix. Oxygenated arterial blood from the mother is delivered into large spaces between the villi (the intervillous spaces) of the placenta and transferred to the fetus through the single umbilical vein. Oxygen-depleted blood travels from the fetus into the chorionic villi through the two umbilical arteries. This blood leaves the intervillous spaces and flows back into the maternal circulation through maternal veins in the basal part of the placenta.

3. The placenta is the means by which the mother provides nutrients and oxygen to the fetus and transfers waste products from the fetus; the placenta also functions as an endocrine organ, producing various hormones.

4. Fetal circulation differs from neonatal circulation in that three shunts—the ductus venosus, the foramen ovale, and the ductus arteriosus—bypass the liver and lungs and separate the systemic and pulmonary circulations of the fetus. Because of the shunts, the umbilical vein carries oxygenated blood and the umbilical arteries carry unoxygenated blood.

Fill in the blank

5. Morula
6. Fertilization
7. Placenta
8. Zygote
9. Amnion, chorion

Multiple choice

10. C. Especially during the embryonic period, drugs ingested by the mother, some viral infections, radiation, and other environmental factors can seriously disturb embryonic development, possibly leading to congenital abnormalities.

11. B. Fertilization restores the cell's genetic component to 46 chromosomes—23 from the spermatozoon and 23 from the ovum.

12. A. HCG in blood and urine can be detected by highly sensitive and specific pregnancy tests even before the first missed menstrual period.

13. A. HPL stimulates the maternal metabolism of protein and fat to ensure adequate amino and fatty acids for the mother and fetus.

True or false

14. True.

15. False. The blastocyst burrows into the endometrium at 8 days after conception.

16. False. The placenta is complete and fetal circulation has developed at 12 weeks' gestation.

17. False. The umbilical cord, which connects the fetus and the placenta, contains two arteries and a single vein.

18. True.

19. False. Most women feel fetal movement between 16 and 20 weeks' gestation.

20. True.

21. True.

CHAPTER 2

Physiologic changes during normal pregnancy

OBJECTIVES   After studying this chapter, the reader should be able to:

1. Distinguish among presumptive, probable, and positive signs of pregnancy.

2. List the major signs and symptoms used to diagnose pregnancy.

3. Discuss physiologic changes that occur in the maternal reproductive, endocrine, neurologic, immune, integumentary, musculoskeletal, cardiovascular, respiratory, gastrointestinal, and urinary systems during pregnancy.

4. Identify the underlying causes for common maternal physiologic changes.

OVERVIEW OF CONCEPTS   Physiologic changes that occur during pregnancy are among the most dramatic that the human body can undergo. They help the patient adapt to pregnancy, maintain health throughout pregnancy, and prepare for childbirth. They also create a safe and nurturing environment for the fetus. Some begin even before the patient becomes aware that she is pregnant.

Physiologic changes associated with pregnancy may range from subtle to overwhelming. Although these changes are normal and necessary, they may be uncomfortable and—especially for the primigravid patient—even frightening. To care for pregnant patients properly, the nurse must understand the physiologic changes of normal pregnancy, when they occur, and how they are likely to affect the patient.

Diagnosing pregnancy   Early pregnancy produces a group of physiologic changes (signs and symptoms) that the health care provider must evaluate before reaching a tentative diagnosis of pregnancy. Some of these changes may be presumptive signs of pregnancy (those that allow an assumption of pregnancy until more concrete signs occur), such as amenorrhea; some may be probable signs of pregnancy, such as abdominal enlargement. Neither presumptive nor probable signs confirm pregnancy because both may be caused by various medical conditions. Positive signs, such as fetal heartbeat and palpable fetal movement, prove pregnancy because they cannot be caused by any other condition. (For more details, see *Presumptive, probable, and positive signs of pregnancy.*)

Changes in body systems

Physiologic changes that help diagnose pregnancy make up only a small number of the changes that occur in a pregnant patient. As the fetus grows and hormones shift, the patient's body systems undergo physiologic changes, primarily to adapt to the fetus and to prepare for childbirth.

Reproductive system

External reproductive structures affected by pregnancy include the labia majora, labia minora, clitoris, and vaginal introitus. These structures enlarge because of increased vascularity; the labia majora and labia minora also enlarge because of fat deposits. Although the structures reduce in size after childbirth, they may not return to their prepregnant state because of loss of muscle tone or perineal injury. In addition, varices may be caused by pressure on vessels in the perineal and perianal areas.

Internal reproductive structures change dramatically to accommodate the developing fetus. Like their external counterparts, these internal structures may not regain their prepregnant states after childbirth.

Ovaries

Once fertilization occurs, ovarian follicles cease to mature and ovulation stops. The chorionic villi, which develop from the fertilized ovum, begin to produce human chorionic gonadotropin (hCG) to maintain the ovarian corpus luteum. The corpus luteum produces estrogen and progesterone until the placenta is formed and functioning. At 8 to 10 weeks of pregnancy, the placenta assumes production of these hormones, and the corpus luteum—no longer needed—undergoes involution (reduction in organ size caused by a reduction in the size of its cells).

Uterus

The nonpregnant uterus is smaller than the size of a fist, measuring approximately 7.5 x 5 x 2.5 cm. Its walls are composed of several overlapping layers of muscle fibers that adapt to the developing fetus and aid in expulsion of the fetus and placenta during labor and childbirth.

The uterus retains the developing fetus for approximately 280 days, or 9 calendar months, and undergoes progressive changes in size, shape, and position in the abdominal cavity.

Enlargement. In the first trimester, the pear-shaped uterus lengthens and enlarges in response to elevated levels of estrogen and progesterone. These changes increase the amount of fibrous and elastic tissue to more than 20 times that of the nonpregnant uterus. Uterine walls become stronger and more elastic. After 12 weeks of pregnancy, the uter-

Presumptive, probable, and positive signs of pregnancy

The following chart lists and describes typical presumptive and probable signs of pregnancy and explains their pregnancy-related and possible other causes. The chart then describes positive signs of pregnancy.

SIGN	DESCRIPTION	PREGNANCY-RELATED CAUSES	POSSIBLE OTHER CAUSES
Presumptive			
Amenorrhea	Absence of menses; usually the first indication of pregnancy in patient with regular menstrual periods.	• Rising levels of human chorionic gonadotropin (hCG) hormone	Anovulation, blocked endo-metrial cavity, endocrine changes, medications (pheno-thiazines), metabolic changes
Nausea and vomit-ing	Onset typically at 4 to 6 weeks, continuing through first trimester or occasionally longer.	• Rising levels of hCG • Emotional stress • Reduced gastric motility, reflux • Altered metabolism	Gastric disorders, infections, psychological disorders (pseudocyesis, anorexia nervosa)
Urinary frequency	Begins during first trimester as uterus enlarges; resolves during second trimester when uterus rises out of pelvis; resumes during third trimester when fetus descends into pelvis.	• Enlarging uterus exerts pressure on urinary bladder	Emotional stress, pelvic tumor, renal disease, urinary tract infection
Breast changes	Enlargement begins early in first trimester. Breasts become tender and may tingle or throb. As pregnancy progresses, nipples enlarge, become more erectile, and may darken. The areolae widen. Veins become more visible.	• Hormonal changes • Growth of secretory ductal system • Increase in glandular tissue	Hyperprolactinemia induced by tranquilizers, infection, prolactin-secreting pituitary tumor, pseudocyesis, premenstrual syndrome
Fatigue	Malaise, general discomfort, lethargy with no apparent cause.	• Unexplained, although progesterone may play a role	Anemia, chronic illness
Quickening	Client's first awareness of fluttering movements in lower abdomen, usually at 16 to 20 weeks.	• Movement of fetus	Excessive flatus, increased peristalsis
Skin changes	May include linea nigra, chloasma, vascular markings, and striae. Because pigment changes may persist, they are not a reliable sign in multigravid clients.	• Increase in melanocyte-stimulating hormone • Increased estrogen • Stretching and atrophy of connective tissue	Cardiopulmonary disorders, estrogen-progestin oral contraceptives, obesity, pelvic tumor
Probable			
Braun von Fernwald's sign (also called Piskacek's sign)	Fullness and irregular softness of fundus near area of implantation. Can be felt at 5 to 6 weeks of pregnancy.	• Local reaction to implantation; increased blood flow to pelvic organs	Uterine tumor
Hegar's sign	Elongation and softening of uterine isthmus may be felt at 6 to 8 weeks via vaginal or rectovaginal examination.	• Increased blood flow to pelvic organs	Excessively soft uterine walls

(continued)

Presumptive, probable, and positive signs of pregnancy *(continued)*

SIGN	DESCRIPTION	PREGNANCY-RELATED CAUSES	POSSIBLE OTHER CAUSES
Probable *(continued)*			
Goodell's sign	Softening of cervix at 6 to 8 weeks.	• Increased blood flow to pelvic organs	Estrogen-progestin oral contraceptives
Chadwick's sign	Bluish coloration of mucous membranes of cervix, vagina, and vulva at 6 to 8 weeks.	• Engorgement caused by increased blood flow to pelvic organs	Hyperemia of cervix, vagina, vulva
McDonald's sign	Easy flexion of fundus onto cervix at 6 to 8 weeks.	• Increased blood flow to pelvic organs	Oral contraceptives, uterine tumor
Ladin's sign	Soft, palpable area on anterior middle portion of uterus near junction of uterus and cervix.	• Increased blood flow to pelvic organs	Oral contraceptives, uterine tumor
Abdominal enlargement	Softening of uterus and fetal growth cause uterus to enlarge and stretch abdominal wall.	• Enlarging uterus	Ascites, obesity, uterine or pelvic tumor
Braxton Hicks contractions	Uterine contractions beginning early in pregnancy and becoming more frequent after 28 weeks.	• Possibly from enlargement of uterus to accommodate growing fetus	Hematometra, uterine tumor
Ballottement	Passive movement of fetus; typically identified at weeks 16 to 18.	• Rebounding of fetus in response to pressure exerted on uterus	Ascites, uterine tumor or polyps
Uterine souffle	Soft, blowing sound synchronous with maternal pulse.	• Increased vascularity as blood flows through placenta	Large ovarian tumor, enlarging myoma
Funic souffle	Sharp, blowing sound synchronous with fetal pulse.	• Increased vascularity as blood flows through umbilical cord	Aneurysm of abdominal aorta, iliac artery, or renal artery
Fetal outline	Fetus may be palpated through uterine wall after 24 weeks.	• Growing fetus	Subserous uterine myoma
Positive pregnancy test	Based on detection of hCG secreted by chorionic villi. Levels of hCG begin to increase 6 to 8 days after conception, peak at 8 to 12 weeks, and then gradually decline.	• Increased levels of hCG	Luteinizing hormone is similar to hCG and may cross react in some pregnancy tests
Positive			
Fetal heartbeat	May be detected as early as week 5 using ultrasound, week 10 using doppler ultrasound, week 12 using fetal electrocardiography, and week 16 using a standard fetoscope	• Fetal cardiovascular development	None
Fetal movement on palpation	May be felt as thump or flutter through abdomen after week 18; may be visible after week 20.	• Fetal growth	None

us typically reaches the level of the symphysis pubis; it then can be palpated through the abdominal wall.

In the second trimester, the corpus and fundus become globe-shaped and, as pregnancy progresses, the uterus lengthens to become oval in shape. The uterine walls become thinner as the muscles stretch; the uterus rises out of the pelvis, shifts to the right, and rests against the anterior abdominal wall. At 20 weeks of pregnancy, the uterus may be palpated just below the umbilicus. As uterine muscles stretch, Braxton Hicks contractions may occur, helping to move blood more quickly through the intervillous spaces of the placenta.

In the third trimester, the fundus reaches nearly to the xiphoid process. Between 38 and 40 weeks of pregnancy, the fetus begins to descend in the pelvis (lightening), which causes fundal height to drop. The uterus remains oval in shape.

Vascular growth. As the fetus grows and the placenta develops, uterine blood vessels and lymphatics increase in number and size. Vessels must enlarge to accommodate the increased blood flow to the uterus and placenta. By the end of pregnancy, an average of 500 ml of blood may flow through the maternal side of the placenta each minute (Cunningham, MacDonald, and Gant, 1989). Maternal arterial pressure, uterine contractions, and maternal position affect uterine blood flow throughout pregnancy.

Cervical changes. The cervix softens and takes on a bluish color during the second month of pregnancy; it becomes edematous and may bleed easily upon examination or sexual activity.

Hormonal stimulation causes the glandular cervical tissue to secrete a thick, tenacious mucus. This mucus forms a plug that blocks the cervical canal and erects a protective barrier against bacteria and other substances that might enter the uterus.

Perhaps the outstanding characteristic of the cervix is its ability to stretch during childbirth, which is possible because of increased connective tissue, elastic fiber, and enfoldings in the endocervical lining.

Vagina

Estrogen stimulates vascularity, tissue growth, and hypertrophy in the vaginal epithelial tissue. Vaginal secretions—white, thick, odorless, and acidic—increase. The acidity of vaginal secretions helps prevent bacterial infections, but it fosters yeast infections, a common occurrence during pregnancy.

Breasts

During the first trimester, increased levels of estrogen and progesterone enlarge the breasts and cause tenderness. The nipples enlarge, become more erectile, and—along with the areolae—darken in color. Sebaceous glands in the areolae become hypertrophic, producing small elevations known as Montgomery's tubercles; the areolae widen.

As blood vessels enlarge, veins beneath the skin of the breasts become more visible and may appear as intertwining patterns over the anterior chest wall. Breasts become fuller and heavier as lactation approaches. Increasing hormones cause the secretion of a yellowish, viscous fluid from the nipples known as colostrum. High in protein, antibodies, and minerals but low in fat and sugar as compared with mature human milk, colostrum may be secreted after the first several months of pregnancy, but it is most common during the last trimester. This secretion continues for 2 to 4 days after delivery and is followed by mature milk production.

Endocrine system

Together with the nervous system, the endocrine system controls metabolic functions that promote maternal and fetal health throughout pregnancy. Estrogen stimulates and temporarily enlarges the pituitary and thyroid glands. Other major endocrine changes occur as well.

Pituitary gland

Two hormones secreted by the anterior pituitary—thyrotropin and adrenocorticotropic hormone (ACTH)—alter maternal metabolism so that pregnancy can progress. Prolactin, another anterior pituitary hormone, increases throughout pregnancy in preparation for lactation.

The posterior pituitary releases two hormones important in pregnancy. Vasopressin (antidiuretic hormone, or ADH) helps regulate water balance through its antidiuretic action; oxytocin stimulates labor and aids in lactation through its effect on breast tissue.

Thyroid gland

Thyroid changes produce a slight increase in basal metabolic rate (BMR), cardiac output, pulse rate, vasodilation, and heat intolerance. As the growing fetus places additional demands for energy on the patient's system, the patient's BMR may increase up to 25% at term. It returns to the prepregnant level within 1 week after childbirth.

Pancreas

Although the pancreas itself undergoes no changes during pregnancy, maternal insulin, glucose, and glucagon levels change. As pregnancy advances, fetal growth and development require increased glucose. The placenta secretes a hormone—human placental lactogen (hPL)—that promotes fat breakdown (lipolysis) and provides the patient with an alternate source of energy.

However, hPL has a complicating effect. Along with estrogen, progesterone, and cortisol, hPL inhibits the action of insulin, which results in an increased need for insulin throughout pregnancy.

Neurologic system

Changes in the neurologic system are poorly defined and incompletely understood. For most patients, neurologic changes are temporary and cease once pregnancy is over.

The patient may experience meralgia paresthetica—tingling and numbness in the anterolateral portion of the thigh that is caused when the lateral femoral cutaneous nerve becomes entrapped in the area of the inguinal ligaments. This is more pronounced in late pregnancy, as the gravid uterus presses on these nerves and as vascular stasis occurs.

In the third trimester, carpal tunnel syndrome may occur when the median nerve of the carpal tunnel of the wrist is compressed by edematous surrounding tissue. The patient may notice tingling and burning in the dominant hand, possibly radiating to the elbow and upper arm. Numbness or tingling in the hands also may result from pregnancy-related postural changes.

Increased metabolism creates the need for greater calcium intake. If the patient ingests insufficient calcium, hypocalcemia and muscle cramps may occur.

Light-headedness, faintness, and syncope may result from vasomotor changes, hypoglycemia, and postural hypotension.

Immune system

Ordinarily, a mature immune system rejects implanted tissue within 2 weeks. During pregnancy, however, the fetus and placenta are protected from the maternal immune system by a mechanism that is not fully understood.

Integumentary system

Skin changes vary greatly among pregnant patients. Skin changes associated with pregnancy include striae gravidarum, pigment changes, and vascular markings.

Striae gravidarum

The patient's weight gain and enlarging uterus, combined with the action of adrenocorticosteroids, lead to stretching of the underlying connective tissue of the skin, creating striae gravidarum in the second and third trimesters. Better known as stretch marks, these streaks develop most often in skin covering the breasts, abdomen, buttocks, and thighs. After delivery, they typically grow lighter.

Pigment changes

Pigmentation begins to change at approximately the eighth week of pregnancy. These changes are more pronounced in such hyperpigmented areas as the face, breasts (especially nipples), axillae, abdomen, anal region, inner thighs, and vulva. Specific changes may include linea nigra and chloasma.

Linea nigra is a dark line that extends from the umbilicus or above to the mons pubis. In the primigravid patient, this line develops at approximately the third month of pregnancy. In the multigravid patient, linea nigra typically appears before the third month.

Called the mask of pregnancy, chloasma refers to irregular, brownish blotches that appear on the cheek bones and forehead. Chloasma appears after 16 weeks of pregnancy and gradually becomes more pronounced until childbirth. Then it typically fades.

Vascular markings

Tiny, bright red angiomas may appear during pregnancy as a result of estrogen release. They are called vascular spiders because of the branching pattern that extends from each spot. Occurring mostly on the chest, neck, arms, face, and legs, they disappear after childbirth.

Palmar erythema, commonly seen along with vascular spiders, refers to well-delineated, pinkish areas over the palmar surface of the hands. Once pregnancy ends and estrogen levels decrease, these changes reverse.

Other integumentary changes

Nevi (circumscribed, benign proliferation of pigment-producing cells in the skin) may develop on the face, neck, upper chest, or arms during pregnancy. Oily skin and acne from increased estrogen may occur. Hirsutism (excessive hair growth) also may occur, but reverses when pregnancy ends.

Musculoskeletal system

The patient's musculoskeletal system changes in response to hormones, weight gain, and the growing fetus. These changes may affect the patient's gait, posture, and comfort.

Skeleton

The enlarging uterus tilts the pelvis forward, shifting the patient's center of gravity. The lumbar and dorsal curves become even more pronounced as breasts enlarge and their weight pulls the shoulders forward, producing a stoop-shouldered stance. Increasing sex hormones (and possibly the hormone relaxin) relax the sacroiliac, sacrococcygeal, and pelvic joints. These changes cause marked alterations in posture and gait. Shoe and ring sizes tend to increase because of weight gain, hormonal changes, and dependent edema. Although these changes may persist after childbirth, they more nearly approach their prepregnant states.

Muscles

In the third trimester, the prominent rectus abdominis muscles separate, allowing the abdomen to protrude at the midline. The umbilicus may flatten or protrude. After childbirth, abdominal muscles regain tone but typically do not return to their prepregnant state.

Cardiovascular system

Pregnancy alters the cardiovascular system so profoundly that, outside of pregnancy, the changes would be considered pathological and even life-threatening. During pregnancy, however, these changes are vital to a positive outcome.

Anatomic changes

The heart enlarges slightly during pregnancy, probably because of increased blood volume and cardiac output. This enlargement is not marked and reverses after childbirth.

Auscultatory changes

Changes in blood volume, cardiac output, and the size and position of the heart alter heart sounds during pregnancy. These changed heart sounds would be considered abnormal in a patient who is not pregnant. For example, many pregnant patients exhibit a systolic ejection murmur over the pulmonic area, which is considered normal during this time.

Cardiac rhythm disturbances, such as sinus arrhythmias, may occur. In the pregnant patient with no underlying heart disease, these arrhythmias do not require therapy, nor do they indicate development of myocardial disease.

Hemodynamic changes

Pregnancy affects heart rate and cardiac output, venous and arterial blood pressure, coagulation, and blood volume.

Heart rate and cardiac output. During the second trimester, heart rate increases gradually until it may reach 10 to 15 beats/minute above the prepregnant rate. During the third trimester, heart rate may increase 15 to 20 beats/minute above the prepregnant rate. The patient may feel palpitations occasionally throughout pregnancy.

Increased tissue demand for oxygen and increased stroke volume raise cardiac output by up to 50% by week 32. A side-lying position reduces pressure on the great vessels, which increases venous return to the heart. Cardiac output peaks during labor, when tissue demands are greatest.

Venous and arterial blood pressure. When the patient lies on her back, femoral venous pressure increases threefold from early pregnancy to term. This occurs because the uterus exerts pressure on the inferior vena cava and pelvic veins, retarding venous return from the legs and feet. The patient may feel light-headed if she rises abruptly after lying on her back. Edema in the legs and varicosities in the legs, rectum, and vulva may occur.

Systolic and diastolic pressures may decrease 5 to 10 mm Hg. Blood pressure reaches its lowest during the second half of the second trimester and then gradually returns to first trimester levels during the third trimester. By term, arterial blood pressure approaches prepregnant levels.

Brachial artery pressure is highest when the patient lies on her back, which causes the enlarged uterus to exert the greatest pressure on the vena cava. This pressure is lowest when she lies on her left side, which relieves uterine pressure off the vena cava.

Coagulation. Blood clots more readily during pregnancy and the postpartal period because of an increase in clotting factors VII, IX, and X.

Blood volume. Total intravascular volume increases during pregnancy, peaking at approximately a 40% increase between week 32 and 34. Volume decreases slightly in week 40 and returns to normal several weeks postpartum. The increase consists of two-thirds plasma and one-third red blood cells, or erythrocytes. The increased blood volume supplies the hypertrophied vascular system of the enlarging uterus, provides nutrition for fetal and maternal tissues, and serves as a reserve for blood loss during childbirth and puerperium.

Hematologic changes

The increase in plasma volume is disproportionately greater than the increase in erythrocytes, which lowers the patient's hematocrit (the percentage of erythrocytes in whole blood) and causes physiologic anemia of pregnancy. The hemoglobin level also decreases. A hematocrit below 35% and a hemoglobin level below 11.5 g/dl indicate pregnancy-related anemia.

The white blood cell (leukocyte) count rises, ranging from 10,000 to 12,000 mm^3. The count may increase to 25,000 mm^3 or more during labor, childbirth, and the early postpartal period.

Fibrinogen—a protein in blood plasma—is converted to fibrin by thrombin and is known as coagulation factor I. In the nonpregnant patient, levels average 250 mg/dl. In the pregnant patient, levels average 450 mg/dl, increasing as much as 50% by term. This increase plays an important role in preventing maternal hemorrhage during childbirth.

Respiratory system

Throughout pregnancy, biochemical and mechanical changes occur in the respiratory system in response to hormonal alterations. As pregnancy advances, these changes facilitate gas exchange, providing the patient with increased oxygen.

Anatomic changes

The anteroposterior and transverse diameters of the rib cage increase, as does its circumference. This expansion is possible because increased progesterone relaxes the ligaments that join the rib cage. As the uterus enlarges, thoracic breathing replaces abdominal breathing.

The upper respiratory tract vascularizes in response to increasing levels of estrogen. The patient may develop respiratory congestion, voice changes, and epistaxis as capillaries become engorged in the nose, pharynx, larynx, trachea, bronchi, and vocal cords. Increased vascularization also may cause the eustachian tubes to swell, leading to such problems as impaired hearing, earaches, and a sense of fullness in the ears.

Functional changes

Changes in pulmonary function improve gas exchange in the alveoli and facilitate oxygenation of blood flowing through the lungs. By the third trimester, increased progesterone may increase the respiratory rate by approximately two breaths/minute.

Tidal volume. Tidal volume (the amount of air inhaled and exhaled) rises throughout pregnancy as a result of increased progesterone and increased diaphragmatic excursion. In fact, the pregnant patient will breathe 30% to 40% more air than she does when not pregnant.

Lung capacity. An elevated diaphragm decreases functional residual capacity (the volume of air remaining in the lungs after exhalation); this decreased functional residual capacity contributes to hyperventilation. Also, vital capacity (the largest volume of air that can be expelled voluntarily after maximum inspiration) increases slightly during pregnancy. These changes, along with increased cardiac output and blood volume, ensure adequate blood flow to the placenta.

Gastrointestinal system

Changes during pregnancy affect anatomic elements in the gastrointestinal system and alter certain functions. These changes are associated with many of the most discussed discomforts of pregnancy.

Anatomic changes

The mouth, stomach and intestines, and gallbladder and liver are affected by pregnancy.

Mouth. The salivary glands become more active, especially in the latter half of pregnancy. The gums become edematous and bleed easily because of increased vascularity. The teeth are unaffected; they lose no minerals to the developing fetus.

Stomach and intestines. As progesterone increases during pregnancy, gastric tone and motility decrease, slowing the stomach's emptying time and possibly causing regurgitation or reflux of stomach contents. The patient may complain of heartburn.

Hormonal changes and mechanical pressure from the enlarging uterus reduce motility in the small intestine. Reduced motility in the colon leads to greater water absorption, which may predispose the patient to constipation. The enlarging uterus displaces the large intestine and puts increased pressure on veins below the uterus, which may predispose the patient to hemorrhoids.

Gallbladder and liver. As smooth muscles relax, the gallbladder empties more sluggishly. This prolonged emptying time, along with increased excretion of cholesterol in the bile caused by increased hormone levels, may predispose the patient to cholesterol crystal formation and gallstone development.

The liver does not enlarge or undergo any major changes during pregnancy. However, some liver function studies show drastic changes, possibly caused in part by increased estrogen levels. These changes would suggest hepatic disease in a nonpregnant patient.

Functional changes

The patient's appetite and food consumption fluctuate. Many women experience nausea and vomiting early in pregnancy. Nausea typically is more pronounced in the morning, beginning at 4 to 6 weeks and subsiding by the end of the first trimester. Some women experience this morning sickness at other hours and beyond the first trimester. Severity varies from a slight distaste for food to severe vomiting.

Although uncomfortable for the patient, morning sickness has no deleterious effects on the fetus. In fact, research suggests that patients who vomit in early pregnancy have a decreased incidence of spontaneous abortion, stillbirth, and premature labor (Klebanoff, Koslowe, and Kaslow, 1985). Morning sickness should be considered abnormal if accompanied by fever, pain, or signs of dehydration.

Once nausea and vomiting cease, the patient's appetite increases as metabolic needs increase. For example, the patient needs more glucose—especially during the second half of pregnancy—to meet increasing energy needs. However, the old adage of "eating for two" is erroneous. (See Chapter 5, Nutrition and diet counseling, for more information.)

Urinary system

The kidneys, ureters, and bladder undergo profound changes in structure and function during pregnancy.

Anatomic changes

As pregnancy advances, the uterus becomes dextrorotated and the ureters and renal pelves become dilated above the pelvic brim, particularly on the right side. In addition, muscle tone decreases, primarily because of the muscle-relaxing effects of progesterone.

These changes retard the flow of urine through the ureters and result in hydronephrosis and hydroureter (distention of the renal pelves and ureters with urine), predisposing the pregnant patient to urinary tract infections.

Hormonal changes cause the bladder to relax during pregnancy, permitting it to distend to hold approximately 1,500 ml of urine. However, hormonal changes and pressure from the growing uterus cause bladder irritation in the early and later months of pregnancy; this manifests as urinary frequency and urgency even if the bladder contains little urine. Bladder vascularity increases and the mucosa bleeds easily.

Functional changes

Pregnancy affects renal tubular resorption, glomerular filtration rate, and nutrient excretion.

Renal tubular resorption. Acting to maintain sodium and fluid balance, renal tubular resorption increases as much as 50% during pregnancy. The sodium requirement increases because the patient needs more intravascular and extracellular fluid. Total body water increases also, to a total of about 7 liters more than in the prepregnant state. The amniotic fluid and placenta account for about half of this amount; increased maternal blood volume and enlargement of the breasts and uterus account for the rest.

Late in pregnancy, changes in posture affect sodium and water excretion. The patient will excrete less when lying on her back because the enlarged uterus compresses the vena cava and aorta, causing decreased cardiac output. This decreases renal blood flow, which in turn decreases kidney function. The patient will excrete more when lying on her left side because, in this position, the uterus does not compress the great vessels.

Glomerular filtration rate and nutrient excretion. The pregnant patient loses increased amounts of some nutrients, such as amino acids, water-soluble vitamins, folic acid, and iodine. Glycosuria (glucose in the urine) may occur as the glomerular filtration rate increases without a corresponding increase in tubular resorptive capacity. Proteinuria (protein in the urine) is considered abnormal in pregnancy. It may occur occasionally during and after difficult labors.

STUDY ACTIVITIES

Short answer

1. Grace Terry, a 32-year-old multigravid patient, is being treated for her second urinary tract infection during her current pregnancy. Which anatomic changes of the urinary tract predispose the pregnant patient to such infections?

_____

_____

2. Why do pregnant patients commonly experience the minor discomfort of heartburn?

_____

3. Ruth St. James, a 28-year-old primiparous patient at 36 weeks' gestation, tells the nurse during a physical assessment that she feels awkward when she walks and that her posture is terrible. How could the nurse explain these alterations in gait and posture to Ms. St. James?

_____

_____

Multiple choice

4. Bonnie Greenwood, age 25, suspects she is pregnant and calls the health center. Ms. Greenwood tells the nurse she is experiencing amenorrhea, urinary frequency, and nausea and vomiting. These signs of pregnancy are:
  A. Presumptive
  B. Probable
  C. Positive
  D. Possible

5. Which findings would be considered positive signs of pregnancy?
  A. Fatigue, skin changes
  B. Quickening, breast enlargement
  C. Fetal heartbeat, fetal movement on palpation
  D. Abdominal enlargement, Braxton Hicks contractions

6. Janice Dill, a 30-year-old primiparous patient at 34 weeks' gestation, comes to the prenatal clinic concerned about the increasing reddish streaks she has developed on her breasts and abdomen. She asks what these skin changes are and whether they are permanent. What should the nurse tell her?

    A. "These streaks are called linea nigra; they'll fade after childbirth."

    B. "These streaks are called hemangiomas; they are permanent changes of pregnancy."

    C. "These streaks are called striae gravidarum, or stretch marks; they'll grow lighter after delivery."

    D. "These streaks are called nevi; they'll fade after the postpartal period."

Fill in the blank

7. The posterior pituitary releases two hormones important in pregnancy; _____ helps regulate water balance through its antidiuretic action, and _____ stimulates labor and aids in lactation through its effect on breast tissue.

8. Thyroid changes in pregnancy produce a slight increase in basal metabolic rate, _____, _____, _____, and heat intolerance.

9. Because the upper respiratory tract vascularizes in response to increasing levels of estrogen, the patient may develop _____, _____, and _____ as capillaries become engorged.

10. Changes in _____, _____, and the _____ and _____ of the heart alter heart sounds during pregnancy.

11. The pregnant patient may experience edema in the legs and varicosities in the legs, rectum, and vulva because the uterus exerts pressure on the _____ and pelvic veins, retarding _____ from the legs and feet.

12. Hormonal changes and mechanical pressure from the enlarging uterus _____ motility in the small intestine; this leads to _____ water absorption, which may predispose the patient to _____.

True or false

13. Maternal arterial pressure, uterine contractions, and maternal position affect uterine blood flow throughout pregnancy.
☐ True   ☐ False

14. The acidity of vaginal secretions helps prevent yeast infections, but it fosters bacterial infections.
☐ True   ☐ False

15. Brachial artery pressure is lowest when the patient lies on her back, which causes the enlarged uterus to exert the least pressure on the vena cava.
☐ True   ☐ False

16. Late in pregnancy, changes in posture affect sodium and water excretion.
☐ True   ☐ False

17. Blood clots less readily during pregnancy and the postpartal period because of a decrease in clotting factors VII, IX, and X.
☐ True   ☐ False

18. The pregnancy-induced increase in plasma volume is disproportionately greater than the increase in erythrocytes, which lowers the patient's hematocrit and causes physiologic anemia of pregnancy.
☐ True   ☐ False

ANSWERS

Short answer

1. As pregnancy advances, the uterus becomes dextrorotated and the ureters and renal pelves become dilated above the pelvic brim. Muscle tone decreases, primarily because of the muscle-relaxing effects of progesterone. These changes retard the flow of urine through the ureters and result in hydronephrosis and hydroureter, predisposing the pregnant patient to urinary tract infections.

2. As progesterone increases during pregnancy, gastric tone and motility decrease, slowing the stomach's emptying time and possibly causing regurgitation or reflux of stomach contents. This reflux causes heartburn.

3. The nurse could explain to the patient that her enlarging uterus tilts her pelvis forward, shifting her center of gravity. The lumbar and dorsal curves of her spine become more pronounced as her breasts enlarge and their weight pulls her shoulders forward, producing a stoop-shouldered stance. Increasing sex hormones (and possibly the hormone relaxin) relax her sacroiliac, sacrococcygeal, and pelvic joints. These normal changes cause marked alterations in her posture and gait.

Multiple choice

4. A. Amenorrhea, urinary frequency, and nausea and vomiting are considered presumptive signs of pregnancy—those that allow an assumption of pregnancy until more concrete signs occur. Presumptive signs do not confirm pregnancy because they may be caused by various medical conditions.

5. C. Fetal heartbeat and fetal movement on palpation are considered positive signs of pregnancy because they cannot be caused by any other condition.

6. C. The patient's weight gain and enlarging uterus, combined with the action of adrenocorticosteroids, lead to stretching of the underlying connective tissue of the skin, creating striae gravidarum in the second and third trimesters. Better known as stretch marks, these streaks develop most often in skin covering the breasts, abdomen, buttocks, and thighs. After delivery, they typically grow lighter.

Fill in the blank
7. Vasopressin, oxytocin
8. Cardiac output, pulse rate, vasodilation
9. Respiratory congestion, voice changes, epistaxis
10. Blood volume, cardiac output, size, position
11. Inferior vena cava, venous return
12. Reduce, greater, constipation

True or false
13. True.
14. False. The acidity of vaginal secretions helps prevent bacterial infections, but it fosters yeast infections.
15. False. Brachial artery pressure is highest when the patient lies on her back, which causes the enlarged uterus to exert the greatest pressure on the vena cava. This pressure is lowest when she lies on her left side, which relieves uterine pressure off the vena cava.
16. True.
17. False. Blood clots more readily during pregnancy and the postpartal period because of an increase in clotting factors VII, IX, and X.
18. True.

CHAPTER 3

Psychosocial changes during normal pregnancy

OBJECTIVES   After studying this chapter, the reader should be able to:

1. Discuss the nurse's role in promoting normal psychosocial adaptation to pregnancy.

2. Identify factors that affect the expectant parents' transition to parenthood.

3. Describe the expectant parents' psychosocial tasks during each trimester of pregnancy.

4. Identify the effects of pregnancy on the couple's relationship and what favors their successful adaptation.

5. Describe the methods that parents can use to prepare siblings for the new family member.

6. Discuss cultural variations that may affect the family's psychosocial experience of pregnancy.

OVERVIEW OF CONCEPTS   Pregnancy and childbirth are psychosocial events that deeply affect the lives of parents and families. Nothing defines the self-concept of most men and women more than the challenge of bearing and raising a child. Pregnancy and childbirth change parents' lives irrevocably, presenting them with a long-term commitment that benefits from intellectual and emotional preparation.

The parents' response to pregnancy and childbirth is affected by psychological, social, economic, and cultural factors and by self-concept and attitudes toward sex-specific and family roles. All of these aspects of childbearing can affect their health and that of their children. Therefore, care of the expectant family presents the nurse with special responsibilities and challenges.

The nurse must facilitate the family's normal adaptation to and integration of the new family member by promoting self-esteem, family integrity, prenatal bonding, conflict resolution, and adaptive coping. To provide appropriate care, the nurse must consider the family's cultural background and avoid imposing personal attitudes about childbearing on others.

Pregnancy: a time of transition

Pregnancy is a time of profound psychological, social, and biological changes that affect the parents' responsibilities, freedoms, values, priorities, social status, relationships, and self-images. The events of the childbearing year (9 antepartal and 3 postpartal months) also may be unpredictable. Although expectant parents can control some events (for example, by obtaining early prenatal care) and can adopt positive attitudes, they cannot control all that happens during that year.

Stress and coping methods

The changes and challenges of pregnancy normally produce stress (psychological and physiologic tension that triggers an adaptive change). Ideally, the pregnant woman will cope realistically with the challenges and adapt to the changes, promoting her health.

Overcrowding, geographic moves, disturbed personal relationships, concerns about the health of the mother or fetus, and economic instability can increase stress during pregnancy. Expectant fathers commonly find the following concerns stressful: the health of the mother and fetus during pregnancy; the neonate's health, normality, and condition at birth; the woman's pain during labor; and unexpected events during childbirth (Glazer, 1989).

First trimester

During the first trimester, the family's key psychosocial challenge is resolution of ambivalence. The mother copes with the common discomforts and changes of the first trimester; the father begins to accept the reality of the pregnancy.

Resolution of ambivalence

The first trimester is known as the trimester of ambivalence because parents experience mixed feelings. Many women have unrealistic ideas about maternal instincts, expecting to feel only loving, happy thoughts about the fetus and motherhood. In fact, most women feel some ambivalence about pregnancy and motherhood (Kitzinger, 1984).

Feelings of ambivalence are inevitable and normal, and partners who discuss them usually can resolve their grief and fears and enjoy the gratifications of expecting a child. When partners share feelings, they may find they are experiencing similar conflicts (Shapiro, 1987).

Coping with common discomforts and changes

In the early weeks of the first trimester, the woman watches for body changes that confirm her pregnancy. Her body image (her mental image of how her body looks, feels, and moves; of her posture, gestures, and physical abilities; and of others' impression of her physical appearance) changes as her breasts enlarge, her menses cease, and she experiences nausea, fatigue, waist thickening, and general weight gain. Depending on her acceptance of the pregnancy, the woman may enjoy or dread these changes.

Preparation for fatherhood

During the first trimester, the father typically finds the pregnancy unreal and intangible. The idea of the fetus may be abstract to him because he cannot observe physical changes in his partner. Accepting the reality of pregnancy is the father's main psychological task in the first trimester (Miller and Brooten, 1983).

Because he is not physically pregnant, the father can choose his degree and type of involvement in the pregnancy. Although each father becomes more involved as the pregnancy advances, his fathering style usually remains consistent (May, 1980).

Because society values a man's provider role, financial concerns remain his major focus throughout pregnancy, and the man may exert tremendous effort to attain financial security. The more secure he feels about his family's economic status, the more open and nurturing he can be with his partner (Muenchow and Bloom-Feshbach, 1982).

Couvade (French for "to brood" or "to hatch") refers to the expectant father's experience of symptoms of pregnancy, including nausea, weight gain, insomnia, restlessness, headaches, inability to concentrate, fatigue, and irritability (Clinton, 1987). Couvade symptoms occur most frequently in fathers who are greatly involved in the pregnancy.

Second trimester During the second trimester, psychosocial tasks include mother-image development, father-image development, coping with body image and sexuality changes, and prenatal bonding. Parents may experience various fears.

Mother-image development

A woman's mother image is a composite of mothering characteristics she has gleaned from role models, readings, and her imagination. Her preoccupation with forming a mother image causes a period of introspection. As a result, she may show less affection, become more passive, or withdraw from her other children, who will react by becoming more demanding. Her partner also may feel neglected during this period.

Father-image development

While the woman develops her mother image, the man begins to form his father image based on his relationship with his father, previous fathering experiences, the fathering styles of friends and family members, and his partner's view of his role in the pregnancy.

Generally, the woman's expectations about her partner's involvement and the quality of their relationship predict the man's role in delivery and child rearing (Reiber, 1976). Some women desire privacy and modesty during childbirth and neither expect nor wish to involve their partners. Others expect their partner's full involvement in tracking fetal movements, attending prenatal visits, and acting as coach, advocate, and primary emotional support during labor.

Coping with body image and sexuality changes

The second trimester often is called a time of radiant health. Physical changes include a heightened sensuality with vasocongestion of the pelvis and increased vaginal lubrication, and 80% of women describe increased sexual gratification, even over prepregnant levels (Colman and Colman, 1977).

The way a woman and her partner view her body's changes will affect her sexual responsiveness and self-image.

Prenatal bonding

A new phase begins at approximately 17 to 20 weeks, when the woman feels fetal movements for the first time. Because fetal movements are a sign of good health and may dispel the fear of spontaneous abortion, the woman almost always experiences the first flutter of movement positively, even when the pregnancy is unwanted.

Prenatal bonding is influenced by the woman's health, developmental stage, and culture, but not necessarily by obstetric complications, general anxiety, or demographic variables, such as socioeconomic level.

This prenatal bonding requires positive self-esteem, positive role models, and acceptance of the pregnancy. Social support improves this attachment (Cranley, 1981), which in turn increases the woman's feelings of maternal competence and effectiveness (Mercer, Ferketich, DeJoseph, May, and Sollid, 1988).

Third trimester During this trimester, psychosocial tasks include adaptation to activity changes, preparation for parenting, partner support, acceptance of body image and sexuality changes, preparation for labor, and development of birth plans. During the third trimester, a key psychosocial task is to overcome fears the woman may have about the unknown, labor pain, loss of self-esteem, loss of control, and death.

Adaptation to activity changes

The growing fetus makes daily activities more difficult for the woman and forces her to slow down. This change can affect her emotional state and her family relationships. Decreased social support for the woman on maternity leave can add to anxiety. Further, her increased dependence during pregnancy and decreased activities outside the home may change the family power structure.

Preparation for parenting

As the woman's body grows larger, the man typically catches up with his partner in anticipating and preparing for the neonate. To prepare for parenting, the couple now may focus on concrete tasks, such as preparing the nursery, making decisions about child care, and planning postpartal events.

Partner support

The couple's ability to support each other through the childbearing cycle is paramount. Relationships that allow flexibility, growth, and risk taking ease role transition.

Acceptance of body image and sexuality changes

Some women are more comfortable with and confident in their bodies during pregnancy, feeling less concerned with each pound of weight gained. Others, however, feel sexually unattractive.

The woman's body image and her partner's feelings affect her sexuality, sometimes diminishing her sexual interest. Some men also experience diminished sexual interest as pregnancy advances. Couples who desire sexual intimacy in the third trimester must be creative, using new positions and techniques. Whether or not the couple remains sexually active, the woman usually desires holding and reassurance.

Preparation for labor

Childbirth education classes can prepare the woman and her partner for labor and delivery. Women who feel supported by their partners during pregnancy and childbirth experience fewer complications and may make an easier postpartal adjustment (May, 1982).

Development of birth plans

A more dependent woman may allow the health care team to make decisions about the birth plans, assuming that their decisions will be the wisest. In contrast, an independent woman may seek health care that is comfortable to her and that fits with her beliefs and knowledge, thus ensuring that her wishes will be honored during labor. A woman who shapes her childbirth experience and who develops realistic expectations of the event has dealt with her fears.

Family and cultural considerations

Throughout the pregnancy, the expectant parents may need to prepare siblings for the new family member and involve the grandparents. Rolfe (1985) suggests that parents share the news of an impending birth positively with their other children and deal with any feelings that arise.

The grandparent-grandchild bond is second in importance only to the parent-child bond. Grandparents provide a sense of family continuity for their grandchildren, sharing family traditions and religious and moral values. They pass on the family history, provide older role models, and, ideally, affirm the vulnerable new parents' self-esteem.

Because the grandparent role is an imposed one, most grandparents have the right to decide what they will offer to grandchildren. Because the parents are in the central position, they must negotiate intergenerational relationships that are comfortable and satisfying for all three generations.

Although each patient has personal beliefs and values, her cultural background may influence her psychosocial adaptation during pregnancy as well as her self-care and health-promotion measures, health-seeking behaviors, and interactions with health care professionals. When caring for a patient from a different culture, the nurse should keep these considerations in mind.

The cultural meanings of pregnancy and parenthood influence a woman's psychosocial experience of the childbearing year and her transition to parenthood. Respecting cultural traditions and beliefs maximizes the patient's social support and personal integrity and the nurse's effectiveness.

STUDY ACTIVITIES

Short answer

1. Corliss and Matthew Hopkins, professionals in their late twenties, are expecting their first child. During the initial prenatal visit at 10 weeks' gestation, the nurse notes that they have many questions about pregnancy and parenthood. What is the Hopkins's key psychosocial adjustment at this stage of the pregnancy? What is Mr. Hopkins's main psychological task at this time?

_____

2. Identify at least four ways that the nurse could facilitate the Hopkins's normal adaptation to and integration of their newest family member.

_____

3. Which factors influence prenatal bonding between a woman and her fetus?

_____

Multiple choice

4. During the second trimester, the father's major psychosocial task is:
   A. Accepting the reality of the pregnancy
   B. Developing a father image
   C. Developing birth plans
   D. Resolving feelings of ambivalence

5. What key psychosocial task must a woman accomplish during the third trimester?
   A. Resolving grief over the loss of old roles
   B. Developing a mother image
   C. Coping with common discomforts and changes
   D. Overcoming fears she may have about the unknown, loss of control, and death

6. *Couvade* refers to:
  A. Vigorous prenatal abdominal massage
  B. The expectant father's experience of symptoms of pregnancy
  C. Continuous maternal nausea and vomiting beyond the first trimester
  D. Overzealous bonding behaviors

Fill in the blank

7. Pregnancy is a time of profound psychological, social, and biological changes that affect the parents' responsibilities, _____, _____, priorities, social status, _____, and self-images.

8. Prenatal bonding requires positive _____, positive _____, and acceptance of the _____.

9. Women who feel supported by their partners during pregnancy and childbirth experience fewer _____ and may make an easier post-partal _____.

10. Although each patient has personal beliefs and values, her _____ background may influence her psychosocial adaptation during pregnancy as well as her self-care and health-promotion measures, _____ behaviors, and _____ with health care professionals.

ANSWERS

Short answer

1. During the first trimester, the family's key psychosocial adjustment is resolution of ambivalence. Accepting the reality of pregnancy is the father's main psychological task in the first trimester.

2. The nurse can facilitate the Hopkins's normal adaptation to and integration of the new family member by promoting their self-esteem, family integrity, prenatal bonding, conflict resolution, and adaptive coping.

3. Prenatal bonding is influenced by the woman's health, developmental stage, and culture; however, it is not necessarily influenced by obstetric complications, general anxiety, or demographic variables, such as socioeconomic level.

Multiple choice

4. B. During the second trimester, the father's major psychosocial task is developing a father image.

5. D. During the third trimester, a key psychosocial task is to overcome fears the woman may have about the unknown, labor pain, loss of self-esteem, loss of control, and death.

6. B. *Couvade* refers to the expectant father's experience of symptoms of pregnancy, including nausea, weight gain, insomnia, restlessness, headaches, inability to concentrate, fatigue, and irritability.

Fill in the blank

7. Freedoms, values, relationships

8. Self-esteem, role models, pregnancy

9. Complications, adjustment

10. Cultural, health-seeking, interactions

CHAPTER 4

Health promotion during the antepartal period

OBJECTIVES

After studying this chapter, the reader should be able to:

1. Discuss general nursing responsibilities during antepartal health assessment.

2. Recognize risk factors that should be assessed during an initial antepartal visit.

3. Calculate the pregnant patient's estimated date of delivery.

4. Outline routine nursing assessments expected during antepartal follow-up visits.

5. Describe nursing interventions for common discomforts of pregnancy.

6. List the danger signs of pregnancy.

OVERVIEW OF CONCEPTS

During the antepartal period, members of the health care team strive to ensure the health of the patient and her fetus. A physician, nurse-midwife, or nurse practitioner may perform the full physical examination, interpret laboratory data, and take pelvimetry measurements. The nurse conducts the initial history, takes vital signs and weight, gathers urine and blood samples, and teaches the patient and family members.

Assessment

Ideally, antepartal assessment begins when a patient seeks health care to confirm a suspected pregnancy and begin prenatal care. During the initial antepartal meeting, the nurse gathers subjective and objective data pertinent to the patient's pregnancy and general health.

Assessment should continue regularly throughout the antepartal period. Traditionally, the patient schedules a routine examination every 4 weeks until the twenty-eighth week of pregnancy, every 2 weeks until the thirty-sixth week, then every week until delivery. However, the number of scheduled examinations depends on the patient's overall condition.

Besides a health history and physical examination, antepartal assessment includes selected laboratory tests. Follow-up care focuses on maintaining the health and well-being of the patient and fetus throughout pregnancy.

Health history

The health history interview should address all pertinent areas of the patient's health—past, present, and potential. The nurse should consider the patient's physical appearance and nonverbal communication as well as her verbal responses to questions.

Biographical data. Record the patient's name, address, telephone number, birth date, and marital status. The patient's age may relate to possible reproductive risks she faces during pregnancy. Investigating the patient's marital status may give the nurse insight into family support systems, sexual practices, and possible stress factors.

Current pregnancy. Ask if the patient menstruates regularly, the typical length of her cycle, the date of her last menstrual period (LMP), and whether the period was normal. If the patient cannot remember the date of her LMP, record it as questionable.

Knowing the date of the LMP is useful in predicting gestational age and estimated date of delivery (EDD). EDD can be calculated using several methods, but Nägele's rule is used most commonly. By Nägele's rule, EDD equals the first day of the last normal menstrual period, minus 3 months, plus 7 days. For example, if the first day of the LMP was September 20, then the EDD will be June 27 of the following calendar year. Nägele's rule is based on a 28-day cycle and must be adjusted if the patient has irregular, prolonged, or shortened menstrual cycles.

Previous pregnancies and outcomes. Discussion and documentation of the patient's previous pregnancies may help the nurse, the patient, and her family anticipate needs and expectations for the current pregnancy. (For more information, see *Documenting previous pregnancies and outcomes.*)

Make note of birth weights, gestational ages, labor outcomes, and neonatal conditions for each of the patient's other children, from the oldest to the youngest. Make special note of any problems or complications she encountered during each pregnancy, labor, and delivery.

If any of the patient's previous pregnancies ended with a miscarriage, stillbirth, or death during the neonatal period, carefully record any contributing factors.

Some risk factors may be linked to ethnic background. Examples include sickle cell disease among Blacks and Tay-Sachs disease among Jews. Refer the couple for genetic counseling, as needed. (For more information, see *Risk assessment for genetic disorders,* page 42.)

Rh factor may raise the risk of complications for some patients. An Rh-negative patient with an Rh-positive partner may need treatment to prevent complications.

Gynecologic history. The patient's gynecologic history may reveal risk factors for the current pregnancy. Determine if the patient used a con-

Documenting previous pregnancies and outcomes

Documentation of a patient's obstetric history should include the number of previous pregnancies (gravidity) and the outcomes of these pregnancies (parity).

The TPAL system uses a single number to indicate gravidity and four numbers to describe parity. The first element, T, stands for the number of term neonates born (37 weeks' gestation or more). The second element, P, stands for the number of preterm neonates born (less than 37 weeks' gestation). The third element, A, stands for the number of pregnancies ending in spontaneous or therapeutic abortion. The fourth element, L, stands for the number of children alive.

For example, a woman who has two living children and was pregnant three times with one pregnancy ending in the birth of a live, full-term infant; one ending in the birth of a premature 35-week gestation infant; and one ending with a spontaneous abortion at six weeks' gestation would be described as gravida 3, para 1112.

Be aware that some institutions use T to refer to the number of term pregnancies, not the number of term neonates; refer to institutional policy.

---

traceptive before becoming pregnant, and how long she used it. Pregnancy that results from contraceptive failure may raise special risks; for example, a failed intrauterine device (IUD) can cause spontaneous septic abortion and should be removed by the physician immediately after verification of pregnancy. Ask if the patient has had recurrent vaginal infections or a sexually transmitted disease, either of which could harm the fetus during development or delivery.

The following factors increase a woman's risk of contracting human immunodeficiency virus (HIV) infection and acquired immunodeficiency syndrome (AIDS):
- having a bisexual male partner
- using illicit intravenous (I.V.) drugs or having a sexual partner who uses such drugs
- having numerous sexual partners
- having a sexual partner with an unknown drug or sexual history
- receiving (or having a sexual partner who received) blood or blood products (especially before HIV safeguards were established in April, 1985).

After a woman contracts HIV and becomes pregnant, she may pass HIV to her neonate at the time of delivery or in breast milk.
Medical history. Collect data about health factors that may be relevant to the current pregnancy.

Previous medical problems. Elicit information about the patient's childhood disease profile, immunizations, past medical conditions and treatments, and any surgical procedures.

Certain medical conditions could place a patient at high risk or jeopardize the pregnancy. These include bleeding disorders, cancer, cardiac disease, diabetes, epilepsy, gallbladder disease, hepatitis, hyper-

Risk assessment for genetic disorders

The health history of the patient and her partner can reveal the risk of genetic disorders and may aid in diagnosing genetic disorders. Risk factors include:
• previous birth of an affected child
• family history of genetic defects
• intrauterine exposure to known teratogens
• part of certain population groups at risk for known genetic disorders
• patient over age 35
• patient's partner over age 40
• history of three or more spontaneous abortions or stillbirths
• consanguinity
• single or multiple congenital abnormalities in a parent or previous offspring
• delayed or abnormal physical or psychological development in a parent or offspring
• mental retardation
• history of failure to thrive in infancy or childhood
• blindness
• deafness
• family history of neoplasms with known hereditary component, such as retinoblastoma

tension, phlebitis, psychiatric problems, renal disease, and recurrent urinary tract infections.

Ask if the patient ever had surgery and, if so, what surgery she had. Previous surgery on the uterus or vagina may have altered their structure, which can complicate delivery. Such patients may require a cesarean delivery.

Inquire whether she has had any X-rays, dental treatments, or surgery since her last menstrual period. X-rays may harm the fetus; some anesthetics may lead to spontaneous abortion.

Exposure to viral or bacterial infections. Determine if the patient has been exposed to or contracted any infections—especially those in the TORCH group—since becoming pregnant. The TORCH group includes *T*oxoplasmosis, *O*ther diseases (chlamydia, group B beta-hemolytic streptococcus, syphilis, and varicella zoster), *R*ubella, *C*ytomegalovirus, and *H*erpesvirus; these infections can harm the fetus.

Ask if the patient has pets at home. Toxoplasmosis, contacted from organisms in cat feces, causes severe congenital anomalies in a fetus infected during the first trimester. Infections contracted from bird and dog parasites may put the patient and fetus at risk as well.

Personal habits. Attempt to determine whether the patient habitually uses substances known to cause or suspected of causing harm to the fetus or to herself.

If the patient smokes, ask how many cigarettes per day. Women who smoke deliver, on average, smaller neonates than those who do not smoke (Naeye, 1981). If the patient does not smoke, ask if she is exposed regularly to a smoke-filled environment, which also presents a risk.

If the patient drinks alcohol, determine how much and how often. A safe level of alcohol intake during pregnancy has not been determined. However, excessive alcohol intake has serious harmful effects on the fetus. The combined effects of alcohol and cigarettes cause a greater number of fetal anomalies than the sum of their individual effects (Brooten, et al., 1987).

Determine how many cups of caffeine-containing coffee, tea, and soda the patient drinks daily. The patient should exercise caution by limiting intake.

Determine if the patient has used marijuana, cocaine, heroin, or other illicit drugs before or since becoming pregnant. These drugs pose serious threats to the health of both patient and fetus. Additionally, the HIV responsible for AIDS can be transmitted via shared needles used to inject drugs.

Medications and allergies. Determine if the patient has taken any prescription or over-the-counter drugs since becoming pregnant; these drugs may adversely affect fetal development. Ask if she has any allergies, especially to medications.

Family health history. Because genetic anomalies and some medical and reproductive conditions are familial, gather family health data. Include the health history of the couple's grandparents, parents, aunts and uncles, and brothers and sisters. Ask whether any member of the patient's family or her partner's family has had any of the following:
• allergies
• anemias
• bleeding disorders
• cesarean delivery
• children born with congenital diseases or deformities
• diabetes mellitus
• heart disease
• hypertension
• kidney problems
• multiple gestations (such as twins)
• pregnancy-induced hypertension (PIH).

Psychosocial assessment. Important areas of psychosocial exploration include the patient's attitude toward her pregnancy, her methods of coping with stress, and how cultural and religious beliefs may affect her pregnancy.

Education and occupation. Educational level may influence the patient's attitude toward pregnancy, the quality of her prenatal care and nutritional intake, her knowledge of neonatal care, and the psychosocial changes that accompany childbirth and parenting.

Identifying the patient's occupation may help detect environmental hazards or exposure to teratogens, such as dry-cleaning fluids or X-rays. A patient who must stand for long periods may develop backache during pregnancy.

Physical assessment

After collecting complete history data, the nurse assists with the physical assessment. The initial examination provides baseline data against which subsequent changes can be evaluated. Follow-up patient visits at regular intervals throughout pregnancy allow the health care team to monitor those changes and detect potential abnormalities.

Weight and height. Record the patient's weight and height. A patient who is underweight or overweight for her height may have poor nutritional habits. Failure to gain weight during pregnancy suggests a serious abnormality. Excessive weight gain—more than 2 lb (0.9 kg) weekly—may result from excessive caloric intake, excessive sodium chloride intake, or PIH.

Vital signs. Record the patient's temperature, pulse, respirations, and blood pressure. Blood pressure normally remains within the patient's prepregnant range. A rise of greater than 30 mm Hg in systolic pressure or 15 mm Hg in diastolic pressure may indicate PIH and should be investigated.

Next, ask the patient to void in preparation for the physical examination. The nurse obtains a urine specimen at this time, which is tested for glucose and protein by dipstick. An empty bladder promotes the patient's comfort during the abdominal and pelvic examinations, which typically are performed by the nurse-midwife, nurse practitioner, or physician.

Maternal status

At each return visit, the nurse asks the patient to describe any changes that have occurred since the previous visit. Compare these changes with those normally encountered by healthy, pregnant women. Question the patient about any symptoms that seem abnormal, such as abdominal pain, vaginal bleeding or discharge, headache, visual disturbances, edema of the face or fingers, or urinary tract pain. (See *Danger signs during pregnancy* for a list of such symptoms.)

On each visit, uterine and fetal growth is monitored by the nurse-midwife or physician and correlated to the estimated gestational age. Fundal height is the characteristic most commonly used to monitor uterine growth.

Fetal status

Document the patient's first report of quickening (fetal movement), which usually occurs between weeks 16 and 20. At each subsequent visit, question the patient about the fetus's activity level. If she reports that the fetus is notably less active, notify the nurse-midwife or physician immediately.

Fetal position is assessed using Leopold's maneuvers. (See Chapter 10, The first stage of labor, for instructions). Fetal presentation may

Danger signs during pregnancy

The nurse should advise the pregnant client to report immediately any of the following signs and symptoms:
- Fever
- Severe headache
- Dizziness, blurred or double vision, spots before the eyes
- Abdominal pain or cramps
- Epigastric pain
- Repeated vomiting
- Absence of or marked decrease in fetal movement
- Vaginal spotting or bleeding (brown or red)
- Rush or constant leakage of fluid from the vagina
- Painful urination or decreased urine output
- Edema of the extremities and face
- Muscle tremors or convulsions

vary during pregnancy but, after week 36, it should remain unchanged until delivery.

Fetal heart tones are evaluated regularly; they can be heard with a Doppler device as early as week 10 and with an ordinary fetoscope as early as week 20. In the case of twins or an obese patient, detection may be delayed.

If suspected abnormalities arise, the nurse-midwife or physician may prescribe special tests to evaluate fetal well-being. For example, the non-stress test and contraction stress test evaluate the oxygen transfer function of the placenta, predicting possible intrauterine asphyxia in high-risk pregnancies. Other tests of fetal well-being include alpha-fetoprotein screening, amniocentesis, chorionic villus sampling, computed tomographic scanning, fetal echocardiography and blood flow studies, fetoscopy, magnetic resonance imaging, and percutaneous umbilical blood sampling.

Diagnostic studies Diagnostic tests that reflect the patient's history and physical findings may include ABO blood group and Rh typing, antibody screening test, complete blood count (CBC), rapid plasma reagent (RPR) test, sickle cell test, rubella antibody test, urinalysis, cervical cultures for sexually transmitted diseases, and Papanicolaou (Pap) test, among others.

The nurse-midwife, nurse practitioner, or physician may decide the patient will benefit from ultrasonography, which displays a two-dimensional echo image of the fetus and surrounding tissues. Ultrasound examination may be ordered to:
- estimate delivery date or "date" the pregnancy
- evaluate fetal growth and condition

• investigate the possibility of ectopic pregnancy, hydatidiform mole, and other anomalies of pregnancy
• determine fetal presentation
• estimate fetal weight
• evaluate fluid volume
• assess placental position and functioning.

Nursing diagnosis

After completing the health history and physical assessment, the nurse analyzes the data and formulates appropriate nursing diagnoses. (See *Selected Nursing Diagnoses: Antepartal period.*) As much as possible, involve the patient in determining appropriate diagnoses, which will increase their usefulness. Also, participation creates a sense of mutual responsibility, preserves the patient's freedom of choice, and fosters her problem-solving ability.

Planning and implementation

The planning phase of the nursing process begins after nursing diagnoses are made. Together, the nurse, other members of the health care team, and the patient set goals and work out ways to implement the plan of care to meet those goals. During the normal antepartal period, nursing goals should include reducing antepartal risks by promoting maternal and fetal well-being, minimizing the discomforts caused by physiologic changes associated with pregnancy, encouraging family adaptation to the addition of a new member, and providing education on antepartal care measures.

Reducing antepartal risks

The nurse must teach the patient and her family about potential risks during the antepartal period and about care required to promote maternal and fetal well-being. These might include teaching about nutrition, exercise, substance abuse, travel, and occupational safety. In addition, without alarming the patient, the nurse should urge her to report promptly any signs that could indicate danger to herself or the fetus. (See *Danger signs during pregnancy,* page 45, for a list of such signs.)

Minimizing discomforts

Discomforts of pregnancy can cause varying amounts of distress for the patient and her family. These discomforts vary with the stage of pregnancy and the size of the uterus. Discuss the patient's comfort level at each antepartal visit and recommend appropriate interventions if she reports problems.

Encouraging family adaptation

Depending on experiences and coping abilities, family relationships may be strengthened or weakened by pregnancy. The nurse intervenes to help the family deal with the changes resulting from pregnancy by being supportive and by providing necessary education for childbirth and parenting.

SELECTED NURSING DIAGNOSES

Antepartal period

The following nursing diagnoses are examples of the problems and etiologies that the nurse may encounter when caring for a client in the antepartal period. To individualize these diagnoses, the nurse would add clarifying signs and symptoms.
- Altered family processes related to inclusion of an additional family member
- Altered nutrition: less than body requirements, related to nausea and vomiting
- Altered sexuality patterns related to fear of harming the fetus during intercourse
- Body image disturbance related to weight gain during pregnancy
- Constipation related to decreased peristalsis
- High risk for injury related to the effect of shifting center of gravity on exercise routine
- Knowledge deficit related to care measures required for optimal pregnancy outcome
- Sleep pattern disturbance related to increased fatigue

Providing education

The nurse instructs the pregnant patient on antepartal care measures in an effort to enhance patient and fetal well-being. Education topics should include rest, breast care, childbirth exercises, clothing, personal hygiene, fetal activity monitoring, preparation for childbirth and parenting, and sexual activity.

Evaluation Evaluation should take place at each antepartal visit. The nurse observes the patient and questions her about problems identified previously. Evaluation statements should reflect actions performed or outcomes achieved for each goal. Examples of evaluation statements for the antepartal period include the following:
- Patient accepts her changing body and has confidence in her partner's acceptance of it.
- Patient and her partner have enrolled in childbirth education classes.
- Patient understands which symptoms could indicate danger to her or her fetus.

Documentation The nurse documents all steps of the nursing process as thoroughly and objectively as possible; this allows more accurate evaluation and better communication between members of the health care team. The nurse must document the nursing activities that are performed. Therefore, documentation for the initial antepartal visit should include minimally:
- the patient's height, weight, and vital signs
- age, occupation, marital status, and social history, including smoking and drug and alcohol use
- number of previous pregnancies and deliveries, and any complications encountered
- relevant data about the patient's past medical history, gynecologic history, and family history
- allergies to medications

- danger signs encountered
- psychological adjustments and areas of concern
- presence and pattern of fetal activity
- patient teaching accomplished
- date of next visit.

The EDD, LMP, and gestation in weeks; fundal height measurement; fetal heart rate and fetal movement patterns; date of quickening; pelvic examination findings; and collection of vaginal specimens for tests are documented by the nurse-midwife or physician who performs these assessments.

Nursing documentation for return prenatal visits includes:
- patient's weight, cumulative weight gain, and vital signs
- danger signals encountered
- patient concerns or symptoms needing evaluation
- prescriptions ordered or laboratory specimens collected
- date of next visit.

STUDY ACTIVITIES

Short answer

1. Tamara Thompson, age 33, has come to the clinic for an initial antepartal visit. During the health history, Ms. Thompson tells the nurse that she has borne three full-term neonates and two preterm neonates, one of whom died shortly after birth; she also had one therapeutic abortion. She confirms that her four children currently are in good health. How would the nurse document her obstetric history using the TPAL system?

_____

2. Ms. Thompson reports that her LMP was May 1. Further questions from the nurse reveal that the period was normal and followed Ms. Thompson's regular 28-day cycle. Using Nägele's rule, calculate the EDD.

_____

3. Josephine Kimbala, a 26-year-old gravida 2, para 1001, comes to the clinic for her initial antepartal visit. She reports that her menstrual cycles have always been irregular; she is uncertain about the date of her LMP. What diagnostic study would the nurse anticipate being ordered to determine Ms. Kimbala's EDD?

_____

4. Ariel Peters, a 27-year-old primigravid patient at 28 weeks' gestation, has completed a routine antepartal examination and wishes to schedule her next appointment. The nurse knows that Ms. Peters has no significant risk factors and has experienced no significant problems during the pregnancy. When should Ms. Peters's next visit occur?

_____

5. How should the nurse respond to Annie Rose, a 23-year old primigravida, who asks what other routine prenatal laboratory tests the nurse-practitioner has ordered besides the sickle cell screening ordered because of her African-American heritage?

_____

6. What subjects are addressed during an initial antepartal health history?

_____

_____

7. When describing the routine, antepartum follow-up visits to Marianne Erickson, a 24-year old primigravida in the clinic for her initial antepartum assessment, how could the nurse explain the usual history and physical assessments that are done at each visit?

_____

_____

_____

8. Identify four general nursing goals that could be integrated into a care plan to facilitate a healthy pregnancy.

_____

_____

Multiple choice

9. At what gestational age range should the nurse advise a prenatal patient to expect quickening?
  A. 10-14 weeks
  B. 12-14 weeks
  C. 16-20 weeks
  D. 24-26 weeks

10. "How early is it possible to hear fetal heart tones with a doppler?", asks a slim multigravida on her first prenatal visit at six weeks gestation. She is anxious to bring her husband in to listen to the baby. What is the nurse's best response?
  A. 8 weeks
  B. 10 weeks
  C. 16 weeks
  D. 20 weeks

Checklist

11. Which of the following signs or symptoms are danger signals of pregnancy that the nurse should investigate for during each visit?

- **A.** ___ Edema of the face and extremities
- **B.** ___ Supine hypotension
- **C.** ___ Leg cramps
- **D.** ___ Severe, continuous headaches
- **E.** ___ Visual disturbances, blurred or double vision
- **F.** ___ Braxton Hicks contractions
- **G.** ___ Fever
- **H.** ___ Urinary frequency and urgency
- **I.** ___ Breast tingling or tenderness
- **J.** ___ Vaginal bleeding or spotting
- **K.** ___ Pain or burning on urination
- **L.** ___ Shortness of breath
- **M.** ___ Muscle tremors or convulsions

ANSWERS

Short answer

1. According to the TPAL system, Ms. Thompson's obstetric history would be documented as gravida 6, para 3214.

2. By Nägele's rule, EDD equals the first day of the last normal menstrual period, minus 3 months, plus 7 days. Therefore, Ms. Thompson's EDD is February 8.

3. Ms. Kimbala's EDD can be determined through ultrasonography, which displays a two-dimensional echo image of the fetus and surrounding tissues.

4. The next visit should occur in 2 weeks. The number of scheduled examinations depends on the patient's overall condition, but the traditional schedule calls for routine examinations every 4 weeks until the twenty-eighth week of pregnancy, every 2 weeks until the thirty-sixth week, then every week until delivery.

5. The nurse would explain to Ms. Rose that the routinely ordered lab tests would also include a CBC, ABO blood group typing and RH typing, antibody screening, a rubella antibody test, an RPR, a urinalysis, a Pap test, and a cervical culture. Any other tests would have to be indicated by history and ordered by the nurse-midwife or physician.

6. The subjects addressed in an initial antepartal health history are the patient's biographical data, current pregnancy, previous pregnancies and outcomes, gynecologic history, medical history, family health history, psychosocial assessment, and education and occupation. Within her medical history, the nurse would assess the patient's weight and height, previous medical problems, exposure to viral or bacterial infections, personal habits, medications, or presence of allergies.

7. The nurse would explain to Ms. Erickson that on her return antepartal visits, she will be asked to describe any changes that occurred since the previous visit. Questions will be asked about any symptoms that seem abnormal such as abdominal pain, vaginal bleeding or irritating discharge, fluid leakage from the vagina, headaches or visual disturbances, swelling of the face or fingers, urinary tract pain, fever, or a change in fetal movement.

Ms. Erickson can expect to have her physical assessment start with her weight, blood pressure, and the collection of a urine specimen for routine testing of protein and glucose. She can expect a regular abdominal exam to monitor uterine and fetal growth through a fundal height measurement. Her fetus's status will be evaluated by Leopold's maneuvers to determine fetal position, and fetal heart tones will be regularly evaluated.

8. During the healthy antepartal period, nursing goals would be to promote maternal and fetal well-being through antepartum risk reduction; to minimize discomforts caused by physiologic changes associated with pregnancy; to encourage family adaptation; and to address the learning needs of the childbearing family by providing on-going education throughout pregnancy.

Multiple choice

9. C. Quickening usually occurs between weeks 16 and 20 depending on the patient's gravidity and obesity.

10. B. Fetal heart tone are regularly evaluated and can be heard with a Doppler device as early as week 10.

Checklist

11. A, D, E, G, J, K, and M are all cardinal danger signs of pregnancy.

CHAPTER 5

Nutrition and diet counseling

OBJECTIVES

After studying this chapter, the reader should be able to:

1. Explain how physiologic changes during pregnancy affect nutrient needs.

2. List nutritional risk factors affecting antepartal nutrition.

3. Discuss the necessary information to be collected during assessment of the pregnant patient's nutritional status.

4. Identify appropriate nutritional goals for the pregnant patient.

5. Describe the nursing interventions to maintain adequate nutrition for the pregnant patient.

6. Address educational needs to assist the pregnant patient towards healthy food choices.

OVERVIEW OF CONCEPTS

The fetus, like every living organism, needs adequate nutrition to thrive. Encouraging the pregnant patient to maintain proper nutrition during pregnancy helps ensure that the nutritional needs of the fetus are met.

Many factors influence the outcome of pregnancy, but few can be controlled as easily by the pregnant patient as nutrition. Many women want to know how to ensure the health of their fetus through proper nutrition. As a result, antepartal diet and nutrition information has increased dramatically during recent years, providing anticipatory guidance for the pregnant patient.

Nutrition and pregnancy

Nutrition before conception and during pregnancy is an important factor in the course and outcome of pregnancy. Even before conception, such factors as degree of body fat, body weight, contraceptive method, and alcohol use can influence nutrition and pregnancy outcome.

Antepartal nutrition

Nutritional deprivation during pregnancy, which adversely affects pregnancy outcome and the fetus, can be avoided through nutritional supplementation. Inadequate weight gain, which frequently is used as a measure of nutrition during pregnancy, also may have adverse effects. *Nutrition supplementation.* Improving the pregnant woman's diet by increasing proper food intake or by adding missing nutritional elements can improve pregnancy outcome. The effects of supplementation depend on the severity of malnutrition. The more undernourished a woman, the greater benefit increased food or added elements will have on her pregnancy outcome.

In the United States, various food programs are available to low-income families who are at high risk for malnutrition. For example, the Special Supplemental Food Program for Women, Infants, and Children (WIC) provides nutrition education as well as coupons for purchasing highly nutritious foods (such as milk, cheese, eggs, iron-fortified cereals, and fruit juices). This national program provides assistance through pregnancy, lactation, and the first 5 years of childhood. Other food programs for eligible families include food stamps obtained from public assistance programs and local food banks when food needs are immediate.

Weight gain during pregnancy. General recommendations that exist for the amount and pattern of weight gain during pregnancy include:

Amount of weight gain. Recommendations for weight gain should take the woman's prepregnancy weight into consideration. For a woman entering pregnancy in her ideal weight range, a gain of 24 to 32 lb (11 to 15 kg) is adequate to meet the needs of the mother and fetus. The weight gain is caused by the weight of the fetus and placenta as well as increased adipose tissue, amniotic fluid, blood volume in the uterus, and fat and duct proliferation in the breasts. The usual recommended gain is 20% of prepregnant weight.

A woman carrying more than one fetus has higher nutrient needs and therefore should gain more weight. The optimal weight gain for a twin pregnancy is about 44 lb (20 kg) for a woman with an ideal prepregnant weight (Pederson, Worthington-Roberts, and Hickok, 1989).

Pattern of weight gain. During the first trimester of pregnancy, a woman normally should gain 3 to 5 lb (1 to 2 kg). Because of nausea and vomiting, however, she may gain no weight during this time. This does not harm the fetus; the weight gain during the first trimester goes largely to maternal changes, such as the growing uterus and breasts and increased blood volume.

During the second and third trimesters, weight gain is essentially linear, averaging 1 lb (0.5 kg) per week. For a woman with more than one fetus, the pattern of weight gain should parallel that for a single fetus until approximately 20 weeks. During the second half of the pregnancy, weight gain should average 1.5 lb (0.7 kg) per week (Pederson, Worthington-Roberts, and Hickok, 1989).

Nutrient needs

During pregnancy, a woman's need for many nutrients increases the recommended dietary allowance (RDA)—the daily amount of a nutrient considered adequate for the needs of most healthy people, depending on sex, age, and reproductive status (for example, pregnant or breast feeding). These nutrients include carbohydrates, fats, and proteins (all energy sources) as well as water, vitamins, and minerals.

RDA Standards

More than 50 nutrients are essential to human life. RDAs have been set by the Food and Nutrition Board of the National Academy of Sciences for 28 nutrients to inform the average, healthy person how much of each to consume daily. RDAs vary for different population groups and are revised periodically to reflect new nutritional knowledge.

Energy. Energy needs increase during pregnancy, and the caloric supply must increase to meet these needs while sparing protein for tissue building. A pregnant woman's energy needs increase 10% to 15%, or about 200 to 300 extra calories/day. (Additional calories may be needed for a woman who is underweight, large-framed, or unusually active).

Carbohydrates. The human body primarily uses blood glucose for fuel; because little transformation is required to turn carbohydrates into glucose, carbohydrates are the preferred energy source. Carbohydrates are found in the diet as starches, sugars, and fiber. All carbohydrates, except fiber, provide 4 calories/g.

Despite the general public's impression that starches and sugars are fattening and unhealthy, both are necessary for a balanced diet. Nutrition experts recommend that 55% to 60% of dietary calories come from carbohydrates. This recommendation holds true during pregnancy.

Fats. Fats are a more concentrated source of calories than carbohydrates, providing 9 calories/g. They are provided mostly through the meat and dairy food groups, although grain products also contain a small amount of fat. Although a small amount of fat (providing 30% or less of total daily calories) is needed, this amount usually can be obtained in normal portions of meat, dairy, and grain products. Therefore, no extra fat is necessary during pregnancy.

Protein. This third source of energy supplies 4 calories/g. Protein is the only energy source for which an RDA exists. It is essential for tissue growth and maintenance, formation of essential body compounds (such as hormones and digestive enzymes), water balance regulation, nitrogen balance, antibody formation, and nutrient transport.

The RDA for protein increases to 60 g for a pregnant woman. Although this increase is significant, the average American woman consumes more than 60 g of protein even when not pregnant. Therefore, many women will not need to increase protein intake further during pregnancy.

Water. Another component essential for human life, water is an important part of the pregnant woman's diet. It is the major component of the fetus, placenta, breasts, and blood.

The human body typically contains 50% to 75% water. Water needs vary according to age, body weight, climate, and activity, but necessary intake is roughly 1 liter of water for each 1,000 calories consumed (NRC, 1989).

Vitamins and minerals. Vitamins are compounds that are needed in small amounts by the body for normal functioning; many serve as coenzymes in cellular reactions. They can be divided into two groups, fat-soluble and water-soluble.

The fat-soluble vitamins—A, D, E, and K—are stored in body fat and usually are found in fat-containing products. Because fat-soluble vitamins can be stored in the body, toxicity is a greater risk with them than with water-soluble vitamins.

Water-soluble vitamins cannot be stored by the body and must be provided daily by the diet. They include the B vitamins and vitamin C. Folic acid (folacin) intake particularly is critical during pregnancy; the RDA for this B vitamin more than doubles, whereas the RDA for other B vitamins and vitamin C increases only slightly. The RDA for folic acid during pregnancy is 400 mcg, compared with 180 mcg for nonpregnant needs.

Minerals are necessary for normal body functioning; they help maintain acid-base and water balance, act as catalysts in cellular reactions, transmit nerve impulses, and contribute to body structures. Calcium needs increase greatly during pregnancy; mineralization of the fetal skeleton requires a large amount of calcium. Although the need for extra calcium is most acute during the last trimester (when the fetal skeleton calcifies), the RDA for calcium throughout pregnancy increases 50%, to a total of 1,200 mg/day.

The RDA for elemental iron during pregnancy is 30 mg/day, twice that for nonpregnant needs. This increase is caused by blood volume increases, and is essential to red blood cell production. The placenta also stores a significant amount of iron. The fetus stores a 6-month supply of iron. The need for iron during pregnancy increases gradually; it is sharpest during the last trimester, when the fetus is storing iron. The body typically absorbs only 5% to 10% of dietary iron. Although this absorption rate doubles during the last half of pregnancy (McGanity, 1987) through unknown mechanisms, dietary intake of iron commonly is insufficient, leading to iron deficiency.

Because of the high dietary intake of iron needed to maintain iron stores during pregnancy (18 to 21 mg/day), and because most patients do not consume iron-rich foods regularly, the NRC (1989) recommends routine supplementation of iron.

With the exception of iron and folic acid, a well-balanced diet needs no supplementation for a healthy pregnant woman; however, the woman may take vitamins and mineral supplements to ensure adequate intake. Whenever possible, nutrient deficiencies should be corrected by dietary changes. Health care professionals who routinely prescribe vitamin and mineral preparations should caution pregnant patients that the supplement is not a substitute for a balanced diet and that oversupplementation can cause problems.

Nursing care   The nurse can identify a pregnant patient's nutritional needs and help her meet them by using the nursing process.

Assessment   Because nutrition is important throughout pregnancy, the nurse should assess it as early as possible and reevaluate it frequently. The initial assessment provides baseline information for the nursing care plan.

The initial and subsequent assessments include a health history, physical assessment, and review of laboratory tests.

Health history

To obtain information about nutritional status review health history data previously collected about the patient's age, medical history, contraceptive history, obstetric history, and personal habits. (See Chapter 4, Health promotion during the antepartal period, for details.)

In addition, gather data on the patient's socioeconomic status, cultural and religious influences, and nutritional intake as they specifically relate to a nutritional assessment.

Socioeconomic status. The patient's occupation, income, educational level, and family may influence her exposure to educational materials, her awareness of community resources, or her knowledge of food and diets. Question the patient about her intake of nutritious foods.

Cultural and religious influences. Find out if the patient's culture or religion affects her through food restrictions, commonly chosen foods, and cooking methods. Cultural and religious factors may determine which foods the patient is likely to include in her diet. Assess whether such factors interfere with proper nutrition.

Nutritional intake. To assess nutritional intake, obtain a diet history from the patient using the dietary recall or dietary record methods. Both can be effective; therefore, use the method best suited to the situation and patient. Perform a diet analysis after obtaining the information.

Physical assessment

Review the patient's vital signs, and determine the appropriateness of her weight for her height. Remember that height-weight tables apply to nonpregnant patients. However, they may be used as a baseline for evaluating the patient's preconception weight and weight gain during pregnancy. If a patient is obviously underweight or overweight, her eating patterns may not be optimal for health.

Although the condition of certain tissues, such as the eyes, skin, hair, and teeth, can give information on nutritional status, physical examination is of limited value. Changes in physical state typically do not occur until a particular deficiency is advanced. Dietary assessment and laboratory tests provide a more accurate view of nutritional status.

Laboratory tests

A few nutritionally related blood tests typically are performed during pregnancy, including hemoglobin levels and hematocrit to identify anemia, mean corpuscular volume (MCV) and mean corpuscular hemoglobin concentration (MCHC) to differentiate folic acid and cobalamin (vitamin B_{12}) deficiencies from iron deficiency anemia. A fasting 1-hour glucose tolerance test (GTT) at 24 to 28 weeks' gestation is used to screen for gestational diabetes, a 3-hour GTT if the 1-hour GTT is elevated.

Nursing diagnosis After reviewing the patient's health history data, diet analysis, physical assessment findings, and laboratory test results, the nurse formulates nursing diagnoses for the patient. (See Selected Nursing Diagnoses: *Nutrition and diet counseling,* page 58.)

Planning and implementation Based on the patient's assessment findings and nursing diagnoses, the nurse establishes goals and then plans and implements interventions to meet the patient's needs.

Basic goals for nutrition throughout pregnancy include:
• adjusting dietary intake to promote appropriate weight gain
• increasing nutrient intake to meet the RDAs for pregnancy
• establishing appropriate food intake patterns for nutrition-related problems, such as anemia and nausea.

Monitor weight gain

Obtain the patient's weight at every prenatal visit and compare it to her prepregnancy weight and her previous antepartal weight measurements.

Characteristically, after the first trimester, a weight gain of 2.5 pounds in one week or 4 pounds in a two-week period is considered excessive. The most common causes of disproportionate weight gain are overeating and fluid retention. Overeating usually results in a overall trend of weight gain that exceeds the norm.

In contrast, a sudden large increase in weight after 20 weeks' gestation may be caused by excess fluid retention. Although some fluid retention is normal, it should occur gradually. A sudden shift in fluid balance can be a symptom of pregnancy-induced hypertension (PIH), especially if blood pressure elevation and proteinuria are present.

Teach about nutrition

When developing a meal plan with the patient, emphasize that the purpose of her diet is to promote fetal health, not to lose weight. Because the term diet may be associated with weight loss, use the term meal plan instead.

Explain which foods will help the patient improve her nutrient intake. Based on the diet analysis, recommend specific foods and portion sizes.

SELECTED NURSING DIAGNOSES

Nutrition and diet counseling

The following nursing diagnoses address representative problems and etiologies that a nurse may encounter when caring for a pregnant client.
- Altered nutrition: more than body requirements, related to excessive caloric intake
- Altered nutrition: less than body requirements, related to inadequate calcium intake
- Altered nutrition: less than body requirements, related to inadequate nutrient intake
- Altered nutrition: less than body requirements, related to nausea and vomiting
- Altered nutrition: less than body requirements, related to strict vegetarianism
- Anxiety related to weight gain
- Constipation related to insufficient fiber intake
- Knowledge deficit related to antepartal nutrition
- Knowledge deficit related to methods of increasing iron intake and absorption during pregnancy
- Knowledge deficit related to blood sugar control through food choices and distribution (for gestational diabetics)
- Knowledge deficit related to nutritional needs
- Knowledge deficit related to nutritional supplements
- Noncompliance with dietary intake recommendations related to desire to remain thin
- Pain related to heartburn and nausea

When developing the patient's meal plan, consider the forces that influence her food choices, including food allergies, food preferences, dietary restrictions related to disorders, and cultural, ethnic, and religious factors. Respect the patient's preferences while helping her select appropriate foods to meet her nutritional needs.

Prevent nutrition-related problems

Teach the iron-deficient patient about iron-rich foods, foods that may increase or decrease iron absorption, cooking techniques to increase iron, and any prescribed iron supplements. Routine iron supplementation has several drawbacks. Iron causes nausea and constipation in one-fifth of women, which contributes to the noncompliance of about one-third of women. Iron-containing multivitamin supplements commonly are prescribed throughout pregnancy however and through 3 months postpartum. Give the patient written instructions to follow at home.

Teach about weight control

Review the patient's beliefs about antepartal nutrition especially if weight control is an identified problem. She may believe the myth that a pregnant woman must "eat for two." To dispel this myth, remind her that the second person for whom she is eating is very small and requires only 150 extra calories a day during the first trimester and 350 during the second and third trimesters. If the patient eats more than that, she may gain more than she needs for her pregnancy and have extra fat to lose after childbirth.

A patient who begins her pregnancy at ideal weight should gain between ½ and 1 pound each week after the first trimester. Overweight patients should gain slightly less, underweight patients slightly more.

Remind the patient to eat three servings of milk, two to three of protein, three to five of vegetables, two to four of fruit, and six to eleven of grains each day. Check portion sizes to ensure she is not over or underestimating serving sizes.

Make referrals

Some patients will need more in-depth nutrition education than a nurse can provide. In these cases, refer the patient to a registered dietitian. Recognized as the nutrition experts in the health-care field, registered dietitians are found in private practices and hospital settings. Suggest that the patient locate one by calling the American Dietetic Association. The patient with financial difficulties may need referral to appropriate social agencies or programs, such as WIC.

Evaluation
State evaluation findings in terms of actions performed or outcomes achieved for each goal. The following examples illustrate some appropriate evaluation statements:
• The patient accurately described her antepartal meal plan.
• The patient agreed to seek financial assistance through WIC to obtain foods for a balanced diet.
• The patient described ways in which she will decrease foods of low nutritional value to help prevent excessive weight gain.

Documentation
When assisting a pregnant patient with nutrition and diet planning, documentation should include:
• appropriateness of prepregnancy weight for height and frame
• current weight
• number of weeks pregnant
• appropriateness of weight gain for number of weeks pregnant
• significant attitudes concerning diet and weight
• significant health history findings
• dietary history
• adequacy of diet
• effects of attitudes on nutritional status
• significant physical assessment and laboratory test data
• patient teaching performed
• nutrition information given to the patient

STUDY ACTIVITIES

Short answer

1. Joan Gabriel, a 25-year-old primigravida, confides in the nurse during her first prenatal visit that she is worried about gaining too much weight. What guidance can the nurse offer Ms. Gabriel regarding the average, expected weight gain during pregnancy? Also identify the components of this weight gain.

_____

_____

2. Describe the expected pattern of maternal weight gain (including weight at conclusion of a full-term pregnancy) for Dawn Scott, a 34-year old gravida 2, para 1001 at thirteen weeks of pregnancy. She had a prepregnant weight of 140 pounds and has a current weight gain of 3 pounds.

_____

3. When teaching a prenatal patient about good nutrition and developing a meal plan, what must the nurse take into consideration that may influence her food choices? How many daily servings from each of the food groups should be recommended?

_____

Multiple choice

4. For the average pregnant woman, energy needs increase 10% to 15% during the second and third trimesters, which can be translated into:
   A. 150 extra calories a day
   B. 200 extra calories a day
   C. 350 extra calories a day
   D. None of the above

5. How much calcium supplementation should the nurse recommend for Hannah Sherwood, a 28-year old gravida 3, para 2002 who has a history of lactose intolerance and states she can't eat any dairy products?
   A. 800 mg
   B. 1,000 mg
   C. 1,200 mg
   D. 1,500 mg

True or false

6. For a woman with a twin pregnancy, the pattern of prenatal weight gain will be double that of a singleton gestation from the onset of the pregnancy.
   ☐ True   ☐ False

7. No extra fats are needed during pregnancy because the recommended amount can be obtained in normal portions of meat, dairy and grains.
☐ True   ☐ False

8. Starches and sugars, sources of carbohydrates in the diet, are generally fattening and unhealthy, especially during pregnancy.
☐ True   ☐ False

9. Protein is essential for tissue growth and maintenance, formation of specify body compounds, water balance regulation, nitrogen balance, antibody formation and nutrient transport.
☐ True   ☐ False

10. Because it's an essential component for human life, a pregnant women should drink approximately one liter of water for each 1,000 calories consumed.
☐ True   ☐ False

11. Calcium needs remain unchanged during pregnancy.
☐ True   ☐ False

12. The absorption rate of dietary iron doubles in the last half of pregnancy.
☐ True   ☐ False

ANSWERS   **Short answer**

1. Recommendations for weight gain take the woman's prepregnancy weight into consideration. For a woman like Ms. Gabriel who enters pregnancy in her ideal weight range, a gain of 24 to 32 pounds is adequate to meet the needs of both her and her fetus. The weight gain is caused by the weight of the fetus and placenta as well as increased adipose tissue, amniotic fluid, blood volume in the uterus, and fat and duct proliferation in the breasts. The usual recommended gain is 20% of prepregnant weight.

2. The expected, ideal gain is 24 to 32 pounds, which is adequate to meet both maternal and fetal needs. Ms. Scott should gain between $\frac{1}{2}$ and 1 pound a week, after the first trimester. Thus, her final weight should be between 164 and 172 pounds.

3. When the nurse is developing the patient's meal plan, influences on food choices that must be considered include: food allergies, food preferences, dietary restrictions related to disorders, and cultural, ethnic and religious factors. The nurse should respect the patient's preferences while helping her select appropriate foods to meet nutritional needs.

4. C. 350 calories are all the extra nourishment that the patient will need in the second and third trimesters.

5. C. 1,200 mg of supplemental calcium should be recommended for Ms. Sherwood because she consumes no dairy products.

True or false

6. False. The optimal weight gain for a twin pregnancy is about 44 pounds. For a woman with more than one fetus, the pattern of weight gain should parallel that for a single fetus until approximately 20 weeks, then 1.5 pounds per week is average.

7. True.

8. False. Despite the public's impression that starches and sugars are fattening and unhealthy, both are necessary for a balanced diet.

9. True.

10. True.

11. False. Calcium needs increase greatly during pregnancy; mineralization of the fetal skeleton requires a large amount of calcium.

12. True.

CHAPTER 6

Selected antepartal complications

OBJECTIVES After studying this chapter, the reader should be able to:

1. Identify common nursing needs of patients experiencing antepartal complications.

2. Recognize the signs and symptoms of selected antepartal complications.

3. Discuss the assessment information to be collected for a patient with an antepartal complication.

4. Interpret significant laboratory and diagnostic test data about the patient with an antepartal complication and her fetus.

5. Describe the maternal, fetal, and neonatal effects for selected antepartal complications.

6. Discuss comfort and support measures for the patient and family.

OVERVIEW OF CONCEPTS A normal pregnancy, even under ordinary circumstances, is accompanied by multiple physiologic and psychological changes. If complications develop, the patient and family can be further challenged. Antepartal complications threaten maternal or fetal health and can interfere with normal fetal development, childbirth, or transition to parenthood.

Antepartal complications that place the mother or fetus at risk can occur throughout the pregnancy. Prior to 20 weeks' gestation, commonly encountered complications include spontaneous abortion, ectopic pregnancy, gestational trophoblastic disease, hyperemesis gravidarum, and incompetent cervix. Some complications result from a mother's previously established medical condition, such as cardiac disease, gestational diabetes mellitus, anemia, or infection; other complications can result from socioeconomic problems such as poverty, limited access to prenatal care, or substance abuse. Still other complications are the direct result of the pregnancy itself and typically present after 20 weeks' gestation, such as in pregnancy-induced hypertension, Rh incompatibility, premature rupture of membranes, or preterm labor and delivery.

Nursing responsibilities

Care of patients with antepartal complications requries experienced, vigilant nursing expertise. The nurse utilizes the nursing process to develop effective strategies to respond to current and potential needs and problems while promoting the patient's health.

Assessment

In order to build a useful, current data base, collect a detailed health history, assist with a thorough physical examination, and obtain appropriate diagnostic studies, as prescribed.

Health history

Begin by assessing the patient's present health status so that it can be evaluated with her personal and family health history. This may uncover a previously undetected problem and suggest the need for specific tests. Next, ask the patient to identify any medical problems for which she is receiving care, such as a cardiac disease or diabetes. Signs and symptoms caused by this problem should be investigated. Also note the effectiveness of the patient's current regimen in managing any previously diagnosed condition.

Collect the patient's past and present obstetric history. Any obstetric problems, including spontaneous abortion or stillbirth, may be related to an undiagnosed or uncorrected condition. Obstetric problems may recur unless the patient is properly tested and treated.

Physical assessment

Obtain the patient's vital signs and weight. Document these baseline data and compare them to preconception measurements to detect significant changes. Then assist with a head-to-toe physical assessment, including a pelvic examination.

Diagnostic studies

Additional assessment data may be ordered from routine prenatal laboratory tests, including coagulation studies, blood glucose levels, electrolyte and cardiac enzyme levels, hepatitis B screening, and HIV assay. Also note the results of any fetal diagnostic studies that were performed (see *Fetal testing*).

Nursing diagnoses

After considering all assessment findings, formulate appropriate nursing diagnoses for the patient. (For a partial list of applicable diagnoses, see Nursing Diagnoses: *Antepartal complications,* pages 66 and 67.)

Planning and implementation

After assessing the patient with antepartal complications and formulating nursing diagnoses, develop and implement a plan of care centered on the following common nursing goals:
• promoting the physical well-being of the patient and her fetus
• preventing or controlling further complications
• preventing sequelae
• providing emotional support to the patient and her family.

Fetal testing

The patient with an antepartal complication may benefit from antepartal testing, which may be noninvasive (occurring outside the body) or invasive (requiring entry into the body). The chart below describes various antepartal tests.

NONINVASIVE TESTS
Ultrasonography
- Determines position of the uterus and cervix, size and position of the developing fetus, area of placental formation, and cord insertion site
- Differentiates between a normal and abnormal fetus
- Determines number of fetuses, congenital abnormality, ectopic pregnancy, and amniotic fluid volume
- Diagnoses fetal death through absence of fetal heart sounds and fetal movements or by identifying overlapping of fetal skull sutures
- Estimates gestational age by
- Provides a baseline that allows meaningful interpretation of fetal growth during the pregnancy

Fetal movement count
- Provides a rough index of fetal health. Wide variations in normal fetal movement exist. However, the pattern of movement should not change greatly during her pregnancy. (Fetal movements normally decrease during fetal sleep periods, when maternal serum glucose levels are low, and during maternal use of tobacco or a central nervous system depressant.)

Biophysical profile (BPP)
- Predicts perinatal asphyxia
- Assesses fetal risks
- Detects fetal anomalies

Nonstress test (NST)
- Assesses fetal well-being
- Reactive (favorable) results show two to three fetal heart rate (FHR) increases of 15 or more beats/minute (bpm), lasting for 15 or more seconds over 20 to 30 minutes. These increases occur with fetal movement. Nonreactive (unfavorable) results occur when the FHR response does not rise by 15 or more bpm over the specified time; they may indicate fetal hypoxia.

INVASIVE TESTS
Chorionic villus sampling (CVS)
- Diagnoses fetal karyotype, hemoglobinopathies (sickle cell anemia, alpha and some beta thalassemias), alpha$_1$-antitrypsin deficiency, phenylketonuria, Down's syndrome, and Duchenne muscular dystrophy

Alpha-fetoprotein (AFP) test
- Predicts open neural tube defects (NTDs), such as spina bifida and anencephaly, and screens for Down's syndrome

Amniocentesis
- Detects genetic disorders
- Diagnoses various fetal defects, including chromosomal anomalies, skeletal disorders, infections, central nervous system disorders, blood disorders, inborn errors of metabolism, miscellaneous metabolic disorders, and porphyrias
- Assesses fetal lung maturity during the third trimester by evaluating the lecithin/sphingomyelin (L/S) ratio in the amniotic fluid

Percutaneous umbilical blood sampling (PUBS)
- Diagnoses fetal blood disorders, such as coagulopathies, hemoglobinopathies, and hemophilias; congenital infections, such as rubella and toxoplasmosis; and chromosomal abnormalities
- Treats Rh isoimmunization through blood transfusions

Oxytocin contraction test (OCT)
- Evaluates the FHR in response to uterine contractions

Nursing care is holistic and encompasses the patient, her fetus, and her family. The nurse monitors trends in the patient's health; teaches about the condition, its management, and effects; promotes adequate rest, exercise, and nutrition; prevents infection; provides support; promotes family well-being; monitors fetal health; and promotes compliance.

Evaluation
Care of the patient with antepartal complications requires a multidisciplinary approach throughout preconception, antepartal, intrapartal, and

NURSING DIAGNOSES

Antepartal complications

The following nursing diagnoses address representative problems and etiologies that a nurse may encounter when providing care for a high-risk antepartal patient. Specific nursing interventions for many of these diagnoses are provided in the "Planning and implementation" sections of this chapter.

Spontaneous abortion
- Anticipatory grieving related to loss of pregnancy
- Denial related to impending loss of pregnancy
- Ineffective family coping: compromised, related to ineffective support as manifested in the partner's expressed frustration with the patient
- Situational low self-esteem related to the inability to maintain pregnancy as manifested by crying and by verbalizing guilt

Ectopic pregnancy
- Anticipatory grieving related to loss of pregnancy
- Decreased cardiac output related to bleeding at the site of ectopic pregnancy rupture
- Denial related to tubal pregnancy as manifested by minimization of symptoms and use of home remedies to relieve symptoms

Gestational trophoblastic disease
- Anxiety related to the unknown
- Knowledge deficit related to necessary follow-up care

Hyperemesis gravidarum
- Fluid volume deficit related to persistent vomiting
- Ineffective management of therapeutic regimen, related to hospitalization for persistent vomiting
- Situational low self-esteem related to persistent vomiting

Incompetent cervix
- Anticipatory grieving related to potential loss of a fetus
- Impaired physical mobility related to prescribed bed rest

- Ineffective family coping: compromised, related to prolonged bed rest of the mother
- Knowledge deficit related to in-home uterine monitoring
- Situational low self-esteem related to diagnosis of incompetent cervix

Cardiac disease
- Activity intolerance related to fluid retention leading to rapid weight gain and edema
- Activity intolerance related to altered cardiac function and decreased tissue oxygenation
- Altered cardiopulmonary tissue perfusion related to decreased cardiac output
- High risk for infection related to altered cardiac status
- Impaired gas exchange related to decreased cardiac output
- Knowledge deficit related to cardiac disease management during pregnancy

Diabetes mellitus
- Activity intolerance related to rapid weight gain and fluid retention
- Altered nutrition related to altered carbohydrate metabolism
- Altered peripheral tissue perfusion related to vascular impairment
- Anxiety related to maternal, fetal, and neonatal effects of diabetes
- High risk for infection related to metabolic and vascular abnormalities
- Knowledge deficit related to the effects of diabetes on pregnancy and future health
- Noncompliance related to specified diet, schedules for serum glucose testing, or insulin administration

Hypertensive disorders
- Constipation related to bed rest
- Impaired physical mobility related to prescribed bed rest
- Ineffective family coping: compromised, related to prolonged bed rest of the mother
- Knowledge deficit related to hypertensive disorder

Anemias
- Altered nutrition: less than body requirements, related to increased need for iron-rich foods
- Altered peripheral tissue perfusion related to inadequate blood supply
- Fatigue related to decreased oxygen-carrying capacity of the blood
- High risk for infection related to altered red blood cells structure and tissue perfusion
- Knowledge deficit related to the effects of anemia on pregnancy

Rh incompatibility
- Fear related to unknown effect of blood incompatibility on the fetus

Infection
- Anticipatory grieving related to potential for congenital anomaly or death of fetus or neonate
- Ineffective individual coping related to possibility of delivering a neonate with a congenital anomaly or fatal infection
- Knowledge deficit related to disease transmission and prevention
- Knowledge deficit related to fetal and neonatal effects of maternal infection
- Noncompliance related to incomplete administration of prescribed medication
- Social isolation related to others' fear of disease transmission

Antepartal complications *(continued)*

Substance abuse
- Altered nutrition: less than body requirements, related to limited food intake from continued substance abuse
- Altered parenting related to performance of neonatal care while under the influence of a substance

- High risk for infection related to self-administered I.V. drugs.
- Knowledge deficit related to fetal effects of substance abuse

Premature rupture of membranes
- High risk for infection related to premature rupture of membranes

- High risk for premature labor and delivery related to uterine irritability

Preterm labor and delivery
- Altered health maintenance related to skipping medication doses
- Knowledge deficit related to in-home uterine monitoring

---

postpartal periods. Goals include maintenance of patient health and safe delivery of a healthy neonate.

Documentation
All steps of the nursing process should be documented as thoroughly and objectively as possible. Thorough documentation allows the care plan's effectiveness to be evaluated; it also makes this information available to other members of the health care team to ensure consistency of care.

Early antepartal complications

Commonly encountered complications of early pregnancy—generally defined as prior to 20 weeks' gestation—frequently involve loss of the fetus and serious threats to maternal health. The nurse must be prepared to recognize signs and symptoms of these early antepartal problems, understand their significance and etiology, and work closely with other members of the health care team to help ensure an optimal outcome for the patient and family.

Spontaneous abortion
Abortion is the termination of a pregnancy at any time before the age of viability. Viability is reached at about 24 weeks' gestation and at a weight of over 500 grams, when the fetus is able to survive in an extrauterine environment. An abortion may be spontaneous, or the pregnancy may be terminated for medical, therapeutic, or other elective reasons.

Because the word "abortion" has negative connotations for many people, a spontaneous abortion is commonly referred to as a "miscarriage." An early spontaneous abortion is one that occurs before 12 weeks' gestation; a late abortion occurs between 12 and 20 weeks' gestation. Births after 20 weeks are considered preterm.

Etiology
A majority of spontaneously aborted fetuses display a problem with implantation or an abnormal genetic or chromosomal makeup that is not

compatible with life; the remaining spontaneous abortions result from maternal causes. The risk of early pregnancy loss is increased in women who have a history of first-trimester pregnancy loss, uterine defects, chronic infections, or cigarette, alcohol, or drug abuse.

Incidence

The exact incidence of spontaneous abortion is difficult to calculate because many early pregnancies are lost for unknown reasons before they are clinically evident. At least 15% of all pregnancies are known to end in spontaneous abortion.

Classification

Abortions can be classified according to gestational age or fetal weight—that is, whether the fetus weighs 500 grams or less—as well as maternal signs and symptoms. (For a complete classification, see *Assessing different types of abortion*).

Assessment

Little can be done to avoid genetic causes of spontaneous abortion. Certain other causes, however, can be prevented. Prepregnancy correction of maternal disorders, immunization against infectious diseases, proper early prenatal care, and prompt treatment of complications may prevent some spontaneous abortions.

A detailed, accurate history focusing on the patient's recent health, menstrual, gynecologic, and obstetric history, contraceptive method used, and possible date of conception is necessary for a complete diagnostic evaluation. In addition to obtaining the health history, gather all pertinent information related to the patient's physical state. Assess the amount and consistency of blood to determine whether any products of conception have been passed. Obtain complete pain information, including location, type, and duration.

A pregnancy may have been terminated for several days before signs and symptoms become definite. Signs and symptoms of spontaneous abortion depend on the development of the implantation site, determined by the length of gestation. Urine, blood, and endocrine studies may be ordered to confirm the diagnosis or rule out the presence of infection.

Nursing diagnoses

After considering all assessment findings, formulate appropriate nursing diagnoses for the patient. (For a partial list of applicable diagnoses, see Nursing Diagnoses: *Antepartal complications,* pages 66 and 67.)

Planning and implementation

A patient with suspected spontaneous abortion should be referred to a physician immediately because emergency medical intervention may be needed to minimize complications. To care for this patient, advise saving all expelled tissues and clots; maintain a calm, confident, and sympathetic manner; alert the physician to pertinent signs and the patient's history (for example, vital signs and amounts of bleeding); and

Assessing different types of abortion

The nurse must assess the different types of abortion accurately to provide adequate nursing care and emotional support.

DEFINITION	PHYSICAL FINDINGS
Threatened	
Appearance of signs and symptoms of possible loss of embryo	*Bleeding:* slight *Cramping:* mild and intermittent *Expelled tissues:* none *Internal cervical os:* closed *Uterus size:* varies according to length of gestation
Inevitable (imminent)	
Signs and symptoms indicate certain loss of embryo	*Bleeding:* slight to moderate *Cramping:* mild and intermittent *Expelled tissues:* none *Internal cervical os:* open *Uterus size:* varies according to length of gestation
Incomplete	
Part of the products of conception retained in the uterus	*Bleeding:* heavy *Cramping:* severe *Expelled tissues:* some *Internal cervical os:* open *Uterus size:* smaller than expected for length of gestation
Missed	
Nonviable fetus and other products of conception retained in uterus for 2 months or longer	*Bleeding:* slight *Cramping:* none *Expelled tissues:* none *Internal cervical os:* closed *Uterus size:* smaller than expected for length of gestation
Septic	
Infection of products of conception and endometrial lining of uterus, which may result from attempted interference early in pregnancy	*Bleeding:* varies; malodorous *Cramping:* varies *Expelled tissues:* varies, depending on whether tissue fragments remain *Internal cervical os:* usually open *Uterus size:* varies but will be tender *Other:* fever

encourage rest. Prepare the patient physically and emotionally for medical interventions, such as a dilatation and curettage (D&C), if indicated.

If the cause of the abortion can be determined and eliminated, the chance for a future normal pregnancy is excellent. If no complications (such as infection or hemorrhage) occur, the abortion probably will have no detrimental physical effects on the patient.

Evaluation

To evaluate nursing care, determine if specific goals were achieved. The following examples illustrate some appropriate evaluation statements:

- The patient has verbalized understanding of the necessity for having a D&C after an incomplete abortion.
- The patient's vital signs and bleeding are within normal limits.
- The patient's family has demonstrated appropriate support and concern.

Ectopic pregnancy

In ectopic pregnancy, the fertilized ovum is implanted in tissue other than the endometrium (lining of the uterus). More than 95% of ectopic pregnancies occur in the fallopian tubes.

Etiology

The majority of extrauterine pregnancies result from impeded progress of the fertilized ovum through the fallopian tube. The primary causes are tubal obstruction and delayed tubal transport.

Incidence

Ectopic pregnancy is the leading cause of maternal death in the first trimester. In the United States, it occurs in 10.8 of every 1,000 pregnancies, and accounts for 11% of all maternal deaths. The majority of ectopic pregnancies occur in women ages 25 to 34.

Common predisposing factors other than age include infertility and a previous ectopic pregnancy. A woman who has had an ectopic pregnancy in one fallopian tube is at increased risk for developing an ectopic pregnancy in the opposite tube. Only 1 in 3 women who experience an ectopic pregnancy will give birth to a live neonate in a subsequent pregnancy.

Classification

Ectopic pregnancies are classified by the site of implantation, such as tubal or ovarian, because the uterus is the only organ capable of maintaining a term pregnancy. Abdominal pregnancies occur once in approximately 15,000 live births and are associated with increased maternal mortality caused by uncontrolled hemorrhage and sepsis.

Assessment

If ectopic pregnancy is suggested or suspected, collect history regarding current signs and symptoms of unruptured versus ruptured ectopic pregnancy (see *Signs and symptoms of ectopic pregnancy*).

Signs and symptoms of ectopic pregnancy

To act decisively, the nurse must be able to distinguish between these signs and symptoms of unruptured and ruptured ectopic pregnancy.

Unruptured
- Unilateral lower abdominal cramps and tenderness
- Menstrual spotting or vaginal bleeding
- Low-grade fever (99° to 100° F [37.2° to 37.7° C])
- Normal pulse
- Nausea and vomiting

Ruptured
- Sudden onset of abdominal pain
- Signs of shock: pallor, tachycardia, and hypotension
- Shoulder pain
- Rapid, thready pulse
- Cold extremities

Complicating ectopic pregnancy diagnosis are the numerous disorders that share many of the same signs and symptoms. These disorders include appendicitis, salpingitis, abortion, ovarian cysts, and urinary tract infections. Because definitive diagnosis is difficult, the condition may become an obstetric emergency if the ectopic pregnancy is not recognized until the tube ruptures.

The most effective diagnosis of an ectopic pregnancy combines three diagnostic tools; serum hCG levels in conjunction with ultrasonography and laparoscopy provide accurate information without using an invasive procedure.

Culdocentesis—aspiration or incision through the posterior vaginal fornix—also may be performed to detect intraperitoneal bleeding. Retrieval of nonclotting blood is a positive indication of ectopic pregnancy or other peritoneal bleeding.

Nursing diagnoses

After considering all assessment findings, formulate appropriate nursing diagnoses for the patient. (For a partial list of applicable diagnoses, see Nursing Diagnoses: *Antepartal complications,* pages 66 and 67.)

Planning and implementation

A patient who exhibits the signs and symptoms of ectopic pregnancy may have decreased cardiac output. Contact the physician immediately when signs and symptoms are presented, and assess vital signs every 15 minutes or as prescribed. As ordered, gather appropriate laboratory data, including Rh factor, blood type, and crossmatch, complete blood count, and serum hCG level.

Administer intravenous (I.V.) fluids, medications, and treatments as prescribed. Observe for signs and symptoms of hypovolemia, which could follow hemorrhage. In addition, determine if an Rh-negative patient is to receive RhIg (immunoglobulin). Also, clarify for the patient and her family, the physician's explanation of cause, management, and expected recovery, including chances for future pregnancies.

Immediately after an ectopic pregnancy is diagnosed, a laparoscopy is generally performed to determine the need for a laparotomy, which may be performed to remove the products of conception, to control blood loss by evacuating blood and clots, and to cauterize bleeding vessels. However, laser surgery is preferred, because it decreases damage to the tube and provides a beneficial hemostatic effect. In many cases, the affected fallopian tube can be repaired and left in place. An advanced ectopic pregnancy, which is typically abdominal, requires a laparotomy as soon as the patient is stable and able to withstand surgery.

An ovarian pregnancy requires the removal of the affected ovary. An adherent fallopian tube also may require removal.

Evaluation

To evaluate nursing care, determine if specific goals were achieved. The following examples illustrate some appropriate evaluation statements:

- The patient's vital signs have remained stable.
- The patient's pain, which resulted from ectopic pregnancy rupture, has been controlled with the prescribed analgesic agent.
- The patient has verbalized feelings over the loss of the pregnancy.

Gestational trophoblastic disease

Gestational trophoblastic disease (GTD) may be benign (hydatidiform mole) or malignant (choriocarcinoma). In GTD, trophoblastic cells covering the chorionic villi proliferate, and the villi undergo cystic changes.

In benign GTD, chorionic villi degenerate and become transparent vesicles that hang in grapelike clusters. These vesicles contain a clear fluid and may involve all or part of the decidual lining of the uterus. Usually no embryo is present because it has been absorbed.

In malignant GTD—a serious, rapidly developing, but rare carcinoma—neoplastic trophoblasts proliferate without cystic villi and may metastasize.

Etiology

The cause of GTD is unknown. Because no specific etiology has been determined, prevention techniques are unknown.

Incidence

GTD is reported to occur in about 1 of every 2,000 pregnancies. Some cases are not recognized because the pregnancy is aborted early and the products of conception are not available for analysis.

Classification

The classification of GTD depends on whether it is localized or disseminated. A benign neoplasm is well localized in the uterus, whereas a malignant neoplasm may metastasize.

A diagnosis of benign GTD does not denote a benign long-term prognosis, nor does a diagnosis of malignant GTD definitely indicate an unfavorable prognosis. For both diagnoses, close medical monitoring and thorough follow-up care are vital. (For more information, see "Planning and implementation" section below.)

Assessment

A specimen of the patient's vaginal discharge (usually brownish red) is sent to the laboratory. The uterus typically is enlarged out of proportion to the weeks of gestation. No fetal heart tones are heard nor can any fetal body parts be palpated. Laboratory studies show a reduced hemoglobin level, hematocrit, and red blood cell count and an increased white blood cell count and sedimentation rate. Human chorionic gonadotropin titers are extremely elevated. Urinalysis probably will show proteinuria. An ultrasound performed after the third month will show grapelike clusters rather than a fetus.

Nursing diagnoses

After considering all assessment findings, formulate appropriate nursing diagnoses for the patient. (For a partial list of applicable diagnoses, see Nursing Diagnoses: *Antepartal complications,* pages 66 and 67.)

Planning and implementation

Monitor the patient's vital signs, vaginal bleeding or discharge, and urine (for proteinuria). Both the patient and her partner will require support when they are given the diagnosis. Be sensitive to the patient's ability to cope, and assess her family support. Be aware of the many options available for dealing with GTD in order to respond to the patient's and family's questions about the procedures and probable outcomes.

Management of GTD involves evacuation of the uterine contents. An induced abortion may be followed by D&C. Tissue obtained from curettage must be examined by a pathologist for residual trophoblastic cells. After the D&C, routine post-operative care is necessary.

Because GTD can be malignant, follow-up care must continue for at least 1 year. If hCG levels remain within normal limits for 1 year, the patient can anticipate a normal subsequent pregnancy. In this instance, probability of a recurrence of GTD is relatively low, especially if the patient is age 40 or younger.

Evaluation

To evaluate nursing care, determine if specific goals were achieved. The following examples illustrate some appropriate evaluation statements:

• The patient understands the need for follow-up monitoring of GTD.

• The patient's family has demonstrated appropriate support and concern.

Hyperemesis gravidarum

Hyperemesis gravidarum, sometimes called "pernicious vomiting," involves dehydration and malnutrition. Because hyperemesis begins as simple nausea and vomiting, a definitive diagnosis can be difficult. The patient's tolerance for nausea and vomiting, the degree of hydration, her electrolyte balance, and her level of disability all affect the diagnosis. Every case of nausea and vomiting during pregnancy can be serious.

Etiology
The cause of hyperemesis gravidarum is not known. Hormonal alterations occur frequently in pregnancy and are questionably related to hyperemesis gravidarum. Progesterone produced by the placenta slows gastric and intestinal motility, which may predispose pregnant patients to emesis. Human chorionic gonadotropin levels also may affect emesis during pregnancy as levels increase proportionately with placental size and the number of fetuses. Emesis is more probable in patients who are pregnant with more than one fetus. Although psychological factors have been implicated in some pregnancy-related nausea and vomiting, no research supports a psychosomatic cause of hyperemesis.

Incidence
Hyperemesis gravidarum occurs in 7 to 16 of every 1,000 pregnant women. Its incidence appears to vary with lifestyle, race, amount of stress, number of gestations, marital status, and age; however, demographic factors are difficult to separate from cultural, sociologic, and environmental ones.

Assessment
Unremitting nausea and vomiting that persist beyond the first trimester are characteristic of hyperemesis gravidarum. Vomitus ranges from undigested food, mucus, and bile early in the disorder to a "coffee-grounds" appearance in later stages.

Continued vomiting leads to dehydration, ultimately decreasing the circulating blood volume (hypovolemia). Laboratory studies may reveal hemoconcentration and, in severe cases, loss of sodium, potassium, and chloride. Signs of progressive dehydration and impending hypovolemia are weight loss, increased pulse rate, decreased blood pressure, changes in skin turgor, and dry mucous membranes. A urine ketodiastick may reveal ketones that indicate dehydration. Persistent dehydration also leads to confusion and coma as well as hepatic and renal failure.

Nursing diagnoses
After considering all assessment findings, formulate appropriate nursing diagnoses for the patient. (For a partial list of applicable diagnoses, see Nursing Diagnoses: *Antepartal complications,* pages 66 and 67.)

Planning and implementation

For the patient with persistent vomiting and decreased fluid intake, expect to administer parenteral fluids, electrolytes, vitamins, and proteins, as prescribed, to counteract dehydration and loss of nutrients. Administer antiemetics, as prescribed, to decrease vomiting and promote rest. Oral intake may be restricted for the first 48 hours, followed by cautious resumption of small, dry meals and then clear liquids. This allows the gastrointestinal system to rest from overstimulation.

Keep the patient's room quiet, pleasant, and well ventilated to promote rest and relaxation. Maintain excellent daily hygiene, especially oral hygiene following vomiting episodes. Limit visitors to promote patient rest.

A patient who appears clinically stable may be managed as an outpatient, with frequent follow-up visits. Hydration with isotonic fluids is essential. In addition, teach the patient how to assist with her own treatment—in nutrition, for example. Teach the patient that small, frequent meals consisting of easily digested, high-carbohydrate foods will help reestablish adequate vitamin and protein levels. Heartburn and reflux esophagitis are common and typically are treated symptomatically.

Antiemetics, a mainstay in treating hyperemesis, also have a mildly sedating effect. These may increase the patient's ability to eat and rest. However, be aware of the nursing implications of such medications.

Evaluation

To evaluate nursing care, determine if specific goals were achieved. The following examples illustrate some appropriate evaluation statements:
• The patient has responded to small, frequent feedings by a reduced emesis.
• The patient has maintained adequate nutritional status and no weight loss.

Incompetent cervix

Incompetent cervix (or premature dilation of the cervix) is characterized by painless dilation of the cervix without labor or uterine contraction. Depending on the length of gestation, spontaneous abortion or premature delivery may result. Up to 40% of all perinatal deaths occur in association with pregnancies that terminate at between 20 and 28 weeks' gestation. Cervical incompetence is a major contributor to those losses.

Etiology

Cervical incompetence may be caused by a previous traumatic delivery or a forceful D&C of the cervix. Other etiologic factors may be congenital, such as a short cervix or an anomalous uterus (such as a double uterus or other altered shape).

Incidence

Incompetent cervix occurs in approximately 1 of every 1,000 deliveries, 1 of 100 abortions, and 1 of 5 habitual abortions (where the patient has had three or more consecutive abortions).

Assessment

The patient with this condition does not have uterine contractions or other signs and symptoms of labor. A pelvic examination reveals other signs and symptoms of a dilated cervix possibly accompanied by a congenital problem, such as a short cervix, a double uterus, or a uterus with an altered shape. The patient may report a previous traumatic delivery, history of incompetent cervix, or a D&C.

Nursing diagnoses

After considering all assessment findings, formulate appropriate nursing diagnoses for the patient. (For a partial list of applicable diagnoses, see Nursing Diagnoses: *Antepartal complications,* pages 66 and 67.)

Planning and implementation

The procedure most frequently used to maintain a pregnancy is the transvaginal cervical cerclage (McDonald procedure), in which a band of nonabsorbable ribbon (Mersilene) is placed around the cervix beneath the mucosa to constrict the opening. The suture works much like the string on a drawstring bag. The key to the procedure's success is placing the suture high enough on the cervix so that it will remain in place.

Cervical cerclage may lead to painful abdominal cramping. A suture that has loosened or has become displaced will not maintain cervical closure. In that case, the suture is clipped and removed when labor begins, and vaginal delivery may proceed.

Provide basic preoperative and postoperative care for the patient undergoing a cerclage of the cervix, paying special attention to vaginal bleeding. Frequently assess the presence and quality of fetal heart tones.

Because incompetent cervix usually is not diagnosed until after one or more abortions, this probably is not the first time the patient and her partner have had to face delivery complications or the loss of a fetus. Therefore, she and her family will need much support.

Evaluation

To evaluate nursing care, determine if specific goals were achieved. The following examples illustrate some appropriate evaluation statements:
- The patient correctly described the potential effects of her condition on herself and her fetus.
- The patient and her family actively participated in planning care, and understand the potential warning signs.

Medical and late antepartal complications

Once the point of fetal viability has been reached—defined as gestational age beyond 20 weeks—has been reached, any early pregnancy complications should have been recognized and resolved. Nursing care now focuses on optimizing maternal and fetal outcomes.

Cardiac disease

Pre-existing cardiac disease places about 1% of pregnant women at risk. Common cardiac diseases affecting pregnant patients include rheumatic heart disease, maternal congenital heart defects, mitral valve prolapse, and peripartum cardiomyopathy.

With any cardiac disorder, cardiac decompensation may occur, challenging maternal and fetal health. Rarely, it may lead to maternal or fetal death. Careful medical, obstetric, and nursing care before and during pregnancy can minimize maternal and fetal risks.

Assessment

Physiologic changes of pregnancy may cause cardiac stress, especially during the second trimester in women with cardiac disease. These changes include increased plasma volume and expanded uterine vascular bed, which increase heart rate 10 to 15 beats/minute by the end of pregnancy and boost cardiac output by about 30% between 28 and 32 weeks' gestation. A patient who experiences cardiac stress needs weekly evaluation and may require bed rest, fluid restrictions, or such drugs as digitalis preparations, diuretics, antiarrhythmics, antibiotics, or anticoagulants (usually heparin).

Cardiac stress may intensify in the third trimester and may be severe enough to cause persistent pulmonary effects, such as crackles, tachycardia, tachypnea, dyspnea, or orthopnea. A patient who experiences severe cardiac stress should adhere to prescribed treatments and should be monitored weekly for changes in pulmonary effects. To prevent complications, she may need to be placed on bed rest.

For a patient with cardiac disease, expect to monitor the results of the CBC, electrolyte levels, and, if complications arise, cardiac enzyme levels.

Nursing diagnoses

After considering all assessment findings, formulate appropriate nursing diagnoses for the patient. (For a partial list of applicable diagnoses, see Nursing Diagnoses: *Antepartal complications,* pages 66 and 67.)

Planning and implementation

The antepartal patient may have decreased cardiac output related to a valvular dysfunction. To monitor her status, obtain her vital signs and weight at each prenatal visit. Obtain an electrocardiogram periodically, as prescribed. Monitor fluid intake and output. If a patient develops pulmonary complications, a pulmonary artery catheter may be inserted to provide pulmonary pressure measurements.

Teach the patient to monitor cardiac status and report significant changes, especially signs and symptoms of potential complications, such as increased limitation of activity; presence of or increase in dyspnea, orthopnea, tachypnea, or edema; development of palpitations; significant increase or decrease in heart rate; and chest discomfort.

Regular examinations and tests are advised. The importance of frequent follow-up visits and continuity of care must be stressed. Also teach the patient with cardiac disease about her condition, its management, and its effects on her preganancy and her fetus. Encourage the patient to rest in the semi-Fowler's or side-lying position. Promote adequate rest and appropriate exercise. Encourage a balanced diet and adequate fluid intake. Also instruct the patient to avoid people with infections.

Evaluation

To evaluate nursing care, determine if specific goals were achieved. The following examples illustrate some appropriate evaluation statements:

- The patient accurately described her condition and its limitations on her health.
- The patient correctly listed the signs and symptoms of cardiac complications during pregnancy.
- The patient endorsed a care regimen that affords her optimum health and functioning.

Diabetes mellitus

The most common endocrine disorder in obstetrics, gestational diabetes mellitus (GDM) occurs in 1 out of approximately every 300 pregnancies. Insulin therapy for diabetes has reduced fetal mortality to less than 5%; however, the risk of congenital anomalies remains high in patients with insulin-dependent diabetes mellitus. Strict control of maternal serum glucose levels before conception and especially during the first trimester can help reduce this risk. Also, careful medical and nursing care can help the patient manage her disorder successfully and deliver a normal, healthy neonate.

This disorder begins or is first diagnosed during pregnancy. A patient with GDM may be asymptomatic except for impaired glucose tolerance. GDM has great implications for pregnancy because even mild diabetes increases the risk of fetal or neonatal morbidity and mortality. GDM may resolve after childbirth or may evolve into impaired glucose tolerance or type I or II diabetes mellitus.

Assessment

All pregnant women experience dramatic changes in carbohydrate, lipid, and protein metabolism. A pregnant diabetic woman is susceptible to hypoglycemia (abnormally low serum glucose level) and hyperglycemia (abnormally high serum glucose level). In some women, however, the growing fetus stresses maternal glucose production and use, disrupting normal carbohydrate metabolism and causing GDM.

If diabetes is not adequately identified and managed before conception and during pregnancy, it increases fetal and neonatal risks. Preconception diabetic management maintains the patient's health and prepares her for pregnancy, allowing fetal development to proceed normally. Blood glucose control throughout pregnancy reduces the risk of congenital anomalies and complications to the same level as that of the general population.

Maternal effects. Uncontrolled diabetes or diabetes associated with vascular damage increases the risk of complications. However, comprehensive health care can control and lessen these risks.

Uncontrolled diabetes causes maternal hyperglycemia, increases the amount of circulating ketones from fatty acid metabolism, and results in ketosis. Decreased gastric motility (a normal change of pregnancy) and hPL's antagonistic effect on insulin further increase circulating glucose, predisposing the patient to increased ketosis. Without treatment, she may become comatose, and she or her fetus may die.

Hydramnios (excess amniotic fluid) occurs in about 10% of pregnant diabetic women. Amniotic fluid volume increases to more than 1,500 ml. Although the exact cause of hydramnios is unknown, it may result from increased maternal and fetal circulating blood sugar, which increases fetal urine in the amniotic fluid. The added fluid may increase maternal discomfort later in pregnancy. Also, it occasionally leads to premature rupture of membranes and premature labor. Although amniocentesis may reduce fluid volume, it is not commonly used for this purpose because it increases the risk of infection, labor stimulation, and placental injury.

The vascular changes of diabetes produce pregnancy-induced hypertension in 20% to 30% of pregnant diabetic patients. Glycosuria predisposes the pregnant diabetic patient to infections, especially moniliasis and urinary tract infections. These non-life-threatening infections usually can be controlled with perineal hygiene, increased fluid intake, and anti-infective agents.

Fetal and neonatal effects. Maternal diabetes may have many adverse effects on the fetus and neonate. It increases the incidence of fetal anomalies and neonatal morbidity and predisposes the neonate to diabetes. Without careful management, it increases the risk of fetal or neonatal death. Neonates born to women with advanced diabetes may display intrauterine growth retardation (IUGR). Neonatal hyperbilirubinemia and hypoglycemia also are possible effects of maternal diabetes.

Neonates born to mothers with poorly controlled diabetes usually have macrosomia (large body size and birth weight), causing cephalopelvic disproportion and uterine dystocia and thereby requiring cesarean delivery. Macrosomia can affect all fetal organs except the brain.

Because selective screening may miss previously undiagnosed diabetes, all pregnant patients should be screened for glucose intolerance with a 1-hour (50-gram) diabetes screening test. If screening reveals glucose intolerance, treatment should begin immediately. (For a list of diagnostic screenings, see *Antepartal diabetic screening,* page 80.)

Antepartal diabetic screening

The following diagnostic tests are used to detect gestational diabetes.
* *Urine glucose testing.* With the use of a urine dipstick (Dextrostix), test the patient's urine for glucose, protein, and ketones at each prenatal visit.
* *Glucose challenge test.* This 1-hour, 50-gram oral glucose screening test is recommended for each pregnant patient at 24 to 28 weeks' gestation. The patient does not need to fast before the test. A blood sample for glucose testing will be drawn 1 hour after she ingests 50 grams of oral glucose solution. If her plasma glucose level is abnormally high, prepare her for a 3-hour oral glucose tolerance test.
* *3-hour oral glucose tolerance test (OGTT).* The OGTT may be used to diagnose gestational diabetes. Advise the patient to eat a high-carbohydrate diet (more than 200 grams daily) for 2 days before this test. She must fast from midnight until the test time. When she arrives for her test, draw a blood sample to obtain a fasting plasma glucose level. Then after she ingests 100 grams of oral glucose solution, blood samples for plasma glucose levels will be drawn at 1, 2, and 3 hours. If two or more of the samples show abnormally high glucose levels, the patient has gestational diabetes. Check her specific institutional levels to accurately identify abnormal values.

Nursing diagnoses

After considering all assessment findings, formulate appropriate nursing diagnoses for the patient. (For a partial list of applicable diagnoses, see Nursing Diagnoses: *Antepartal complications,* pages 66 and 67.)

Planning and implementation

For a patient with diabetes during pregnancy, provide her with information about the disease, its effects on her and her fetus, and the recommended treatment. Reassure the patient that careful antepartal management can prevent fetal and neonatal problems.

Instruct the diabetic patient and her family about the importance of dietary modifications during pregnancy, glucose monitoring and, if applicable, about insulin therapy. Review the signs and symptoms of hypoglycemia and hyperglycemia. Recommendations for close glucose monitoring and dietary management should be reinforced. Teach the patient about acceptable glucose values and the need for frequent prenatal plasma glucose monitoring. If insulin is indicated, provide information and guidance about home glucose monitoring and insulin administration.

The nurse provides the patient with specific nutritional guidelines and, if necessary, referrals to a dietitian. The patient should be encouraged to balance appropriate exercise with rest and to avoid potential infections.

Fetal monitoring also becomes an important component in the evaluation of fetal well-being. Daily fetal movement counts, which can be done by the patient at home, are a valuable tool. In addition, nonstress tests, contraction stress tests, oxytocin challenge tests, ultrasonography, and biophysical profiles may be ordered to determine fetal health.

A key element in diabetic management during pregnancy is the patient's compliance with health care recommendations. Encourage the patient to participate in the planning of her prescribed regimen.

Evaluation

To evaluate nursing care, determine if specific goals were achieved. The following examples illustrate some appropriate evaluation statements:

- The patient accurately monitored her blood glucose levels at home.
- The patient accurately described her condition and its limitations on her health.
- The patient planned nutritious meals with the assistance of a dietitian.

Hypertensive disorders

Hypertension is the third leading cause of maternal mortality in the United States, preceded only by hemorrhage and infection. About 7% of all pregnancies are affected by hypertension; 6% to 10% of perinatal deaths are associated with hypertensive episodes. Pregnancy-induced hypertension (PIH) affects major body systems, including the kidneys, lungs, liver, and uterus.

The American College of Obstetricians and Gynecologists accepts the following terms in association with gestational hypertension: preeclampsia and eclampsia, chronic hypertension, PIH, chronic hypertension with superimposed preeclampsia, and transient hypertension.

PIH is characterized by hypertension, proteinuria, and generalized edema. It has two basic forms: preeclampsia (a nonconvulsive form) and eclampsia (a convulsive form). This syndrome may develop at any point after 20 weeks' gestation or in the early postpartal period. (Hypertension occurring before 20 weeks' gestation usually is associated with GTD.) Typically, the syndrome appears in the last trimester and disappears after 42 postpartal days. PIH may be difficult to distinguish from hypertensive states that predate the pregnancy. In addition, a definitive diagnosis of PIH may be impossible unless the patient's blood pressure returns to baseline after pregnancy.

Chronic hypertension is present and observable before the pregnancy and is diagnosed by 20 weeks' of gestation or extends 42 days after delivery. Chronic hypertensive disease may occur alone or with superimposed PIH.

Etiology

The exact cause of PIH is unknown; however, geographic, ethnic, racial, nutritional, immunologic, and familial factors may play a role in its development. (See *Predisposing factors for PIH,* page 82.)

Assessment

Note the length of gestation in the patient with a hypertensive disorder because PIH typically occurs after 20 weeks' gestation. Also ascertain

Predisposing factors for PIH

Factors that predispose a pregant patient to PIH include:
- *Primigravidity.* Most women who develop PIH are pregnant for the first time. The incidence is especially high in those under age 17 or over age 35.
- *Multiple gestation.* The incidence of PIH increases with the number of fetuses.
- *Vascular disease.* Especially associated with PIH are diabetes mellitus, hypertensive renal disease, and essential hypertension.
- *Gestational trophoblastic disease (hydatidiform mole).* The hypertensive syndrome usually appears before 20 weeks' gestation if associated with GTD.
- *Malnutrition or dietary deficiencies.* Deficiencies in proteins and in water-soluble vitamins frequently are associated with the development of PIH.

if the patient had elevated blood pressure, proteinuria, or edema in her face, hands, feet, or legs in any previous pregnancies. Inquire about visual disturbances, headaches, epigastric pain, irritability, or muscle tremors.

Physical examination will disclose the three classic signs of PIH: elevated blood pressure, proteinuria, and edema. When caring for a patient with preeclampsia in the hospital setting, obtain a daily weight, measure urine output, as prescribed, and assess for proteinuria using a reagent strip.

Evaluate the patient for edema in her legs, hands, and face by depressing her skin over a bony prominence. In pitting edema, a depression remains in the skin and subcutaneous tissue after the pressure has been removed.

Assessment of deep tendon reflexes (DTRs) may indicate hyporeflexia or hyperreflexia. Elicit the patellar (knee-jerk), biceps, and ankle reflexes.

Nursing diagnoses
After considering all assessment findings, formulate appropriate nursing diagnoses for the patient. (For a partial list of applicable diagnoses, see Nursing Diagnoses: *Antepartal complications,* pages 66 and 67.)

Planning and implementation
Bed rest is prescribed for the patient with a hypertensive disorder. Encourage a left lateral position to increase uterine and renal perfusion. Increased renal perfusion facilitates diuresis. Other positions—such as the supine position—may compromise renal and uterine blood flow through compression of the vena cava and aorta.

Mild preeclampsia. Nursing care is aimed at improving or stabilizing the patient. The patient may remain at home as long as edema and proteinuria do not increase. A physician, nurse-midwife, or nurse practitioner must assess the patient at least weekly to determine changes in her condition. Carefully instruct the patient and her family about the signs that indicate a deterioration in her condition, such as severe headache, rapid rise in blood pressure, epigastric pain, hyperreflexia (muscle twitching), edema, decreased urine output, or visual disturbances. Instruct the patient to report such signs to the physician immediately. The patient usually remains on bed rest and must maintain a well-balanced, high-protein and high-fiber diet.

Severe preeclampsia. Treatment includes in-hospital bed rest in a left lateral position. Keep the environment quiet, with minimal stimulation and dim lighting, and follow these procedures:

• Assess the patient's vital signs and DTRs at least every 4 hours; record her weight daily; measure urine output every 1 to 4 hours according to the patient's status. The patient should maintain a high-carbohydrate, low-fat, 70- to 100-g protein diet with 2 g of sodium daily.

• Administer sedatives, as prescribed; monitor regularly for signs of labor and fetal well-being.

If the patient's condition improves within 3 to 5 days (for example, if urine output increases or weight decreases by .9 lb [2 kg] or more), further therapy will depend on the fetus's gestational age.

If no improvement is noted, hyperreflexia occurs, the fetus is full term at 38 weeks' gestation, or the lecithin/sphingomyelin (L/S) ratio is appropriate, the physician may elect delivery. Nursing care for the patient with severe preeclampsia has the following aims:

• preventing eclampsia and seizures
• ensuring maternal survival with minimal morbidity
• ensuring birth of as mature a neonate as possible
• avoiding significant postdelivery complications
• educating the patient.

Provide the same monitoring and care that the patient received before she was hospitalized. In addition, prepare emergency equipment as soon as the patient is admitted in case eclampsia occurs. Emergency equipment should include medications, suctioning apparatus, tongue blade, and padded side rails on the patient's bed. Keep emergency anticonvulsant and antihypertensive medications available; these include magnesium sulfate, methyldopa, hydralazine, and propranolol hydrochloride.

Eclampsia. Eclampsia is a complication of PIH. It is preceded by the signs of severe preeclampsia and one or both of the following:

• tonic (normal tone of muscles) and clonic (alternating between involuntary muscle contraction and relaxation in rapid succession) seizures
• hypertensive crisis, in which blood pressure is elevated to such a degree that the patient has an increased chance of developing a cerebrovascular accident or shock.

Tonic-clonic seizures are followed by hypotension and collapse and, in many cases, nystagmus, muscle twitching, and coma. Oliguria or anuria also may occur. Disorientation and amnesia delay immediate recovery. The nurse's first priority during seizures is to ensure a patent airway, provide adequate oxygenation, and notify the physician immediately.

Evaluation

To evaluate nursing care, determine if specific goals were achieved. The following examples illustrate some appropriate evaluation statements:

- The patient kept all appointments for prenatal care and laboratory tests.
- The patient reported a change in her condition as soon as it occurred.
- The patient's family demonstrated appropriate support and concern.

Anemias

Two commons forms of anemia may complicate the antepartal period: iron deficiency anemia and folic acid deficiency anemia. *Iron deficiency anemia* results from an inadequate supply of iron for optimal formation of RBCs, producing smaller (microcytic) cells. Insufficient iron stores lead to a depleted RBC mass and, in turn, to a decreased concentration of hemoglobin, which normally transports oxygen throughout the body.

Also known as megaloblastic anemia, pernicious anemia of pregnancy, or macrocytic anemia, *folic acid deficiency anemia* is rare in the United States. Women with multiple gestation and those with hemoglobinopathies or other hemolytic disorders are especially susceptible to developing folic acid deficiency anemia. (For more information, see *Maternal, fetal, and neonatal effects of anemias.*)

Etiology

Pregnancy greatly increases the body's need for iron, and a pregnant patient may not have adequate iron stores to meet this increased need. Furthermore, pregnancy-induced hemodilution can exacerbate an anemia. Without iron supplementation, the patient may develop iron deficiency anemia.

The body uses folic acid to break down proteins and to form nucleic acids and heme for hemoglobin. A deficiency may result from inadequate intake of animal protein and uncooked fresh vegetables, malabsorption, or a metabolic abnormality. When deficiency occurs, immature RBCs fail to divide and are released as enlarged cells (megaloblasts). Because they are fragile, many cells are destroyed before they are released into the bloodstream.

During pregnancy, the need for folic acid increases. This places the pregnant patient at risk for folic acid deficiency.

Assessment

Anemia is diagnosed by blood tests after a thorough health history and physical examination. When iron deficiency anemia is present, the hemoglobin level is below 11 g/liter, and the hematocrit drops below 32%.

Maternal, fetal, and neonatal effects of anemias

Iron deficiency anemia and folic acid deficiency anemia can produce various maternal, fetal, and neonatal effects as described in the chart below.

ANEMIA	MATERNAL EFFECTS	FETAL AND NEONATAL EFFECTS
Iron deficiency anemia	• Poor tissue integrity • Tissue damage at birth • Antepartal or postpartal infection with impaired healing • Excessive bleeding after delivery, which may seriously compromise cardiovascular status	• Spontaneous abortion, stillbirth, or small-for-gestational-age neonate • Intact fetal iron stores • Fetal distress from hypoxia during third trimester of pregnancy and labor, when hemoglobin fails to carry sufficient oxygen to the mother and fetus
Folic acid deficiency anemia	• Urinary tract and other infections • Bleeding complications during delivery • Pancytopenia (reduction of all cellular components of the blood) resulting from immature red blood cell production	• Spontaneous abortion and abruptio placentae complications

For an anemic patient, monitor the results of hemoglobin electrophoresis, CBC, folic acid levels, and serum iron measurements. Folic acid deficiency anemia gradually produces clinical findings, such as decreased hemoglobin levels despite sufficient iron intake, GI distress (including anorexia, nausea, and vomiting), fatigue, weakness, and pallor. In advanced stages, dyspnea and edema may appear.

A patient with iron deficiency anemia may tire easily and be susceptible to infection and postpartal bleeding. Even minimal blood loss during childbirth may cause an already anemic patient to experience decreased blood pressure or dizziness. Other signs and symptoms may include weakness, headache, shortness of breath on exertion, anorexia, pica (craving to eat nonfood substances), irritability, pallor, tachycardia, palpitations, and excessive bleeding of the gums.

Nursing diagnoses
After considering all assessment findings, formulate appropriate nursing diagnoses for the patient. (For a partial list of applicable diagnoses, see Nursing Diagnoses: *Antepartal complications,* pages 66 and 67.)

Planning and implementation
Administer supplemental iron to an anemic patient before conception to maintain normal hemoglobin concentration, and continue it during pregnancy. Daily oral doses of 200 mg of elemental iron, supplied in 1 g of ferrous sulfate or 2 g of ferrous gluconate, provide the necessary requirements for a pregnant patient with anemia. Divided doses help prevent or decrease adverse GI effects, such as nausea and constipation.

To prevent folic acid deficiency anemia, the patient should take 0.8 mg of folic acid daily supplements during pregnancy. To treat folic acid deficiency anemia, she should receive 1 mg of folic acid daily. Frequently, folic acid is also found in prenatal multivitamins. Because iron deficiency anemia almost always coexists with folic acid deficiency anemia, the patient also should receive iron supplements.

Depending on the patient's disorder or problem, provide information its effects and treatments. Stress the importance of compliance with iron supplementation.

The patient may need an increased intake of iron-rich foods. To help such a patient, evaluate her food preferences, needs, and restrictions, and estimate the nutritional value of the foods she eats. These are incorporated into a balanced diet—generally a high-iron, high-fiber diet—that fulfills nutritional requirements, meets food preferences, and is economical. Furthermore, taking iron pills with citrus juice increases their absorption.

Encourage the patient to eat foods high in folic acid. Depending on the patient's underlying disorder, make specific dietary recommendations with the assistance of a registered dietitian.

Evaluation

To evaluate nursing care, determine if specific goals were achieved. The following examples illustrate some appropriate evaluation statements:

• The patient accurately described her condition and the potential effects on herself and her fetus.
• The patient planned nutritious meals that were rich in iron.

Rh incompatibility

Hemolytic disease of the newborn, also called erythroblastosis fetalis, is a progressive disorder of the fetal blood and blood-forming organs characterized by hemolytic anemia and hyperbilirubinemia. The more severe forms of isoimmune hemolytic disease are associated with $Rho(D)$ group incompatibility. Since immunization with prophylactic $Rho(D)$ human immunoglobulin (RhIg) such as Rhogan began, the incidence of severe hemolytic disease of the newborn has been reduced drastically.

Etiology

Hemolytic diseases of the newborn, such as erythroblastosis fetalis, hydrops fetalis, and icterus gravis, were found to be linked to the Rh factor. These hemolytic disorders, which lead to the hemolysis of fetal RBCs, are caused by maternal antibodies. Approximately 90% of clinical cases of hemolytic diseases in neonates followed maternal sensitization (isoimmunization) by Rh antigens. The Rh-negative mother was sensitized by her fetus's Rh-positive RBCs, inherited from the Rh-positive father.

Maternal isoimmunization can also be caused by a transfusion with Rh-positive or D^u-positive blood or by the presence of aberrant antibodies in the transfusion unit. This type of isoimmunization is rare, however, because typing and crossmatching are performed routinely before blood administration.

Incidence

Almost 65% of the neonates of Rh-incompatible couples are Rh positive. The risk of maternal sensitization is less than may be expected. Factors involved include antigenicity, the amount of antigen infused, and the mother's immunologic response to the antigen. Some patients have a greater antigenic response to the Rh factor. The risk of isoimmunization increases with the number of pregnancies if treatment with RhIg is not instituted.

Maternal effects from Rh incompatibility have not been identified; however, severe Rh incompatibility results in erythroblastosis fetalis. When fetal blood reacts to the Rh-positive antibodies of the mother, fetal RBCs are destroyed (hemolysis) and fetal hemolytic anemia results. The released blood pigments, or bilirubin, are transported across the placenta, processed by the maternal liver, and excreted in the bile. When the amount of pigments is greater than the maternal liver can process, the neonate will be icteric (jaundiced) at birth. Hyperplasia of the bone marrow and extramedullary (spleen) hematopoiesis occur as fetal compensatory mechanisms to offset fetal anemia, which can lead to cardiac decompensation, cardiomegaly, hepatomegaly, and splenomegaly. A syndrome of generalized edema and ascites known as "hydrops fetalis" may result, with the fetus at increased risk for intrauterine or early neonatal death.

The placenta of the seriously affected fetus is enlarged. The amniotic fluid may be stained a yellowish color from bile pigments. Following delivery, the neonate with erythroblastosis becomes icteric because the neonate cannot excrete the bile pigments resulting from RBC hemolysis. Icterus neonatorum (jaundice in the neonate) can occur soon after birth in severe cases.

Generalized pigmentation of brain cells (kernicterus) commonly develops when the serum bilirubin rises to toxic levels that can lead to death. Serious abnormalities, such as choreoathetoid cerebral palsy, may develop and persist if the neonate survives.

Rh hemolytic disease of the neonate occurs in approximately 1 out of 150 to 200 full-term pregnancies in the United States. With intrauterine (fetal) transfusions, that number can be reduced significantly. Amniocentesis studies, early delivery of affected fetuses, and exchange or replacement transfusions have decreased the mortality rate.

Complete recovery can be expected in neonates who do not develop kernicterus. If hyperbilirubinemia is treated promptly and effectively, most neonates recover without residual effects or sequelae.

Assessment

Gather data on previous pregnancies, especially those that ended in early abortion. Note any blood replacement therapy or any RhIg therapy the patient has received previously.

The physical assessment may not be significant for a patient with Rh incompatibility, but diagnostic studies are important. Blood type for ABO and Rh factor is established early in pregnancy to identify a patient at risk for isoimmune hemolytic disease. Maternal isoimmunization is probable when antibody screening tests on maternal serum at around 20 weeks' gestation are positive. If the first test is negative, it should be repeated at 32 to 36 weeks' gestation. For the indirect Coombs' test, the level of maternal antibodies and the titer indicate the degree of maternal sensitization. If the titer reaches 1:16, an amniocentesis to measure the amount of bilirubin in the amniotic fluid is performed after 36 weeks' gestation.

Nursing diagnoses
After considering all assessment findings, formulate appropriate nursing diagnoses for the patient. (For a partial list of applicable diagnoses, see Nursing Diagnoses: *Antepartal complications,* pages 66 and 67.)

Planning and implementation
Prophylaxis for Rh isoimmunization requires the use of RhIg. RhIg is not a treatment for isoimmunization because it has no effect against antibodies present in the maternal bloodstream. It provides passive immunity, which is transient and therefore will not affect a subsequent pregnancy. RhIg also prepares RBCs containing the Rh antigen for destruction by phagocytes before the patient's immune system is activated to produce antibodies (active immunity). Antibodies formed by an active immune response remain within the individual's bloodstream, presumably for life.

RhIg given to an $Rh_O(D)$-negative patient who already is sensitized would accomplish nothing. Therefore, RhIg is recommended only for Rh-negative patients at risk for developing Rh isoimmunization. It should not be given to an Rh-positive patient because the Rh antibodies could destroy her Rh-positive RBCs.

Rh sensitization also is possible during pregnancy if the cellular layer separating the maternal and fetal circulations is disrupted and fetal blood enters the maternal bloodstream. The cellular layer may be disrupted during amniocentesis or by abruptio placentae.

For the patient who is $Rh_O(D)$ negative and RhD^u negative and who has not already formed Rh antibodies, RhIg administered at about 28 weeks' gestation and again within 72 hours after delivery can help prevent Rh isoimmunization.

Evaluation
To evaluate nursing care, determine if specific goals were achieved. The following examples illustrate some appropriate evaluation statements:
• The patient correctly described the potential effects of her condition on herself and her fetus.

• The patient and her family actively participated in planning care during and after the pregnancy.

Infection

Throughout pregnancy, the patient should take measures to avoid infection. If infection occurs despite these measures, the patient should be evaluated and promptly treated to prevent maternal and fetal complications. The most potentially harmful infections during pregnancy are TORCH, HIV, and genitourinary infections.

The acronym TORCH refers to toxoplasmosis, other infections (including Chlamydia, group B beta-hemolytic streptococcus, syphilis, and varicella zoster), rubella, cytomegalovirus, and herpesvirus type 2 infections. These infections can cause major congenital anomalies or death of the embryo or fetus.

HIV infection causes acquired immunodeficiency syndrome (AIDS), a life-threatening disease that affects the body's immune system, rendering it susceptible to opportunistic infections. In the first 6 months of 1988, women accounted for more than 10% of reported HIV cases. The percentage may be higher because many women who carry the virus can be asymptomatic.

Genitourinary infections include urinary tract infections, sexually transmitted diseases (STDs), and gynecologic infections. Some of these infections, such as gonorrhea and herpes, can be passed to the fetus as the fetus traverses the birth canal.

Assessment

For a patient with an infection, laboratory data can reveal culture results, antibody titers, and immune status to identify the specific organisms. An abnormally high white blood cell count signals infection.

Nursing diagnoses

After considering all assessment findings, formulate appropriate nursing diagnoses for the patient. (For a partial list of applicable diagnoses, see Nursing Diagnoses: *Antepartal complications,* pages 66 and 67.)

Planning and implementation

The patient with an infection will need to learn about the causes of infections, transmission routes, and prevention techniques. Describe the signs and symptoms of common infections, help the patient identify predisposing factors, and encourage the patient to seek medical help if she suspects infection. Stress that all of this information is confidential.

Care for the patient with an infection involves all family or household members in controlling the infection, ensuring satisfactory health for these individuals, and protecting the caregivers. To accomplish these goals, educate the family about the infection, its risks, and preventive measures. These measures may include:

• sexual abstinence during the active phases of the disease
• use of a condom during sexual intercourse, as recommended by health care professionals

- simultaneous treatment of the patient and her partner
- evaluation for reinfection, as indicated by health care professionals
- careful adherence to perineal hygiene measures
- careful attention to proper disposal of body fluids and contaminated needles
- thorough hand washing after contact with infected areas and before contact with the neonate and others.

For the patient with an infection, help the couple identify the needs of the neonate as a member of their family; help them identify ways to handle society's fear of disease transmission; and encourage them to obtain information about the disease so that they can prevent transmission.

Evaluation

To evaluate nursing care, determine if specific goals were achieved. The following examples illustrate some appropriate evaluation statements:

- The patient correctly described the potential effects of her condition on herself and on her child.
- The patient and family demonstrated correct infection control measures.

Substance abuse

When a pregnant woman abuses illegal drugs or alcohol, it can affect her as well as her child. She may suffer physical, psychological, social, and economic consequences. In addition, she may have a spontaneous abortion or premature delivery, or she may develop PIH, hemorrhage, or abruptio placentae.

A pregnant substance abuser is likely to neglect prenatal care because she fears admonishment from health care professionals, lacks the self-esteem to make personal health care a priority, or views prenatal care as unimportant and unnecessary. Yet such a patient has a greater need for care because of possible exposure to HIV, STDs, hepatitis, malnutrition, and infection from injection sites—as well as the increased risk of hypertension, antepartal bleeding, abruptio placentae, spontaneous abortion or stillbirth, and preterm labor. These factors and risks may arise from poor health, inadequate nutrition, infection, shared needles, multiple sex partners, and drug abuse and its effects.

First-trimester substance abuse has teratogenic effects and increases the risk of spontaneous abortion. Use of cocaine may cause abnormalities in chromosomal structure or numbers and congenital anomalies, such as genitourinary malformations. Substance abuse may cause problems for the neonate as well, including IUGR, premature birth, withdrawal symptoms, and fetal alcohol syndrome.

Assessment

A careful, open-ended history regarding each pregnant patient's potential use and abuse of alcohol, illicit drugs, and cigarettes must be collected. Urine drug testing provides information about substances abused. Biophysical profile testing later in pregnancy assists with fetal health evaluation.

Nursing diagnoses
After considering all assessment findings, formulate appropriate nursing diagnoses for the patient. (For a partial list of applicable diagnoses, see Nursing Diagnoses: *Antepartal complications,* pages 66 and 67.)

Planning and implementation
When a pregnant substance abuser seeks health care, obtain baseline data and suggest ways to correct any health deficits, such as referring her to a drug rehabilitation program to control her substance abuse or providing nutrition counseling and information about prescribed vitamin and iron supplements. Encourage the patient to keep scheduled appointments.

The pregnant substance abuser needs early prenatal care to decrease the risk of congenital anomalies in her neonate. Offer her firm support and reassurance during follow-up visits. If she appears for care late in the pregnancy or misses appointments, continue to provide sensitive care at every opportunity during the antepartal, intrapartal, and postpartal periods. Stress confidentiality and the importance of keeping her and her baby healthy. Help the patient recognize that substances affect her fetus. If appropriate, inform the patient that her neonate may undergo withdrawal.

For a patient with an opiate or heroin addiction, a controlled substance withdrawal method with methadone administration, although controversial, may be recommended. "Cold turkey" withdrawal is not recommended during pregnancy because of the risk of fetal seizures, fetal hypoxia, and fetal death as well as the risk of preterm labor and delivery. A patient receiving methadone also participates in group counseling sessions. A multidisciplinary approach provides comprehensive physical, psychological, social, and economic care to the pregnant substance abuser.

When evaluating the patient's dietary habits, also assess her financial status to determine if she has enough money to buy food. Such a patient may spend more money on drugs than on basic needs. If necessary, consult a social worker, who will determine the patient's eligibility for food stamps and Women, Infants, and Children assistance. The patient should also see a nutritionist or dietitian regularly.

The patient may benefit from neonatal care instruction during individual counseling sessions or from frequent home follow-up visits by the public health nurse.

Evaluation

To evaluate nursing care, determine if specific goals were achieved. The following examples illustrate some appropriate evaluation statements:

• The patient correctly described the potential effects of her condition on herself and her child.
• The patient kept appointments for prenatal care and laboratory tests.

Premature rupture of membranes

Premature rupture of membranes (PROM) is any rupture of the amniotic sac before onset of labor, independent of length of gestation. It presents a challenge because of the divergent opinions surrounding its treatment. It is associated with maternal morbidity and mortality, primarily because of increased incidence of infection. Fetal and neonatal risks include sepsis, preterm delivery, anoxia, respiratory distress syndrome, umbilical cord prolapse, and traumatic delivery.

Etiology

The etiology of PROM usually is unknown. Many conditions predispose a woman to this disorder, including incompetent cervix, amnionitis, placenta previa, fetal malpresentation, hydramnios, multiple gestation, and trauma. A complication of PROM, infection also may be a cause.

Incidence

Between 3% and 19% of all deliveries are preceded by PROM. The percentage is significantly higher in preterm pregnancies.

Assessment

A pelvic examination discloses whether PROM has occurred. Using aseptic technique, a physician, nurse-midwife, or specially prepared nurse uses a sterile speculum to observe the cervix. Direct observation of amniotic fluid seeping from the cervical os confirms PROM. If this fluid is not visible, the practitioner may elect to test with nitrazine paper, which will indicate an alkaline substance by turning blue. (The vaginal area normally is acidic and amniotic fluid is alkaline.)

Nitrazine paper has about a 95% accuracy rate. False-negative results may occur if several hours have elapsed since rupture of the membranes or if the vaginal area has been contaminated with blood, urine, or antiseptic solutions.

Other tests to determine if fluid is amniotic include a smear on a clean slide (amniotic fluid makes a distinctive ferning pattern when it dries) and a staining technique to identify fetal fat cells. Because no laboratory or clinical test is foolproof, however, a combination of tests is necessary for an accurate diagnosis.

Ultrasound may be useful in identifying PROM if oligohydramnios (a scant amount of amniotic fluid) can be identified on the scan. Once a diagnosis of PROM has been confirmed, the age of the fetus must be determined, and ultrasound can be useful in this area.

Nursing diagnoses
After considering all assessment findings, formulate appropriate nursing diagnoses for the patient. (For a partial list of applicable diagnoses, see Nursing Diagnoses: *Antepartal complications,* pages 66 and 67.)

Planning and implementation
An inaccurate diagnosis of PROM may lead to unnecessary induction of labor, cesarean delivery, or preterm delivery. Therefore, the physician must make every effort to make an accurate diagnosis of the disorder.

Management of PROM usually involves two distinctly different approaches based on the assessment of risks to both mother and fetus. In active management, labor is induced and, if not effective, a cesarean delivery is performed. In expectant management, no action is taken to speed the onset of labor except in cases of amnionitis or fetal distress. During this time, the patient is placed on bed rest and is observed for signs and symptoms of infection.

Respiratory distress syndrome (RDS) develops in 10% to 40% of neonates born to patients with PROM. Neonatal sepsis is identified in approximately 10% of neonates, and amnionitis occurs in 4% to 30%. Other neonatal complications include asphyxia, malpresentation, and umbilical cord prolapse. Maternal complications include cesarean delivery and endometritis (inflammation of the uterus lining), occurring in 3% to 30% of patients with PROM. Maternal mortality related to PROM is rare. Neonatal mortality is caused by RDS in 30% to 70% of cases; infection accounts for 3% to 20%.

About 28% of patients who experience PROM prior to 37 weeks' gestation develop infections, which are potentially severe. Procedures to identify infection include maternal serum C-reactive protein and fetal movement studies, frequent maternal temperatures, and frequent nonstress tests.

Evaluation
To evaluate nursing care, determine if specific goals were achieved. The following examples illustrate some appropriate evaluation statements:
• The patient reported a change in her condition as soon as it occurred.
• The patient's family demonstrated appropriate support and concern.

Preterm labor and delivery
Preterm delivery is defined as any delivery, regardless of the neonate's birth weight, that occurs between 20 and 37 weeks after the patient's last menses. Preterm labor and delivery has been a significant cause of perinatal morbidity and mortality for many years. Advances in technology have enhanced medical management of small neonates, but no significant decrease in low-birth-weight, preterm neonates has been documented. The problem of preterm delivery is one of the most significant to be overcome in attempting to improve the outcome of pregnancy.

Etiology

Many factors can contribute to the onset of preterm labor and delivery, including pneumonia, appendicitis with sepsis, other acute infections, multiple gestation, poverty, smoking, alcohol and drug abuse, grand multiparity (five or more previous births), teenage pregnancy, and uterine anomalies. Psychological trauma also may be a contributing factor, as well as adverse events or chronic stress during the second and third trimesters.

Incidence

Preterm labor and delivery accounts for 5% to 10% of all births. Although the percentage is relatively small, this condition accounts for most neonatal deaths. The incidence almost doubles for African-American patients.

Maternal age under 19 or over 34 also is a significant factor. A previous preterm labor and delivery is associated with a risk of recurrence of 17% to 30%, with the incidence increasing significantly after two or more preterm labors and deliveries.

Women in lower socioeconomic groups have an increased incidence of preterm labor and delivery. This may be related to nutritional status, knowledge deficit, inadequate prenatal care, and many other factors during pregnancy.

Assessment

The early symptoms of preterm labor are so subtle that they may be overlooked by the patient and the medical and nursing staffs. Because of missed early symptoms, fewer than 25% of patients in preterm labor are candidates for long-term therapy to prevent preterm births. Such therapy is contraindicated in PROM (30% to 40%), advanced cervical dilation (4 cm or more), maternal hemorrhage, and evidence of severe fetal compromise (decelerations in fetal heart rate).

Because the onset of preterm labor is insidious, a primary goal of obstetric care is to prevent it. Many of the factors contributing to preterm labor are reliable indicators and can be used to identify the patient at risk. Patient education is of utmost importance. (For more information, see *Identifying the patient at risk for preterm labor.*)

If the membranes are intact, the physician or nurse-midwife performs a digital pelvic examination of the cervix. Cervical changes may indicate that labor is proceeding; nevertheless, in some cases the physician or nurse-midwife may choose to wait for progressive cervical changes before beginning therapy.

Because urinary tract infections commonly are associated with preterm labor, a urinalysis should be performed to determine whether bacteria are present.

Identifying the patient at risk for preterm labor

Several factors in the development of preterm labor are of reliable, predictive value. Any factor from the high-risk category or any two from the moderate-risk category call for increased antepartal surveillance.

HIGH-RISK CATEGORY
History factors
- Cone biopsy
- Uterine anomaly
- At least one abortion during the second trimester
- Exposure to diethylstilbestrol (DES)
- Preterm delivery
- Preterm labor

Factors in current pregnancy
- Placenta previa
- Hydramnios
- Abdominal surgery
- More than one fetus present
- Cervical dilation

- Effacement greater than 50%
- Uterine irritability
- Substance abuse

MODERATE-RISK CATEGORY
Socioeconomic factors
- Low socioeconomic status
- Age: less than age 19 or over age 34
- Single parent
- Work outside the home
- Height: less than 5' 3" (160 cm)
- Weight: less than 100 lb (45 kg)
- Cigarettes: more than 10 daily

History factors
- Febrile illness
- Pyelonephritis

- First trimester abortion (fewer than 3)
- Less than 1 year since last delivery

Factors in current pregnancy
- Bleeding after 12 weeks' gestation
- Weight gain less than 7 lb (3.2 kg) by 22 weeks' gestation
- Albuminuria
- Hypertension
- Bacteriuria
- Weight loss of 5 lb (2.3 kg)
- Febrile illness
- Fetal head engaged at 32 weeks' gestation

Nursing diagnoses
After considering all assessment findings, formulate appropriate nursing diagnoses for the patient. (For a partial list of applicable diagnoses, see Nursing Diagnoses: *Antepartal complications,* pages 66 and 67.)

Planning and implementation
Management of preterm labor begins with bed rest in the lateral decubitus position and external uterine monitoring of fetal status. Tocolysis (inhibition of uterine contractions) is a primary tool in caring for a patient with preterm labor.

Tocolytic drugs may be used to inhibit labor until term, interrupt labor long enough to transport the mother to a high-risk health care facility, or inhibit labor until prenatal steroids are effective in increasing fetal lung maturity. They are 60% to 88% effective.

Absolute contraindications to tocolytic drugs include severe PIH, severe bleeding from any cause, chorioamnionitis, fetal death, a fetal anomaly that is incompatible with life, and severe fetal growth retardation. Relative contraindications include mild chronic hypertension, stable placenta previa, uncontrolled diabetes mellitus, fetal distress, and cervical dilation greater than 5 cm.

Other tocolytic drugs include beta-adrenergic agents (isoxsuprine hydrochloride, ritodrine, and terbutaline sulfate), which inhibit the contractility of the myometrium. Magnesium sulfate, used to treat hypertensive episodes in pregnancy, is gaining use as a tocolytic. It has fewer adverse effects than beta-adrenergic agents and can be used in conjunction with beta-adrenergics or when they are contraindicated. Absolute contraindications to magnesium sulfate include myasthenia gravis, impaired renal function, and recent myocardial infarction.

Tocolysis in conjunction with close uterine contraction monitoring can significantly reduce the incidence of preterm labor. A lightweight, highly sensitive tocodynamometer allows outpatient monitoring of uterine activity. This in-home monitoring capability is provided with an intensive perinatal nursing service that incorporates 24-hour nurse availability, daily transmission of recorded uterine activity, weekly physician update, and ongoing patient teaching and reinforcement of the treatment plan. The cost of these programs varies, but many are covered under health insurance plans. Monitoring usually is initiated at around 20 weeks' gestation and continues until 36 weeks' gestation.

Evaluation

To evaluate nursing care, determine if specific goals were achieved. The following examples illustrate appropriate evaluation statements:
• The patient has exhibited proper use of an in-home uterine monitor.
• The patient has shown an understanding of preterm labor warnings.

STUDY ACTIVITIES

Short answer

1. Debra Solomon, a 38-year-old primigravida at 28 weeks' gestation, has a blood pressure of 148/92 mm Hg during a routine prenatal visit. Her baseline blood pressure has been between 100/68 and 110/72. Ms. Solomon admits a past medical history of labile blood pressure that did not require medication. The nurse should assess Ms. Solomon for which signs and symptoms that would indicate PIH?

_____

2. During the completion of her prenatal visit at 24 weeks' gestation, Alejandra Loyola, a 26-year-old primigravida, is to be scheduled for a 1-hour glucose challenge test at her next return visit in 4 weeks. How can the nurse prepare Ms. Loyola for this test, and why is it routinely recommended for all pregnant women?

_____

_____

3. Josephine O'Neill, a 21-year-old primigravida and a known cardiac patient, is counseled by the nurse during her initial prenatal exam at 6 weeks' gestation. The nurse explains to Ms. O'Neill that self-monitoring is important, especially for the cardiac patient during pregnancy. What signs and symptoms of potential complications should Ms. O'Neill be told to report to the physician?

_____

4. Briefly state the nursing goals that are common to all high-risk antepartal patients.

_____

5. What are the dangers of continued vomiting in a patient with hyperemesis gravidarum, and what should the nurse assess in a patient with this complaint?

_____

6. What is the purpose of an alpha-fetoprotein (AFP) test?

_____

7. List three possible maternal and three fetal or neonatal effects of diabetes during pregnancy.

_____

_____

8. List the factors that predispose a woman to PIH.

_____

9. How is iron deficiency anemia of pregnancy diagnosed? (State the appropriate laboratory values.)

_____

10. Identify all the infections that are characterized in the acronym TORCH and state why they are significant during pregnancy.

_____

True or false

11. Ectopic pregnancy is the leading cause of maternal death in the first trimester.
☐ True   ☐ False

12. GTD is malignant and metastasizes quickly.
☐ True   ☐ False

13. Hyperemesis gravidarum is strictly psychogenic in origin.
☐ True   ☐ False

14. Incompetent cervix is characterized by painless dilation of the cervix without labor or uterine contraction.
☐ True   ☐ False

15. First-trimester substance abuse has teratogenic effects on the fetus and increases the risk of spontaneous abortion.
☐ True   ☐ False

16. "Cold turkey" withdrawal is recommended during pregnancy when the patient is an opiate or heroin addict, because of the serious fetal effects of these drugs.
☐ True   ☐ False

17. Women in lower socioeconomic groups have an increased incidence of preterm labor.
☐ True   ☐ False

18. Maternal mortality related to PROM is of great concern and determines the need for aggressive medical management.
☐ True   ☐ False

ANSWERS   **Short answer**

1. The nurse should ask Ms. Solomon if she has experienced visual disturbances, headaches, epigastric pain, irritability, or muscle tremors. In addition, a physical examination may disclose the three classic signs of PIH: elevated blood pressure, proteinuria, and edema.

2. The nurse should explain that the 1-hour (50-gram) diabetes screening test is recommended for each pregnant patient at 24 to 28 weeks' gestation. Ms. Loyola should be advised *not* to fast before the test. A blood sample for glucose testing will be drawn 1 hour after she ingests 50 grams of oral glucose solution. If her plasma glucose level is abnormally high, she can expect a 3-hour oral glucose tolerance test.

The reason for this routine screening is that all women experience dramatic changes in carbohydrate, lipid, and protein metabolism during pregnancy. A pregnant woman is normally more susceptible to both hypoglycemia and hyperglycemia. Yet for some women, the growing fetus stresses maternal glucose production and use, disrupting normal carbohydrate metabolism and causing GDM. If diabetes is not adequately identified and managed during pregnancy, it increases fetal and neonatal risks.

3. Ms. O'Neill should report increased limitation of activity; the presence of or increase in dyspnea, orthopnea, tachypnea, or edema; development of palpitations; significant increase or decrease in heart rate; and chest discomfort.

4. Common nursing goals include promoting the physical well-being of the patient and her fetus, preventing or controlling further complications, preventing sequelae, and providing emotional support to the patient and her family.

5. Continued vomiting leads to dehydration, ultimately decreasing the circulating blood volume (hypovolemia). Persistent dehydration also leads to confusion and coma as well as hepatic and renal failure. The nurse should assess the patient with persistent vomiting for signs such as weight loss, increased pulse rate, decreased blood pressure, changes in skin turgor, and dry mucus membranes.

6. The purposes of an AFP test is to predict open neural tube defects, such as spina bifida and anencephaly, in the fetus and to screen for Down's syndrome.

7. Maternal effects of diabetes, which are determined by the severity of the disease, include the possibility of developing increased ketosis (which may lead to her coma and death without proper treatment); hydramnios (which may lead to maternal discomfort, PROM, or premature labor); PIH; and glycosuria (which predisposes the patient to moniliasis and urinary tract infections).

Maternal diabetes also may have many adverse effects on the fetus and neonate. Increased incidence of fetal anomalies and neonatal morbidity and predisposing the neonate to diabetes. Without careful management maternal diabetes increases the risk of fetal or neonatal death. Neonates born to diabetic mothers may have macrosomia and are more likely to develop neonatal hyperbilirubinemia and hypoglycemia after birth.

8. Factors that predispose a woman to PIH include primigravidity, multiple gestation, vascular disease, GTD (hydatidiform mole), and malnutrition or dietary deficiencies.

9. Iron deficiency anemia is diagnosed with a hemoglobin level below 11 g/liter and the hematocrit below 32%.

10. The acronym TORCH refers to toxoplasmosis, other infections (such as chlamydia, group B beta-hemolytic streptococcus, syphilis, and varicella zoster), rubella, cytomegalovirus, and herpesvirus type 2 infections. These infections can cause major congenital anomalies or death of the embryo or fetus.

True or false
11. True.
12. False. GTD may be either benign (hydatidiform mole) or malignant (choriocarcinoma).
13. False. The cause of hyperemesis gravidarum is not known. It may be caused by hormonal alterations, such as changes in progesterone or human chorionic gonadotropin levels. Although some believe that hyperemesis is related to psychosomatic causes, research has failed to demonstrate this.
14. True.
15. True.
16. False. "Cold turkey" withdrawal is not recommended during pregnancy because of the risk of fetal seizures, fetal hypoxia, and fetal death as well as preterm labor and delivery.
17. True.
18. False. Maternal mortality related to PROM is rare. Neonatal mortality is caused by RDS in 30% to 70% of cases and caused by infection in 3% to 20%.

CHAPTER 7

Physiology of labor and childbirth

OBJECTIVES
After studying this chapter, the reader should be able to:

1. Identify the physiologic changes that commonly precede the onset of labor.
2. Describe the physiology associated with uterine contractions, cervical effacement, and dilation.
3. Explain the mechanisms associated with fetal cardinal movements.
4. Recognize the four stages of labor and describe the maternal physiologic changes that occur in each stage.
5. Define the five essential factors of labor and briefly identify how each affects the physiology of labor and childbirth.
6. Briefly discuss selected fetal physiologic responses to labor.

OVERVIEW OF CONCEPTS
Impending labor and childbirth typically trigger both excitement and apprehension in a pregnant patient. Whether the patient is about to give birth for the first time (primipara) or is experienced from previous childbirth (multipara), she will have many physical and psychological needs. To meet these needs, the nurse must understand the labor process and how it affects the mother and fetus.

Premonitory signs and symptoms of labor
Although several theories of labor onset have been proposed, the exact mechanism is still unknown. Instead of a single initiating factor, several maternal, fetal, and placental factors probably interact to start labor.

Certain premonitory signs and symptoms typically precede the onset of true labor. Some of these signs and symptoms may occur up to 3 weeks before labor onset; others coincide with the beginning of labor. These signs and symptoms of premonitory labor include lightening, increased Braxton Hicks contractions, weight loss, the nesting instinct, the loss of the mucus plug, increased vaginal secretions, the presence of bloody show, and spontaneous rupture of membranes.

Lightening
Lightening occurs as the fetus settles lower in the pelvis. In primiparas, lightening normally occurs 2 to 3 weeks before labor begins; in multiparas, it may not occur until labor actually begins. This downward fetal movement allows the patient to breathe more deeply.

Braxton Hicks contractions
Throughout pregnancy, the uterus undergoes a series of painless, irregular contractions known as Braxton Hicks contractions. These help prepare for labor by causing subtle, nonprogressive cervical changes late in pregnancy.

Weight loss
A weight loss of 1 to 3 lb, representing water loss, may result from changes in electrolyte concentrations of body fluids, related to hormonal shifts in the last few days before labor onset.

Nesting instinct
In the last few days before labor onset, the patient may experience a burst of energy known as the "nesting instinct." She may feel compelled to ensure that everything is ready for the neonate's arrival. The nurse should caution such a patient against overexertion.

Vaginal and cervical changes
Increased vaginal secretions resulting from congestion of vaginal mucous membranes may occur. The cervix undergoes prelabor changes, and the mucus plug—which protects the cervix throughout pregnancy—becomes dislodged. At the same time, some of the cervical capillaries rupture; blood mixes with the mucus, producing what is known as "bloody show." Normally, only a few drops of blood mix with the mucus plug. Any larger amount of vaginal bleeding must be reported to the physician or nurse-midwife.

Spontaneous rupture of membranes (SROM)
At term, approximately 12% of all pregnant patients experience SROM before labor begins. Within 24 hours, labor then will begin in the majority of these patients. A patient who does not deliver within 24 hours after SROM at term is considered to have prolonged rupture of membranes, a condition that puts her and the fetus at increased risk for infection.

When the rupture occurs, the amniotic fluid may flow profusely or it may dribble. Testing of vaginal discharge with nitrazine paper allows the examiner to distinguish between the two conditions. Amniotic fluid is alkaline (pH 7.2), which turns yellow nitrazine paper a deep blue upon contact. Other tests that determine amniotic fluid include microscopic examination of a sample of the fluid for a characteristic ferning pattern and visualizing the cervix with a sterile speculum to observe fluid leakage.

Mechanisms of labor For most patients, labor follows a consistent pattern. As uterine contractions intensify, the cervix effaces and dilates. Propelled by uterine contractions and the patient's bearing-down efforts, the fetus descends through the birth canal via its cardinal movements.

Cervical effacement and dilation

Myometrial activity of the uterus leads to full cervical effacement and dilation. Effacement refers to a progressive shortening of the vaginal portion of the cervix and thinning of its walls as it is stretched by the fetus during labor. Effacement is described as a percentage, ranging from 0% (noneffaced and thick) to 100% (fully effaced and paper-thin). The fully effaced cervix becomes continuous with the lower uterine segment.

Cervical dilation refers to progressive enlargement of the cervical opening, the os, from less than 1 cm to about 10 cm (full dilation) to allow passage of the fetus from the uterus into the vagina. Because uterine muscle fibers remain shortened even after a contraction ceases, the uterine cavity progressively decreases in size. These actions force the fetus downward on the cervix. Cervical dilation results from this pressure—referred to as fetal axis pressure—plus the upward pulling of longitudinal muscle fibers over the fetus. Typically, effacement and dilation occur more quickly in multiparas than in primiparas.

Cardinal movements

Cardinal movements refer to the typical sequence of positions assumed by the fetus during labor and childbirth (see *Cardinal movements of labor* for illustrations of these positions).

Stages of labor Labor consists of four distinct stages. Understanding what occurs during each stage will help the nurse anticipate and meet the patient's needs in labor.

First stage of labor

The first stage of labor is divided into latent, active, and transitional phases. Cervical dilation and fetal descent begin during the latent phase, then accelerate during the active and transitional phases. In total, the first stage of labor, including the three phases, ranges between 3.3 and 19.7 hours for primiparas and 0.1 to 14.3 hours for multiparas (see *Parameters for phases of the first stage of labor,* page 104, for specific information).

Second stage of labor

The second stage begins with complete cervical dilation and ends with birth. Intense contractions occur every 3 to 4 minutes and last 60 to 90 seconds. For primiparas, this stage averages 1 hour; for multiparas, 24 minutes. In either case, a second stage longer than 2 hours is considered abnormal.

Cardinal movements of labor

For a fetus in the vertex (crown or top of head) presentation, labor follows a typical sequence. Inset boxes show the relationship of the fetal skull to the maternal pelvis.

1. Engagement, descent, flexion. The widest diameter of the head passes the level of the pelvic inlet; as the fetus moves downward toward the ischial spines, the head flexes on the chest.

2. Internal rotation. The anteroposterior diameter of the head comes into line with the anteroposterior diameter of the pelvic outlet caused by twisting of the neck. The shoulders remain oblique. This occurs during the second stage.

3. Extension. The head extends from the perineum after passing under the symphysis pubis in response to uterine contractions, resistance of the pelvic floor, and maternal bearing-down efforts.

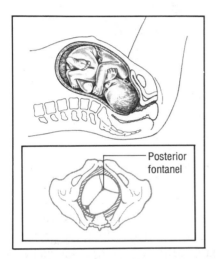

Posterior fontanel

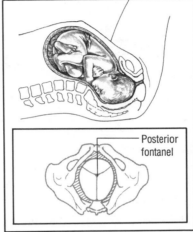

Posterior fontanel

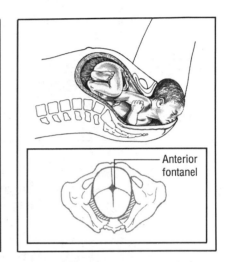

Anterior fontanel

4. External rotation (restitution). The head rotates 45 degrees back to its original position established during engagement.

5. External (shoulder) rotation. The head rotates an additional 45° to align the shoulders with the anteroposterior diameter of the pelvis. The anterior shoulder passes under the symphysis pubis; the posterior shoulder follows.

6. Expulsion. The rest of the body is easily delivered by lateral flexion once the shoulders pass over the perineum.

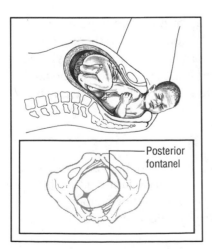

Posterior fontanel

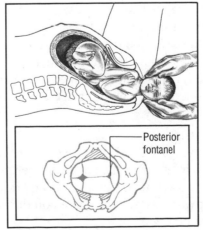

Posterior fontanel

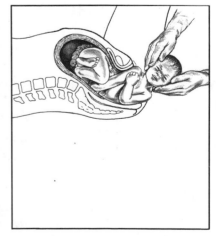

Parameters for phases of the first stage of labor

During the first stage of labor, the nurse must be able to monitor normal progress for primiparas and multiparas. By observing trends in contraction patterns, the nurse can anticipate the patient's needs and identify potential problems.

PHASE	HOURS IN LABOR (AVERAGE/LIMITS OF NORMAL)	CERVIX (DILATION/ EFFACEMENT)	CONTRACTION PATTERN (FREQUENCY, DURATION, INTENSITY)	STATION
Latent	• Primipara: 8.6 hours/<20 hours • Multipara: 5.3 hours/<14 hours	0 to 3 cm/0% to 50%	Occur every 5 to 10 minutes and last 15 to 30 seconds; mild to palpation	-2/0
Active	• Primipara: 4.9 hours/12 hours • Multipara: 2.2 hours/5 hours	4 to 7 cm/50% to 75%	Occur every 3 to 4 minutes and last 45 to 60 seconds; moderate to palpation	-1/0
Transition	• Primipara: 0.84 hour/3 hours • Multipara: 0.36 hour/1 hour	8 to 10 cm/ 75% to 100%	Occur every 2 minutes and last 60 to 90 seconds; strong to palpation; shortest but most intense phase	0/+1

The beginning of this stage is characterized by an increase in bloody show, rupture of membranes (if this has not already occurred), intense rectal pressure, and a bearing-down reflex with each contraction. At this time, the patient assumes an active role and pushes with each contraction. As the fetus approaches the perineal floor, the perineum bulges and flattens. The head appears at the vaginal opening as the labia spread.

Fetal head

To prevent maternal lacerations and damage to the fetus's intracranial area, the birth attendant must control the speed at which the head passes the perineum. When necessary, applying pressure over the perineum can maintain flexion of the head.

Once the head emerges, the physician or nurse-midwife must check for the umbilical cord. If the cord is loose around the neck, it should be slipped over the head. If the cord is very tight, fetal hypoxia may occur; therefore, the birth attendant must clamp and cut the cord while it is still around the neck. The oral and nasal pharynx then are suctioned with a bulb syringe to remove secretions that may be blocking the airway.

Shoulders

Following external rotation of the head, the shoulders pass through the pelvic inlet. After the head emerges, the birth attendant applies slight downward traction to free the anterior shoulder. After it emerges, gentle upward traction is applied on the head to allow the posterior shoulder to emerge.

Body and extremities

Once the shoulders emerge, the rest of the body, which is narrower than the shoulders, slides out with little or no traction needed.

Third stage of labor

The third stage begins immediately after birth and ends with the separation and expulsion of the placenta. Strong but usually less painful contractions continue during this stage; their frequency may decrease to every 5 minutes. Normally, the placenta emerges about 5 minutes after the neonate's delivery.

Placental separation

Placental separation usually begins within minutes after birth. After the neonate is delivered, the uterus consists of an almost solid mass of muscle with walls several centimeters thick above its lower segment. The fundus lies immediately below the umbilicus.

Signs indicating placental separation include lengthening of the umbilical cord, a sudden gush of dark blood from the vagina, and a change in uterine shape from disklike to globular (which the nurse can palpate or see as a visible bulge above the symphysis). The patient may have a sensation of vaginal fullness.

Placental delivery

The placenta is expelled through one of two mechanisms. In the Schultze mechanism, the central portion of the placenta separates from the uterine wall before the outside edges do. Then the central portion folds or buckles outward, away from a retroplacental hematoma. When the placenta is expelled, the shiny fetal side (commonly called "shiny Schultze") is visible.

In the Duncan mechanism, the placental edges separate first, followed by the central portion. Then the central portion rolls up and is expelled sideways, so that the rough-surfaced maternal side (commonly called "dirty Duncan") is visible. In the Duncan mechanism, separation may be incomplete, leaving placental fragments that may lead to infection or bleeding.

Immediately after delivery, the placenta is evaluated carefully for completeness, and the patient is assessed for excessive bleeding or a relaxed uterus.

Fourth stage of labor

Beginning with delivery of the placenta and extending through the first hour after childbirth, the fourth stage allows the patient's body to adjust to the postpartal stage. She should be assessed carefully for uterine atony with a subsequent postpartal hemorrhage. Ideally, the patient and her partner should now hold and examine the neonate and begin bonding.

Factors affecting labor

Successful labor and childbirth require coordination of five essential factors, sometimes termed the "five p's":
- passenger (the fetus)
- passageway (the pelvis)
- powers (uterine contractions and bearing-down efforts)
- placental position and function
- psychological response.

For the fetus to move successfully through the pelvis, the contractions and bearing-down efforts must be of adequate intensity and frequency, the placenta must be properly positioned and provide adequate oxygen to the fetus, and the patient must be psychologically prepared. Problems involving any of these essential factors may jeopardize safe labor and childbirth and require medical or surgical intervention.

Fetus

Fetal factors affecting labor and childbirth include size and shape of the head, lie, attitude, presentation, position, and station.

Head

The skull is composed of several small, thin, and incompletely developed bones, which eventually fuse to form the rigid cranial cavity characteristic of the adult. The skull bones are connected by flexible, membrane-occupied spaces called sutures. During labor, the skull bones are pressed together and may overlap (molding), reducing the size of the head and facilitating passage through the unyielding pelvis (see *The fetal skull and its adaptation to birth* for illustrations).

Lie

Fetal lie refers to the position of the fetal spine in relation to the maternal spine. When the two spines are parallel, the fetus is in a longitudinal lie; when perpendicular, a transverse lie. When the fetal spine is at an angle between the parallel and perpendicular position, the fetus is in an oblique lie. A longitudinal lie is required for a vaginal birth, otherwise surgical intervention is necessary.

Attitude

Fetal attitude refers to overall body flexion or extension, which determines the relationship of fetal parts to one another. The usual fetal attitude in the uterus is vertex, with the head flexed so that the chin rests against the chest, with the legs and arms folded in front of the body and the back curved slightly forward.

Position

Fetal position refers to the relationship of the presenting part to the front, back, or side of the maternal pelvis. It is established by determining three factors: a landmark on the fetal presenting part, whether this landmark faces the right or left side of the maternal pelvis, and whether the landmark faces the front, back, or side of the maternal pelvis (for more information, see *Determining fetal position,* page 108).

The fetal skull and its adaptation to birth

At birth, the skull is composed of several thin, incompletely developed bones connected by membranous joints called sutures, which intersect at areas called fontanels. Responding to pressure exerted by the maternal pelvis and the birth canal during labor and delivery, sutures allow the cranial bones to shift, molding the head and easing the passage of the fetus. The type of molding that occurs is determined by fetal attitude—the overall degree of body flexion or extension.

Skull characteristics

In the normal fetus, the skull includes the landmarks and diameters shown in the illustrations below. The diameter measurements are averages for term neonates; individual measurements vary with fetal size, attitude, and presentation.

- *Biparietal diameter:* measured between the parietal eminences; the widest transverse diameter of the head; 9.5 cm.
- *Bitemporal diameter:* measured between the lateral sides of the temporal bones; the shortest transverse diameter of the head; 8 cm.
- *Occipitofrontal diameter:* measured from the external occipital protuberance to the glabella; 11.5 cm.
- *Occipitomental diameter:* measured from the external occipital protuberance to the chin; 12.5 cm.

- *Suboccipitobregmatic diameter:* measured from the underside of the occipital bone to the middle of the bregma; the anteroposterior diameter that presents when the head is well flexed; 9.5 cm.
- *Submentobregmatic diameter:* measured from the junction of the neck and lower jaw to the middle of the bregma; the diameter that presents in face presentations when the head is fully extended; 9.5 cm.
- *Verticomental diameter:* measured from the chin to the middle of the sagittal suture; seen in brow presentations; 13.5 cm. A normal-sized head cannot pass through a normal-sized pelvis in this position.

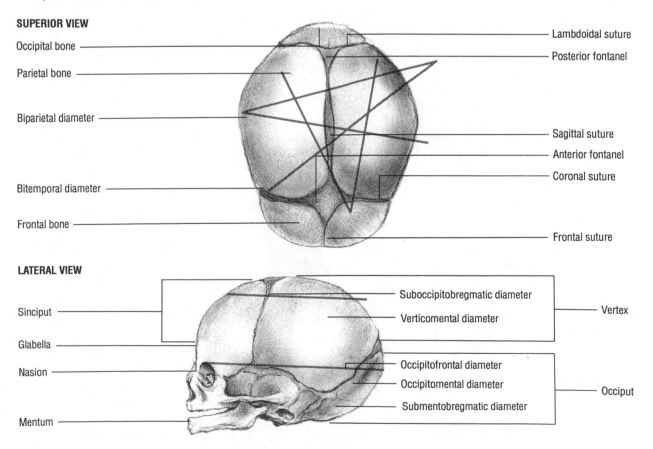

SUPERIOR VIEW

Occipital bone — Lambdoidal suture — Posterior fontanel

Parietal bone

Biparietal diameter — Sagittal suture — Anterior fontanel — Coronal suture

Bitemporal diameter

Frontal bone — Frontal suture

LATERAL VIEW

Sinciput — Suboccipitobregmatic diameter — Verticomental diameter — Vertex

Glabella

Nasion — Occipitofrontal diameter — Occipitomental diameter — Submentobregmatic diameter — Occiput

Mentum

Determining fetal position

Fetal position is determined by the relationship of a specific presenting part to the front, back, or side of the maternal pelvis. A notation system identifies three features: a landmark on the presenting part (O for occiput, M for mentum, S for sacrum, A for acromion process, and D for dorsal); whether this landmark faces the right (R) or left (L) side of the pelvis; and whether the landmark faces the front (A for anterior), the back (P for posterior), or a side (T for transverse) of the pelvis. Thus, for a fetus with the occiput (O) as the presenting landmark, positioned facing the left side (L) and front (A) of the maternal pelvis, the nurse would identify the position as LOA.

LEFT OCCIPUT POSTERIOR (LOP)

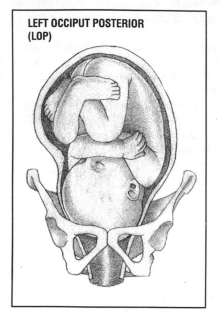

LEFT OCCIPUT TRANSVERSE (LOT)

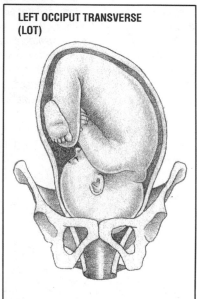

LEFT OCCIPUT ANTERIOR (LOA)

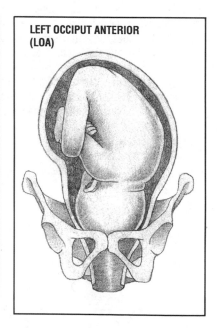

RIGHT OCCIPUT POSTERIOR (ROP)

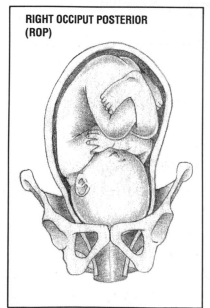

RIGHT OCCIPUT TRANSVERSE (ROT)

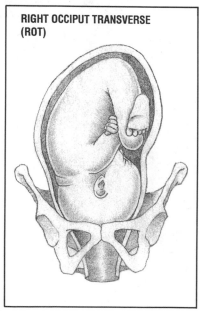

RIGHT OCCIPUT ANTERIOR (ROA)

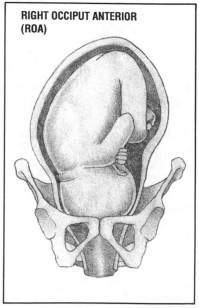

Presentation

Fetal presentation refers to the manner in which the fetus enters the pelvic passageway. Presentation is classified according to the presenting part—the portion of the fetus that enters the pelvic passageway first—as:

- cephalic (head-first)
- breech (buttocks-first)
- shoulder
- compound.

(See *Classifying fetal presentation,* pages 110 and 111, for illustrations and descriptions of these presentations.)

Approximately 95% of all births occur with the fetus assuming a cephalic presentation. Unless the fetus is in this presentation, cesarean delivery may be necessary. Three to four percent of all term pregnancies involve breech presentation. In most cases, the cause of breech presentation cannot be pinpointed; however, numerous maternal, placental, and fetal predisposing factors have been found, such as hydramnios (excessive amniotic fluid), placenta previa, or prematurity.

Station

Fetal station refers to the relationship of the presenting part to the maternal ischial spines. The ischial spines, located at midpelvis, form the narrowest portion of the pelvis through which the fetus must pass. When the largest diameter of the presenting part (usually the biparietal diameter of the head) is level with the ischial spines, the fetus is at station 0.

Successful vaginal birth requires progressive fetal descent. Lack of this progressive descent may indicate cephalopelvic disproportion or an inappropriately short or tangled umbilical cord. In such cases, cesarean delivery may be necessary.

Pelvis

The passageway through which the fetus must travel during labor consists of the pelvis and soft tissues. Pelvic types and diameters affect labor and childbirth. The pelvis is partly ligamentous and partly bony. Although there are four basic pelvic types—gynecoid, android, anthropoid, and platypelloid—a patient usually has features of two or more types.

The true pelvis contains three levels, or planes: the pelvic inlet, the midpelvis, and the pelvic outlet. Diameters measured in these three planes indicate the amount of space available for the fetus during birth.

The pelvis has four major diameters: the anteroposterior diameter of the inlet; the bi-ischial (or transverse) diameter of the midpelvis; the suprapubic angle with its bituberous diameter of the outlet; and the posterior sagittal diameter of all the three planes, somewhat determined by the curve and length of the sacrum.

Classifying fetal presentation

Fetal presentation may be broadly classified as cephalic, shoulder, compound, or breech. Cephalic presentations comprise almost all deliveries. Of the remaining three, breech deliveries are most common.

Cephalic

In the head-down presentation, the position of the fetus may be further classified by the presenting skull landmark, such as vertex, brow, sinciput, or face.

Vertex

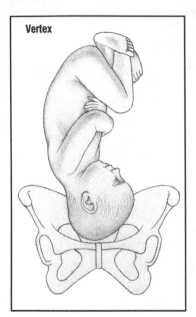

Brow

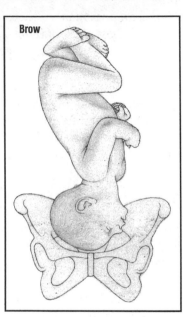

Sinciput

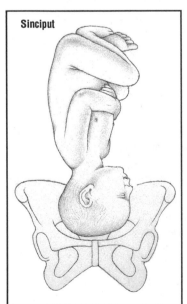

Face

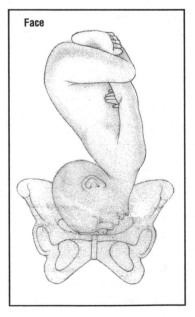

Shoulder

Although a fetus may adopt one of several shoulder presentations, examination cannot differentiate among them; thus, all transverse lies are called shoulder presentations.

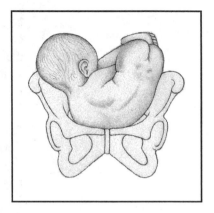

Compound

In this presentation, an extremity prolapses alongside the major presenting part so that two presenting parts appear in the pelvis at the same time.

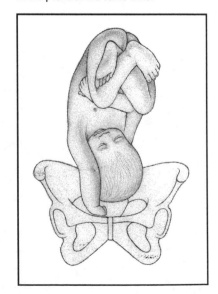

Classifying fetal presentation *(continued)*

Breech

In the head-up presentation, the position of the fetus may be further classified as frank, where hips are flexed and knees remain straight; complete, where knees and hips are flexed; footling, where the knees and hips of one or both legs are extended; kneeling, where knees are flexed and hips remain extended; and incomplete, where one or both hips remain extended and one or both feet or knees lie below the breech.

Frank

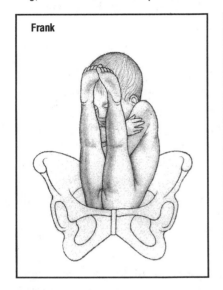

Complete

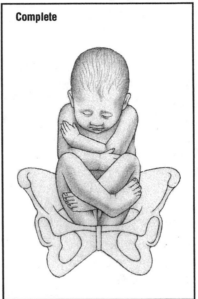

Footling

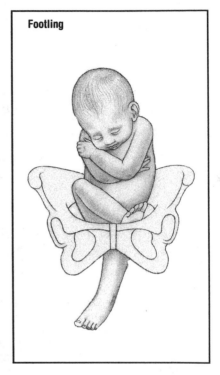

Kneeling

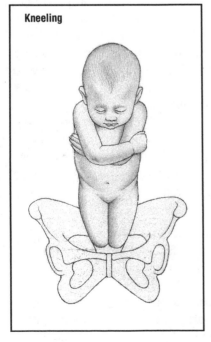

Incomplete

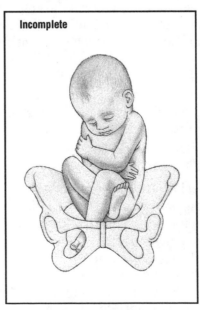

Contractions and bearing-down efforts

Uterine contractions and bearing-down efforts are also known as "the powers." Involuntary uterine contractions and voluntary bearing-down efforts must be adequate in intensity and frequency.

Uterine contractions

Coordinated and effective uterine contractions promote fetal descent and rotation, cervical effacement and dilation, separation and expulsion of the placenta, and constriction of the uterine vasculature to prevent postpartal hemorrhage.

A uterine contraction occurs in three phases: increment, acme, and decrement (see *Phases of a uterine contraction*).

During labor, the nurse evaluates the duration, frequency, and intensity of contractions. The duration of a contraction refers to the time between the beginning and end of the contraction. Duration usually ranges from 15 to 30 seconds in early labor to 60 to 90 seconds in later stages. The frequency of contractions is measured from the beginning of one contraction to the beginning of the next. In early labor, frequency ranges from 20 to 30 minutes; in the later stages, it ranges from 2 to 3 minutes. The intensity of a contraction refers to its strength during the acme phase. Intensity can be measured directly with an intrauterine catheter and indirectly by palpation or external monitoring.

Bearing-down efforts

Once uterine contractions have fully effaced and dilated the cervix, the second stage of labor begins and the patient's voluntary bearing-down efforts take over. The diaphragm and abdominal muscles are contracted to increase intra-abdominal pressure. This maternal action, which applies pressure to the uterine walls, adds to the pressures from uterine contractions and aids fetal descent and expulsion. The patient also experiences a great involuntary urge to push as the head of the fetus descends and pushes against the sacral and obturator nerves.

Positions for labor. Position during labor can affect the frequency and intensity of contractions. For a patient in the supine position, contractions may be less intense but more frequent. For one in the lateral position, contractions tend to be more intense but less frequent. Remaining upright by walking, standing, or sitting may shorten a patient's labor.

Placental position and function

Throughout pregnancy and during labor, the fetus depends on the placenta for oxygenated blood and nutrients. Placental malposition or malfunction can hinder labor and childbirth and may compromise the well-being of the fetus.

In most cases, the placenta is attached to the upper uterine segment. However, 1 in every 200 to 300 pregnancies involves placenta previa—implantation of the placenta in the lower uterine segment, where it partially or totally covers the cervical opening, the os. Besides blocking the os, placenta previa causes the placenta to separate from

Phases of a uterine contraction

As shown in this diagram, a uterine contraction occurs in three phases: increment (building up), acme (peak), and decrement (letting down). Between contractions is a period of relaxation. The two most important features of contractions are frequency and duration. Frequency refers to the elapsed time from the start of one contraction to the start of the next contraction. Duration is the elapsed time from the start to the end of one contraction.

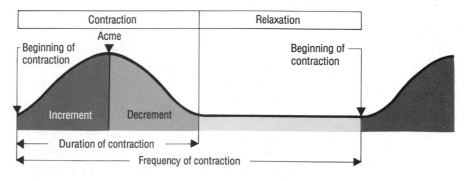

the uterine wall partially or totally as the cervix dilates, typically causing maternal hemorrhage and fetal compromise.

Another serious mechanical complication, abruptio placentae, occurs in about 1 in 250 pregnancies. The placenta prematurely separates from the uterine wall prior to or during labor, causing fetal death unless prompt surgical intervention occurs.

Uteroplacental insufficiency caused by maternal factors such as poor nutrition or pregnancy-induced hypertension impairs the ability of the fetus to withstand the rigors of labor by compromising fetal oxygenation.

Psychological response

The role that a pregnant woman's mental and emotional state plays in labor and childbirth has received increasing attention. There appears to be a relationship between anxiety and the length and difficulty of labor. For example, high epinephrine levels triggered by maternal anxiety can lead to diminished uterine activity and longer labors. Severe pain or distress-related thoughts may create an inefficient labor.

The importance of an appropriate psychological response to the physiologic and emotional demands of labor may be influenced by the patient's preparation for labor, support systems, and coping mechanisms.

Maternal systemic response to labor

Labor produces significant changes in many body systems. Understanding these changes will help the nurse provide better care for the patient during labor.

Cardiovascular system

In the first and second stages of labor, cardiovascular system changes primarily affect blood pressure. Cardiac output increases dramatically between contractions as labor progresses. Contractions during the first stage of labor also raise blood pressure readings slightly. Because of these expected fluctuations, the nurse should assess blood pressure readings between contractions so that they will be the most reliable ones.

Contractions in the second stage raise systolic and diastolic readings an average of 30 mm Hg and 25 mm Hg, respectively. Between contractions, blood pressure may remain elevated by 10 mm Hg systolic and 5 to 10 mm Hg diastolic. Also, the patient's voluntary bearing down efforts increase blood pressure and cardiac output.

The patient's position during labor also can affect blood pressure. Approximately 90% of patients at term experience supine hypotensive syndrome (when the gravid uterus compresses the vena cava in the supine position), although only 10% to 15% exhibit signs and symptoms, such as light-headedness. Factors that may increase a patient's risk of supine hypotensive syndrome include dehydration, hypovolemia, obesity, multiple gestation, and hydramnios.

Other factors that may alter blood pressure during labor include anxiety, pain, and certain medications. For example, hypotension may result from administration of a narcotic, such as meperidine (Demerol), because of its vasodilating effects.

A slow, progressive rise in pulse rate typically occurs during labor. Factors that may exacerbate this rise include pain, anxiety, hemorrhage, infection, certain medications (such as tocolytics), dehydration, increased cardiac output, and decreased plasma volume.

Gastrointestinal system

During labor, gastric motility and absorption decrease, and gastric emptying time (the time required for the stomach to empty) increases. Solid foods usually are withheld during labor to prevent the risk of aspiration if an emergency arises and general anesthesia is needed. For similar reasons, some physicians advocate giving the patient antacids to neutralize gastric acid either during labor or immediately before anesthetic administration. Because they do not alter gastrointestinal absorption of fluids, sipping water or chewing ice chips is allowed during labor.

Respiratory system

Both during and between contractions, oxygen consumption increases progressively throughout labor. By the second stage of labor, a patient's oxygen consumption may be twice that before onset of labor. This dramatic increase is especially likely in an unmedicated patient experiencing extreme anxiety. Resulting hyperventilation can lead to respiratory alkalosis, hypoxia, or hypocapnia. The nurse must monitor the patient for signs of such problems and intervene promptly to avoid endangering the fetus.

Hematopoietic system

The normal leukocyte count of 5,000 to 11,000 mm^3 may increase to about 25,000 mm^3 during labor. This rise occurs particularly during prolonged labor, perhaps due to strenuous muscle activity or increased stress. Other significant hematologic changes include increased plasma fibrinogen levels and decreased plasma glucose levels and blood coagulation times.

Renal and urologic system

During labor, decreased sensory perceptions may impair the patient's ability to feel bladder fullness and the urge to void. Also, compression of the ureters by the uterus may impede urine flow. Either of these factors can lead to urinary stasis and, if bladder fullness is profound, possibly impede fetal descent. For this reason, the nurse should encourage the patient to empty her bladder every 2 hours during labor.

Pressure from the presenting part (as the fetus enters the pelvis) may interfere with its blood and lymph drainage, leading to tissue edema. During labor, trace amounts of protein in urine commonly occur. However, levels above trace amounts should alert the nurse to the possibility of pregnancy-induced hypertension.

Fluid and electrolyte balance

Labor can have several effects on the patient's fluid and electrolyte balance. Increased muscular activity increases body temperature, which in turn causes fluid and electrolyte loss through diaphoresis. Increased respiratory rate and resultant hyperventilation increase fluid loss through evaporation. Vomiting, which may occur during the transitional phase of active labor, also can cause fluid and electrolyte loss. For these reasons, careful monitoring of fluid intake and output is essential during prolonged labor to prevent dehydration and related problems.

Fetal systemic response to labor

Understanding the normal fetal response to labor helps the nurse quickly identify variations from normal and intervene promptly to prevent further complications.

Cardiovascular system

The normal fetal heart rate ranges from 120 to 160 beats/minute. A rate greater than 160 beats/minute is considered tachycardia; a rate of 120 or less, bradycardia. Normal rhythm is fairly constant, with the baseline reflecting a fluctuation of ±5 to 10 beats over a selected time interval. (See Chapter 8, Fetal assessment in labor, for a description of the changes.)

Fetal blood pressure is one of several factors responsible for ensuring an adequate exchange of gases and nutrients to and from the fetal capillaries and the intervillous space. Adequate placental and fetal reserve ensures that the fetus can withstand the stresses of anoxia brought on by uterine contractions.

Respiratory system

The fetus's breathing activity decreases sharply during labor.

Acid-base status

During pregnancy, the fetus is at risk for both respiratory and metabolic acidosis. Because a major role of the placenta is to function as a fetal lung, any conditions interrupting normal blood flow to or from the placenta will increase fetal $PaCO_2$ and decrease fetal pH.

The technique of monitoring fetal scalp capillary blood pH indicates how adequately tissues are being supplied with oxygen. Because the blood pH is influenced by respiratory and metabolic factors, both rapid (respiratory) and prolonged (metabolic) changes can be detected. During the first stage of labor, the fetal scalp capillary blood pH is approximately 7.35; during the second stage, approximately 7.25. Values below 7.2 indicate fetal distress.

Fetal activity

Fetal behavioral states that are present during pregnancy continue during labor. The fetus periodically changes from quiet to active sleep states, in spite of ruptured membranes and uterine contractions that progressively increase in frequency, duration, and intensity.

Vital signs

During the fetus's quiet sleep state, which normally lasts about 40 minutes, the heart rate variability may decrease. A decrease in heart rate variability lasting more than 40 minutes, however, may indicate fetal hypoxia and requires further investigation.

STUDY ACTIVITIES

Short answer

1. Grace Forsythe, a 25-year-old primigravida, asks the nurse during her routine prenatal visit, "Are there ways to know that my body is getting ready for labor to start?" List at least four premonitory signs and symptoms of labor onset that the nurse could describe for Ms. Forsythe.

---

2. During the active phase of the first stage of labor, what parameters would the nurse expect her patient, Jewel Edwards, a 20-year-old multigravida, to experience? Describe this active phase in terms of the dilation and effacement of the cervix and the expected contraction pattern, as well as the anticipated range of labor duration.

---

3. In the early phases of her labor, Jill O'Reilly is encouraged by the nurse to walk and sit in a comfortable rocking chair rather then lie flat in bed. How does position influence labor progress, and what benefit is there in persuading Ms. O'Reilly to stay upright?

---

4. Juanita Costello, an 18-year-old primigravida, is not coping well with her labor. She is crying with each contraction and thrashing about in bed, despite the fact she is only 4 cm dilated. The patient had been extremely anxious during her admission, when she was evaluated in very early labor. Ms. Costello was unaccompanied and confided in the nurse that she was afraid of what was going to happen to her. What effect does a patient's psychological response have on her labor progress?

---

5. Describe four purposes of effective uterine contractions during labor and childbirth.

---

6. Identify the major diameters of the pelvis that are significant for permitting fetal travel through this passageway.

---

7. Name the three phases of a uterine contraction. What parameters of a contraction does the nurse evaluate during labor?

---

8. Briefly describe how maternal blood pressure is normally affected during the first stage of labor and how the nurse accommodates for this.

Multiple choice

9. During a childbirth education class, the nurse-educator explains descent, flexion, internal rotation, extension, external rotation, and expulsion. What are these also known as?

    A. Typical maternal positional changes in labor
    B. The progressive stages of labor
    C. Cardinal movements
    D. Cervical changes associated with the first and second stages of labor

10. Sandy James, a 32-year-old multipara, is admitted to the birthing room after her initial examination reveals her cervix to be 8 cm, completely effaced (100%), and at 0 station. What phase of labor is Ms. James in?

    A. Active phase
    B. Latent phase
    C. Expulsive phase
    D. Transitional phase

11. The bearing-down reflex refers to:

    A. Fetal axis pressure
    B. Premonitory sign of spontaneous rupture of membranes
    C. Natural mechanism for triggering maternal pushing efforts
    D. Maneuver to prevent maternal perineal lacerations during expulsive efforts

12. Signs of placental expulsion include all but which of the following?

    A. Lengthening of the umbilical cord
    B. Rupture of amniotic membranes
    C. Sudden gush of dark blood from the vagina
    D. Change in uterine shape from disklike to globular

13. During the fourth stage of labor, the patient should be assessed carefully for:

    A. Uterine atony
    B. Complete cervical dilation
    C. Placental expulsion
    D. Umbilical cord prolapse

True or false

14. Placental malposition or malfunction can hinder labor and childbirth and compromise fetal well-being.
    ☐ True   ☐ False

15. Maternal gastric motility and absorption increases during labor, while gastric emptying time decreases.
    ☐ True   ☐ False

16. The flexibility of the fetal skull bones to allow the skull to adapt to the pelvic passageway is a process known as "molding."
    ☐ True   ☐ False

17. The most common fetal presentation is the breech presentation.
    ☐ True   ☐ False

ANSWERS   **Short answer**

  1. Premonitory signs and symptoms include lightening, increased Braxton Hicks contractions, weight loss, the nesting instinct, the loss of the mucus plug, increased vaginal secretions, the presence of bloody show, and the spontaneous rupture of membranes.

2. During the active phase, the cervix dilates from 4 to 7 cm and effaces 50% to 75%. Contractions occur every 3 to 4 minutes; they last 45 to 60 seconds and are of moderate intensity. This phase averages 2.2 hours and rarely exceeds 5 hours for a multigravida such as Ms. Edwards.

3. Position during labor can affect the frequency and intensity of contractions. For a patient in the supine position, contractions may be less intense but more frequent. The lateral position tends to make contractions more intense but less frequent. Remaining upright by walking, standing, or sitting may shorten Ms. O'Reilly's labor.

4. The role that a pregnant woman's mental and emotional state plays in labor and childbirth is an essential factor in successful childbirth experience. There appears to be a relationship between anxiety and the length and difficulty of labor. For example, high epinephrine levels triggered by maternal anxiety can lead to diminished uterine activity and a longer labor. Severe pain or distress-related thoughts may create an inefficient labor. Juanita's response may be influenced by her lack of preparation for labor, lack of support systems, and lack of coping mechanisms.

5. Coordinated and effective uterine contractions promote fetal descent and rotation, cervical effacement and dilation, separation and expulsion of the placenta, and constriction of the uterine vasculature to prevent postpartal hemorrhage.

6. The pelvis has four major diameters: the anteroposterior diameter of the inlet; the bi-ischial diameter of the midpelvis; the suprapubic angle with the bituberous diameter of the outlet; and the posterior sagittal diameters of all 3 planes, somewhat determined by the length and curve of the sacrum.

7. The three phases of a uterine contraction are the increment, the acme, and the decrement. During labor, the nurse evaluates the duration, frequency, and intensity of the contraction.

8. In the first stage of labor, changes in the mother's cardiovascular system primarily affect blood pressure. Contractions during the first stage of labor raise the blood pressure readings slighlty. Because of these expected fluctuations, the nurse should assess blood pressure readings between contractions so that they will be the most reliable.

Multiple choice

9. C. Fetal cardinal movements are the typical sequence of positions assumed by the fetus during labor and childbirth.

10. D. The transitional phase of labor extends from 8 to 10 cm; it is the shortest but most difficult and intense for the patient.

11. C. The bearing-down reflex triggers active maternal pushing efforts to deliver the neonate.

12. B. Rupture of membranes occurs during or before the delivery of the neonate.

13. A. Uterine atony should be carefully assessed for during the fourth stage.

True or false

14. True.

15. False. During labor, gastric motility and absorption decrease, while gastric emptying time increases. This is why solid foods are usually withheld during labor.

16. True.

17. False. Approximately 95% of all births occur with the fetus assuming a cephalic presentation.

CHAPTER 8

Fetal assessment in labor

OBJECTIVES

After studying this chapter, the reader should be able to:

1. Recognize factors that affect uteroplacental-fetal circulation.
2. Explain the physiology that regulates the fetal heart rate.
3. Describe various techniques for fetal monitoring.
4. Discuss the basic concepts associated with reading and interpreting baseline fetal heart rate differences, variability, and significant periodic changes.
5. Explain the importance of proper documentation of monitor findings, using correct terminology.

OVERVIEW OF CONCEPTS

Early and informed nursing judgments about fetal heart rate (FHR) data can be crucial to performing timely and appropriate nursing interventions to protect fetal well-being. The nurse must understand the physiologic balance between mother and fetus that is necessary to maintain fetal health and the various conditions that threaten this balance. A familiarity with the basic principles and techniques used to evaluate FHR and uterine contraction patterns, using both direct and indirect electronic fetal monitoring equipment, is essential. Nursing responsibilities associated with fetal monitoring include appropriate interpretation, documentation, and patient education as well as the legal responsibilities to maintain the health of the mother and fetus.

Physiologic basis of fetal monitoring

Fetal monitoring provides data about fetal status during the intrapartal period. Hypoxic or nonhypoxic stress on the fetus produces characteristic FHR patterns detectable through electronic monitoring techniques. To detect such patterns accurately, the nurse must understand basic physiologic principles of uteroplacental-fetal circulation and FHR regulation.

Uteroplacental-fetal circulation

During labor, fetal well-being depends on effective oxygen exchange from the maternal circulation through the placenta to the fetus. Any condition or factor that disrupts this circulatory route can compromise fetal well-being.

Placental blood flow is reduced by any condition that decreases maternal cardiac output. During labor, uteroplacental-fetal circulation can be affected by maternal position, uterine contractions, alterations in placental surface area, anesthetics, maternal hypertension or hypotension, and cord compression. The nurse's primary goal is to maintain adequate maternal circulation and perfusion to the placenta so that the fetus can receive the necessary oxygen and nutrients.

Fetal heart rate regulation

The FHR is regulated by the fetal sympathetic and parasympathetic divisions of the autonomic nervous system as well as by its chemoreceptors (sensory nerve cells) and baroreceptors (pressure-sensitive nerve endings in the walls of the large systemic arteries). The normal range of the FHR is 120 to 160 beats/minute.

Through the fetus's vagal reflex, the parasympathetic nervous system controls the FHR and is responsible for its beat-to-beat (moment-to-moment) changes. When the vagal reflex is stimulated, the FHR decreases. Conversely, stimulation of the sympathetic nervous system increases the FHR. The autonomic nervous system receives information on maternal blood pressure and oxygen status from chemoreceptors and baroreceptors, which help the fetal system to stabilize its blood pressure.

Fetal and uterine monitoring

Careful monitoring of fetal and uterine functions during labor helps the nurse identify problems before they cause serious complications. Available monitoring methods include manual techniques (fetal heart auscultation and uterine palpation) and internally or externally applied devices for electronic fetal monitoring (EFM).

Fetal monitoring

The nurse can monitor the FHR through auscultation, using a fetoscope or an ultrasound stethoscope (Doppler blood flow detector), or through EFM. Each method carries distinct advantages and disadvantages.

Fetoscope and ultrasound stethoscope

Auscultating the FHR during labor traditionally has been considered sufficient monitoring for the low-risk patient and fetus. The fetoscope is a special stethoscope that enhances the nurse's ability to hear the fetal heartbeat.

In contrast, the ultrasound stethoscope uses ultra-high-frequency sound waves to detect fetal heartbeats. The ultrasound stethoscope can be useful as early as the tenth week of gestation.

According to the national practice standards established by the Association of Women's Health, Obstetric, and Neonatal Nurses (AWHONN), the nurse should perform fetal auscultation for the low-risk patient in labor every 60 minutes during the latent phase and every 30 minutes during the active phase of the first stage of labor, and

Advantages and disadvantages of external and internal electronic fetal monitoring

ADVANTAGES	DISADVANTAGES
External EFM	
• Can be employed at any time, regardless of whether the patient is in active labor • Is noninvasive and easy to apply • Provides a continuous picture of the fetal heart rate pattern and uterine contraction pattern, as well as demonstrates the fetal response to labor • Identifies the baseline fetal heart rate and alterations, such as bradycardia or tachycardia; also identifies periodic changes, such as accelerations and decelerations.	• Is difficult to use if patient is obese or is very vigorous in labor • Sounds other than fetal heart "artifacts" can be electronically misinterpreted and falsely recorded • Tracing may be erratic if fetus is active or changes positions • Graphic printout does not give information about fetal heart variability (the most important indicator of fetal well-being) or the quality and intensity of the uterine contraction
Internal EFM	
• Allows greater maternal freedom of movement in bed or permits ambulation with a special halter device •Assesses fetal heart variability and provides an accurate measurement of the intensity of contractions and baseline uterine tone • Free of artificial "sounds" • Permits direct access to amniotic fluid, if needed for intrauterine cultures.	• Requires cervical dilation and ruptured membranes for application • Necessitates a skilled examiner to apply internal equipment • Sterile, disposable equipment is costly yet essential • Risks of maternal or fetal morbidity are associated with the use internal equipment because of its invasive nature

Adapted from Carlton, L.L. (1990). "Basic intrapartum fetal monitoring". In Martin, Jean (Ed). *Intrapartum Management Modules.* Baltimore: Williams & Wilkins, pp. 160-161.

every 15 minutes during the second stage. For the high-risk patient, the nurse performs fetal auscultation/monitoring every 30 minutes during the latent phase and every 15 minutes during the active phase of the first stage, and every 5 minutes during the second stage.

Employing intermittent fetal auscultation through the ultrasound stethoscope is regarded as comparable to the more sophisticated EFM techniques, especially for the low-risk patient, in determining fetal well-being.

Electronic fetal monitoring

Electronic fetal monitoring can be used externally (outside the uterus) through equipment placed over the patient's abdomen. Alternately, EFM can be used internally, placed in direct contact with the fetal scalp to establish a continuous and more accurate record of the FHR and its relationship to uterine contractions. A heart rate pattern that is within EFM guidelines is a reliable indicator of fetal well-being.

Every method for EFM has advantages and disadvantages that the nurse should understand (see *Advantages and disadvantages of external and internal electronic fetal monitoring*). When this technology is used

Indications for electronic fetal monitoring

For many patients, electronic fetal monitoring (EFM) offers advantages over other monitoring methods. High-risk maternal, fetal, pregnancy, and uterine factors that typically call for EFM are listed below.

Maternal factors
- Diabetes
- Pregnancy-induced hypertension
- Hypertension
- Cardiac disease
- Renal disease
- Previous stillbirth

Fetal factors
- Abnormal heart rate on auscultation
- Meconium staining
- Intrauterine growth retardation
- Rh disease

Pregnancy factors
- Third-trimester bleeding
- Premature rupture of membranes
- Pre-term labor
- Post-term labor
- Amnionitis
- Hydramnios or oligohydramnios

Uterine factors
- Induction or augmentation of labor
- Regional anesthesia
- Multiple gestation (more than one fetus)
- Failure of labor to progress

accurately and appropriately, EFM is the most reliable means currently available for assessing fetal status in utero. (For more information, see *Indications for electronic fetal monitoring.*)

Uterine activity monitoring

Like any muscle, the uterus can contract and relax. Its normal resting tone (or baseline tone) is 5 to 15 mm Hg. In the first stage of labor, when the uterus contracts, the tone rises to 50 to 75 mm Hg. During the second stage of labor, when the patient is not pushing, it may rise to 75 to 100 mm Hg with contractions.

Contractions that occur at 3-minute intervals dilate the cervix most effectively and allow sufficient time for the fetus and uterine muscle to reoxygenate. Contractions that occur less than 2 minutes apart or last longer than 90 seconds generally reflect increased uterine activity.

Increased uterine activity can become hyperstimulation, which reduces perfusion to the placenta and can lead to fetal distress. In response to uterine hyperstimulation and subsequent hypoxias, the fetus typically displays a prolonged deceleration or late decelerations of the heart rate. Therefore, the nurse must monitor uterine activity as closely as the FHR. Uterine activity can be monitored externally by using palpation or, alternately, using an electronic dynamometer or tocodynamometer. Internally, contractions can be monitored directly in utero with an intrauterine pressure catheter. Telemetry also can be used to monitor the patient in labor.

Reading a fetal monitor strip

The monitor strip is divided into two sections. The top section shows the fetal heart rate (FHR), measured in beats/minute (bpm). The nurse reads the strip horizontally and vertically. When the strip is read horizontally, each small square represents 10 seconds. Between each vertical dark line are six squares, representing 1 minute. When the strip is read vertically, each square represents an amplitude of 10 bpm.

The bottom section shows uterine activity (UA), measured in mm Hg. Again, the nurse reads the strip horizontally and ver-

tically. When the strip is read horizontally, each small square represents 10 seconds, with the space between each vertical black line representing 1 minute. When the strip is read vertically, each square represents 5 mm Hg of pressure.

The baseline FHR, the "resting" heart rate, is assessed between uterine contractions and when no fetal movement is occurring. The baseline FHR—normally 120 to 160 bpm—serves as a reference for subsequent heart rate readings taken during contractions.

BASELINE FETAL HEART RATE

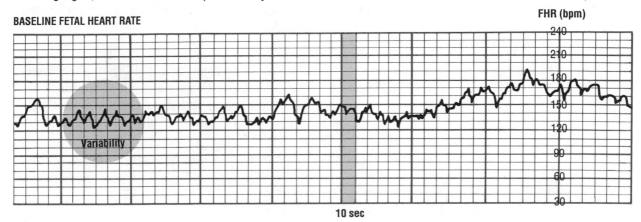

UTERINE ACTIVITY

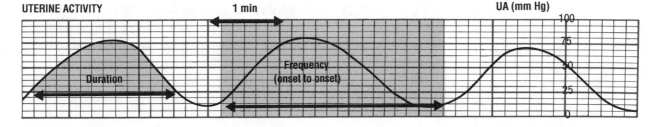

Fetal heart rate patterns   Labor and delivery put stress on even the healthiest fetus. Accurate interpretation of an electronic monitor strip of fetal heart patterns can help the nurse determine when a fetus has crossed the line from normal stress to distress.

A fetus coping well with the stress of labor typically will exhibit a reassuring FHR pattern; a fetus in distress invariably will demonstrate an abnormal pattern. Fetal distress may reveal itself in various combinations of symptoms: an increasing baseline in FHR may indicate that the fetus is attempting to compensate for decreased oxygen reserves; periodic changes, such as late decelerations, indicate placental insufficiency and the need for prompt intervention. (For more information, see *Reading a fetal monitor strip.*)

Baseline fetal heart rate

The starting point for all fetal assessment is the baseline FHR. Accurate baseline FHR determination serves as a reference for all subsequent FHR readings taken during labor. The proper time for establishing the baseline FHR is between uterine contractions and when no fetal movement is occurring.

Initially, the nurse establishes the baseline FHR by examining approximately 15 minutes of the FHR on the monitor strip. Once a baseline FHR is established, it does not change unless a new rate is present for 15 minutes. In a full-term fetus, baseline FHR normally ranges between 120 and 160 beats/minute. Deviations from the normal baseline FHR include tachycardia and bradycardia. (For more information, see *Variations on baseline fetal heart rate.*)

Variability

Variability refers to the beat-to-beat changes in FHR that result from the interaction of the sympathetic nervous system, which speeds up the FHR, and the parasympathetic nervous system, which slows the FHR. It is considered the most important indicator in clinical assessment of fetal well-being.

Variability has two components—long-term and short-term. Long-term variability refers to the larger periodic and rhythmic deviations above and below the baseline FHR. This can be determined through either external or internal EFM.

Short-term variability represents actual beat-to-beat fluctuations in the FHR and the balance between the sympathetic and parasympathetic nervous systems. Short-term variability is considered the most reliable single indicator of fetal well-being. This can be monitored only through internal EFM by direct contact with the fetus through the placement of a small wire electrode just under the scalp. (For more information, see *Factors associated with fetal heart rate variability,* page 128.)

Periodic changes

Transient accelerations or decelerations from the baseline FHR are called periodic changes and are caused by uterine contractions and fetal movements. They represent the normal rhythmic fluctuations from the fetal resting pulse.

Accelerations

Transient accelerations in the FHR normally are caused by fetal movements and uterine contractions. This type of acceleration typically indicates fetal well-being and adequate oxygen reserve. Accelerations also may be caused by partial umbilical cord compression.

Decelerations

Periodic decelerations from the normal baseline FHR are classified as early, late, or variable, depending on when they occur and their waveform shape. (For more information, see *Common decelerations.*)

Variations on baseline fetal heart rate

FHR bpm

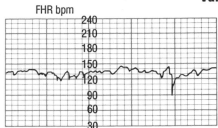

Baseline FHR 130 bpm

By properly interpreting baseline fetal heart rate (FHR), the nurse can determine much about fetal well-being. This chart presents possible causes, clinical significance, and nursing interventions associated with baseline tachycardia (FHR above 160 beats/minute [bpm] persisting for more than 15 minutes) and baseline bradycardia (FHR below 120 bpm persisting for more than 15 minutes). The strip on the left shows representative baseline FHR; variations on baseline are shown in the charts below.

VARIATIONS ON BASELINE	POSSIBLE CAUSES	CLINICAL SIGNIFICANCE	NURSING INTERVENTIONS
Baseline tachycardia FHR bpm 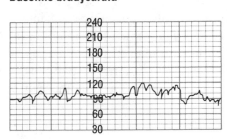 Baseline FHR 170 bpm	• Early fetal hypoxia • Maternal fever • Parasympathetic agents, such as atropine and scopolamine • Beta-sympathomimetic agents, such as ritodrine and terbutaline • Amnionitis (inflammation of the inner layer of the fetal membrane—the amnion) • Maternal hyperthyroidism • Fetal anemia • Fetal heart failure • Fetal cardiac arrhythmias	Persistent tachycardia without periodic changes usually does not adversely affect fetal well-being—especially when associated with maternal fever. However, tachycardia is an ominous sign when associated with late decelerations, severe variable decelerations, or absence of variability.	Intervene to alleviate the cause of fetal distress and provide supplemental oxygen (7 to 8 liters/minute), as prescribed. Also administer I.V. fluids, as prescribed.
Baseline bradycardia Baseline FHR 100 bpm	• Late fetal hypoxia • Beta-adrenergic blocking agents, such as propranolol, and anesthetics • Maternal hypotension • Prolonged umbilical cord compression • Fetal congenital heart block	Bradycardia with good variability and without periodic changes is not a sign of fetal distress if the fetal heart rate remains above 80 bpm. However, bradycardia caused by hypoxia is an ominous sign when associated with loss of variability and late decelerations.	Intervene to alleviate the cause of fetal distress. Administer supplemental oxygen (7 to 8 liters/minute), start an I.V. line, and administer fluids, as prescribed.

Factors associated with fetal heart rate variability

Considered the most important indicator in clinical assessment, variability is described as normal, increased, decreased, or absent.

Factors which cause increased variability
- Fetal movement
- Occiput posterior positioning
- Typical response upon entering second stage
- Initial response to uterine hyperstimulation

Factors which cause decreased variability
- Analgesia or anesthesia during labor
- Certain fetal arrhythmias
- Quiet fetal sleep
- Persistent fetal hypoxia and acidosis
- Breech presentation

Also known as a reflex bradycardia, prolonged decelerations can occur in response to sudden stimulation of the vagal system by a vaginal examination, electrode application, uterine hyperstimulation, regional anesthesia, and maternal pushing efforts in the second stage. They may persist for several minutes or longer. During decelerations, the FHR exhibits normal or increased variability. The vagal reflex itself may be caused by sudden hypoxemia with or without accompanying acidosis.

When prolonged decelerations occur, the nurse first must assess for cord prolapse or imminent delivery. If the patient is receiving oxytocin, discontinue the drug as prescribed and perform or assist with a vaginal examination. If the examination reveals a pulsating cord, intervene using traditional techniques. (See *Cord prolapse* in Chapter 13, Intrapartal complications and related obstetrical interventions.)

Alternately, if the deceleration is the result of uterine hypertonus, drugs, or maternal pushing, stay with the patient and ask another nurse to call the physician. Then stop the oxytocin, turn the patient on her left side, tell her to stop pushing, administer oxygen by mask, and increase the I.V. fluid rate as prescribed.

In most cases, the deceleration corrects itself within 10 minutes, and the fetus resuscitates itself within 30 to 60 minutes after deceleration ends. During recovery, the FHR shows baseline tachycardia and a few late decelerations. Because tachycardia is a compensatory mechanism that aids fetal reoxygenation, it is a reassuring sign after a prolonged deceleration. The late decelerations verify that the fetus has just experienced hypoxia; they disappear as the fetus recovers.

Common decelerations

Decelerations—periodic decreases in fetal heart rate (FHR) — are caused by uterine contractions and fetal movements. This chart illustrates early, late, and variable decelerations, and then lists their possible causes, clinical significance, and appropriate nursing interventions.

Early deceleration

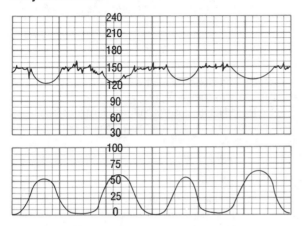

Possible causes
- Compression of the fetus's head

Characteristics
- Descent, peak, and recovery of deceleration waveform mirror the contraction
- Begins early in the contraction with normal FHR variability
- Exhibits uniform waveform shape that mirrors the contraction

Clinical significance
- Is benign
- Indicates head compression at 4 to 7 cm dilation

Nursing interventions
- Reassure the patient that the fetus is not at risk. No other intervention is necessary. (Early deceleration is unaffected by maternal oxygen administration or position changes.)

Late deceleration

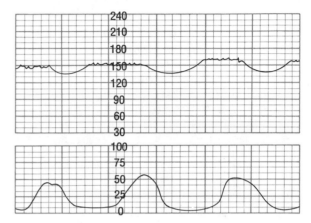

Possible causes
- Uteroplacental-fetal circulatory insufficiency caused by decreased blood flow during contractions or a mechanical defect in placental function, such as abruptio placentae
- Uterine hyperactivity caused by excessive oxytocin infusion
- Maternal hypotension or maternal supine hypotension syndrome

Characteristics
- Deceleration waveform begins about 30 seconds after the contraction begins
- Lowest point of deceleration waveform occurs after the peak of the contraction
- Recovery occurs after the contraction ends; descent and return are gradual and smooth, typically U-shaped
- Usually repetitive with each contraction

(continued)

Common decelerations *(continued)*

Late deceleration *(continued)*
Clinical significance
- Indicates uteroplacental-fetal insufficiency
- May lead to fetal hypoxia and acidosis, if underlying cause is not corrected

Nursing interventions
- Turn the patient on her left side to increase placental perfusion and decrease contraction frequency.
- Increase the I.V. fluid rate to increase intravascular volume and placental perfusion, as prescribed.
- Administer oxygen by mask at 8 to 10 liters/minute to increase fetal oxygenation, as prescribed.
- Notify physician or nurse-midwife.
- Assess for signs of the underlying cause, such as hypotension and uterine tachysystole.
- Take other appropriate measures, such as discontinuing oxytocin, as prescribed.
- Explain the rationales for nursing interventions to the patient and her support person.

Variable deceleration

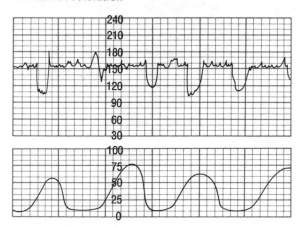

Possible causes
- Umbilical cord compression causing decreased fetal oxygen perfusion

Variable deceleration *(continued)*
Characteristics
- Deceleration waveform shows abrupt onset and recovery
- Waveform shape varies and may resemble the letter U, V, or W
- FHR commonly decreases to 60 beats/minute
- Can be mild, moderate or severe

Clinical significance
- Is most common deceleration pattern in labor because of contractions and fetal movement
- May indicate cord compression
- Is well tolerated if the fetus has sufficient time to recover between contractions and if the deceleration does not last more than 50 seconds
- Can lead to hypoxia

Nursing interventions
- Help the patient change positions. No other intervention is necessary, unless fetal distress is present.
- Assure the patient that the fetus tolerates cord compression well.
- Assess the deceleration pattern for reassuring signs: baseline FHR not increasing, short-term variability not decreasing, abrupt beginning and ending of decelerations, and deceleration duration of less than 50 seconds.
- If assessment does not reveal reassuring signs, notify the physician or nurse-midwife; then start I.V. fluids and administer oxygen by mask at 8 to 10 liters/minute, as prescribed.
- Explain the rationales for nursing interventions to the patient and her support person.

Nursing responsibilities   According to nursing practice standards, the nurse using EFM when caring for a patient in labor is held legally responsible for any procedures performed. This means that the nurse is responsible for recognizing abnormal fetal heart patterns and uterine activity, intervening appropriately, and notifying the physician or nurse-midwife whenever necessary. To meet this responsibility, the nurse must have received the special preparation needed to perform EFM procedures and interpret results.

The nurse can be held liable for preparing a patient for a procedure to which she did not consent. Therefore, once the physician has explained the procedure and informed consent has been obtained, make sure the patient fully understands the procedure that will be performed.

If a nonreassuring FHR pattern occurs, standards of care dictate that the nurse notify the physician or nurse-midwife and then intervene appropriately to prevent further deterioration of fetal status. If the physician does not respond in a timely fashion, the nurse must follow the policy established by the health care facility. In most cases, this means informing the nurse-manager, who can intervene as necessary.

Patient teaching and support

As simply as possible, explain to the patient how evaluating FHR and uterine contractions can identify possible sources of danger to the fetus. Emphasize that a normal FHR is a highly reliable indicator of fetal well-being. EFM allows constant tracking of the FHR; even the nurse who is not in the room can view the tracing on the central display at the nursing station and evaluate the data. Also, describe how EFM can assist the patient during labor and delivery by helping her time the frequency and duration of contractions.

Patient teaching should include anticipating any possible situations that may cause undue anxiety about EMF. The patient should hear the fetal heartbeat and understand that the normal heart rate varies. If the belt moves, the fetal heart tracing may change and the patient may think the heart rate is too fast or slow. Therefore, the nurse should demonstrate how moving the belt can cause a false FHR reading. Turning off the microphone on the monitor will eliminate distracting noises.

Despite the advantages of EFM, the nurse should remember that the patient is the focus of the care. She needs to feel that the nurse is monitoring and concerned about her, not a machine.

Documentation

The monitor strip is considered a vital part of the medical record. Therefore, the nurse must document all assessments, procedures, and interventions on the monitor strip as well as on the chart according to facility policies. If time is short, make the monitor strip the primary place to document because it provides a chronological record of events.

Documentation checklist for fetal monitoring

When assessing the fetal monitor strip and documenting findings, the nurse should ask these questions:
- What is the frequency of contractions?
- How long do the contractions last?
- What is their intensity?
- What is the baseline fetal heart rate (FHR)?
- Is the baseline FHR within the normal range? If not, is baseline tachycardia or bradycardia present?
- Are long-term and short-term variability present?
- Are accelerations present?
- Are decelerations present? If so, are they early, late, variable, or prolonged?
- Based on the monitor readings, have appropriate nursing interventions been performed and documented?
- What was the outcome of the interventions?
- Was the physician or nurse-midwife notified? At what time? What was the response and the subsequent fetal status?

Every health care facility should have a manual of terms and abbreviations for EFM. To avoid legal difficulties, use only these terms on the chart and the monitor strip in documenting fetal assessments and interventions. Call the deceleration or any periodic change by its specific name in charting and include all communication with the physician or nurse-midwife. (For a list of points to cover when documenting EFM tracings, see *Documentation checklist for fetal monitoring.*)

STUDY ACTIVITIES

Short answer

1. Jan Roberts, a 26-year-old primigravida, is admitted to the labor and delivery area in active labor at full-term gestation. She is accompanied by her husband, who plans to be her labor coach. During an initial nursing assessment, Ms. Roberts reveals she is a gestational diabetic and has been followed closely during her pregnancy for pregnancy-induced hypertension. She also reports that her membranes ruptured spontaneously on her way to the hospital and that the fluid was "green" (meconium-stained). On pelvic examination, Ms. Roberts is found to be 5 cm, completely effaced, and 0 station. Identify at least four significant factors in Ms. Roberts's history and pelvic exam that would be indications for continuous, internal electronic fetal monitoring.

2. What are the benefits of this kind of fetal assessment for Ms. Roberts?

3. During the preparation for the insertion of the internal EFM, Ms. Roberts's physician provides her with information on the procedure and an informed consent of the plan to use continuous fetal monitoring. Once this is obtained by the physician, what nursing responsibilities are involved?

_____

4. What teaching and support should the nurse anticipate that Ms. Roberts may need?

_____

_____

5. After several hours, the nurse notes the onset of subtle, persistent late decelerations on the fetal monitor strip. What is the clinical significance of this periodic change in fetal heart rate? List the appropriate nursing interventions associated with this type of FHR pattern.

_____

_____

6. Briefly discuss the guidelines the nurse should use for documenting Ms. Roberts's care at this time.

_____

_____

Fill in the blank

7. During labor, uteroplacental-fetal circulation can be affected by

_____, _____, alterations in _____, _____, maternal _____ or _____ and cord _____.

8. The fetal heart rate (FHR) is regulated by the fetal _____ and _____ divisions of the autonomic nervous system as well as its _____ (sensory nerve cells) and _____ (pressure-sensitive nerve endings in the walls of the large systemic arteries).

9. The nurse can monitor the FHR through auscultation, using a _____ or an _____ , or through _____ .

10. According to AWHONN guidelines, the nurse should perform fetal auscultation for the low-risk patient every _____ minutes during the latent phase and every _____ minutes during the active phase of the first stage of labor, and every _____ minutes during the second stage. For the high-risk patient, the nurse should assess FHR every _____ minutes during the latent phase and every _____ minutes during the active phase of the first stage, and every _____ minutes during the second stage.

11. In a full-term fetus, baseline FHR normally ranges between _____ and _____ beats/minute.

Matching related elements

Indicate which type of periodic change is associated with the following characteristics of periodic fetal heart rate patterns (note that there may be more than one answer per characteristic):

12. ___ Most common type of periodic change

A. Accelerations

13. ___ Benign, not sign of fetal distress

B. Early decelerations

14. ___ Usually well tolerated, if fetus has sufficient time to recover between contractions

C. Variable decelerations

15. ___ May lead to fetal hypoxia and acidosis

D. Late decelerations

16. ___ Has abrupt onset and recovery in relation to the contraction pattern

17. ___ Usually begins about 30 seconds after the contraction begins

18. ___ Caused by fetal head compression

19. ___ FHR commonly decreases to 60 beats/minute

20. ___ Should be treated with oxygen therapy

21. ___ Caused by uteroplacental insufficiency

22. ___ Caused by umbilical cord compression

True or false

23. A significant disadvantage of auscultation is that it cannot be used to assess the most important sign of fetal well-being: short-term, beat-to-beat variability.
☐ True   ☐ False

24. Contractions that occur at 3-minute intervals dilate the cervix most efficiently and allow sufficient time for the fetus and uterine muscle to reoxygenate.
☐ True   ☐ False

25. The proper time for establishing a baseline FHR is at the peak of the uterine contractions.
☐ True   ☐ False

26. The starting point for all fetal assessment is identifying any significant periodic changes.
☐ True   ☐ False

ANSWERS **Short answer**

1. Three significant factors in Ms. Roberts's history that indicate the need for continuous, internal EFM are her gestational diabetes, pregnancy-induced hypertension, and the green (meconium-stained) amniotic fluid. In addition, on pelvic examination, she has documented cervical dilation and ruptured membranes, which allows for the internal placement of EFM.

2. Electronic fetal monitoring placed internally, in direct contact with the fetal scalp, establishes a continuous and more accurate record of the FHR and its relationship to uterine contractions. When the nurse uses this technology accurately and appropriately, EFM is the most reliable means currently available for assessing fetal status in utero.

3. After the physician obtains informed consent, it is the nurse's responsibility to make sure that the patient fully understands the procedure that will be performed. According to nursing practice standards, the nurse using EFM when caring for a patient in labor is held legally responsible for any procedures performed.

4. The nurse should explain to Ms. Roberts, as simply as possible, how evaluating FHR and uterine contractions can identify possible sources of danger to the fetus, emphasizing that a normal FHR pattern is a highly reliable indicator of fetal well-being. EFM can assist Ms. Roberts during labor by helping her time the frequency and duration of her contractions. Further patient teaching should include anticipatory guidance regarding all possible situations that may cause Ms. Roberts anxiety, including normal variations in fetal heart rate patterns and the distraction of the monitor equipment noise. Also, the nurse can show Ms. Roberts the equipment and explain its application and functions.

5. Late decelerations indicate uteroplacental-fetal insufficiency and may lead to fetal hypoxia and acidosis if the underlying cause is not corrected. Appropriate nursing interventions include turning Ms. Roberts on her left side to increase placental perfusion and decrease contraction frequency, increasing the I.V. fluid rate to increase intravascular volume and placental perfusion, administering oxygen by mask at 8 to 10 liters/minute to increase fetal oxygenation, notifying the physician or nurse-midwife of the need for further evaluation, and explaining the purposes of the interventions to Ms. Roberts and her coach.

6. The monitor strip is considered a vital part of the medical record. Therefore, the nurse must document all assessments, procedures, and interventions on the monitor strip as well as on the chart (according to facility policies). To avoid legal difficulties, the nurse should use only approved terms and abbreviations for EFM on the chart. The nurse should call the deceleration or any periodic change by its specific name in the charting and include all communication with the physician or nurse-midwife. The nurse should document the outcomes of the interventions as well.

Fill in the blank

7. Maternal position, uterine contractions, placental surface area, anesthetics, hypertension or hypotension, compression.
8. Sympathetic, parasympathetic, chemoreceptors, baroreceptors
9. Fetoscope, ultrasound stethoscope, electronic fetal monitoring
10. 60, 30, 15; 30, 15, 5
11. 120, 160

Matching related elements

12. C
13. B
14. C
15. D
16. C
17. D
18. B
19. C
20. D, C
21. D
22. C

True or false

23. True.
24. True.
25. False. The proper time for establishing the baseline FHR is between uterine contractions and when no fetal movement is occurring.
26. False. The starting point for all fetal assessment is the baseline FHR. Accurate baseline FHR determination serves as a reference for all subsequent FHR readings taken during labor.

CHAPTER 9

Comfort promotion during labor and childbirth

OBJECTIVES

After studying this chapter, the reader should be able to:

1. Describe the locations and characteristics of pain typically felt during each stage of labor.

2. Identify factors that affect a patient's responses to pain during labor.

3. Describe the physical and psychological benefits of support from family and friends to the patient in labor.

4. Describe techniques that promote comfort during labor.

5. List analgesic and anesthetic agents used to reduce labor pain and discuss their characteristics, administration routes, and adverse effects.

OVERVIEW OF CONCEPTS

Few women experience painless labor. Pain experienced during normal labor follows a predictable cycle of peaks and valleys. Despite its predictable course, however, each patient perceives labor pain as a unique, personal experience based on her physical condition, pain tolerance, and psychological background. The nurse must collaborate with other health care providers to assess the patient's perception of pain and the degree of comfort achieved through therapy. Because childbirth is a stressful experience, steadfast support by the nurse can help ease emotional stress and physical discomfort during this time. The nurse plays a key role by helping the patient's primary support person function effectively. The nurse also provides direct support, as needed, to the patient and to involved family members.

Pain during labor

Even though each patient responds to pain uniquely, nursing interventions can help reduce pain perception and alter pain response for most patients. To intervene properly, the nurse should understand the type of pain typically experienced during labor, physical and psychological factors that influence pain perception, and how observation of behavior patterns can clarify a patient's response to pain.

During the first stage of labor, pain results primarily from cervical effacement and dilation. At 0 to 3 cm of cervical dilation, the patient may describe the pain as an ache or discomfort; at 4 to 7 cm, as moderately sharp; at 7 to 10 cm, as severe, sharp, and cramping.

During the second stage of labor, pain results from friction between the fetus and birth canal and from pressure on the perineum, bladder, bowel, and uterine ligaments.

During the third stage of labor, pain results from ischemia caused by contraction of uterine blood vessels. Uterine contractions may perpetuate pain after the placenta has been expelled.

Many factors affect a patient's perception of and ability to cope with pain. These factors may be physiologic, social, or psychological. They include parity; fetal size and position; certain medical procedures, such as labor induction; anxiety; fatigue; the degree of childbirth education; cultural influence; and coping mechanisms.

Support during labor

Support from trusted family members or friends can help an individual gain, regain, and use personal strength during difficult or challenging periods that demand extra energy and resources. Several people may be available to assist a patient during labor. Her partner, family members, friends, and health care professionals all care about her physical and emotional needs. Whatever their cultural, social, economic, or religious background or configuration, most family members who assist the woman in labor will need the nurse's support and guidance.

Patients who have a continuous support person during labor can benefit physically and psychologically. Research has found that women with a constant companion during labor have shorter labors, fewer obstetric complications, reduced feelings of pain and anxiety, less use of labor-inducing drugs and anesthesia, more positive feelings about the birth experience, and better coping behaviors than those without a support person.

Although labor and childbirth almost always are associated with pain and anxiety, patients vary in the degree of pain they experience, their tolerance for the pain, and the cultural beliefs that affect their perception of and ability to cope with pain, as well as their verbal and nonverbal responses to pain. Regardless of who the patient selects as support person, important considerations include the person's ability to provide support and the patient's and family's satisfaction with that support.

The partner's support can be invaluable to a patient in labor. The partner may assist the patient by communicating her needs to health care professionals. The partner also can show concern for the patient's needs by being supportive, available, and reliable. These feelings should be accompanied by physical actions and by verbal and nonverbal communication.

Nursing care To provide care for the patient in labor, the nurse must be familiar with various nonpharmacologic and pharmacologic pain-relief methods and provide care for the patient and her family. During labor and delivery, the nurse should administer sensitive and appropriate care based on the particular needs of the patient and her family. This requires a twofold effort: applying clinical knowledge to assess labor progress, and using personal skills to assess the patient's and family's needs during this physically and emotionally stressful time.

Assessment

Assessment of a patient experiencing labor pain includes three parts. First is the health history, which investigates any medical factor that could affect the safety or efficacy of pain-reducing pharmacologic agents, ongoing questions about the patient's pain perception, and assessment of the patient's and family's needs and support. Second is physical assessment, which includes the patient, the fetus, and labor progress. Third is follow-up assessment, performed after implementing pain-relief measures to determine their effectiveness.

Health history

Review the patient's medical history, asking specifically about medication allergies and any medical or obstetric problems that could affect the choice of pain-relief methods. Determine how much the patient knows about childbirth and pain-relief measures, ask about previous experiences with pain and pain-relieving agents, and assess the patient's current pain level and cultural or emotional reaction to it.

Consider the patient's obstetric history when assessing the need for pain-relief measures. Pertinent assessment topics include the length of previous labors, the patient's perception of previous labor pain, pain-relief measures used in previous labors, and the patient's perception of those measures' effectiveness.

Assess the patient's knowledge of relaxation techniques, positioning, and pharmacologic options for pain relief. Determine patient preferences and desires for labor and delivery and identify who will function as the patient's main support. Assess the patient's reaction to her partner, if he is present. Is he helpful and supportive? Is his anxiety level disturbing to the patient?

Also explore the patient's birth culture and its influence on labor and delivery. Birth culture refers to a set of beliefs, values, and norms surrounding the birth process and shared to various degrees by members of a cultural or ethnic group. The birth culture may influence the patient's prenatal diet, her response to labor, preferred positions for childbirth, activity restrictions, and family members' roles during childbirth.

Physical assessment

When evaluating possible implementation of comfort promotion or pain-relief measures, consider maternal coping, labor progress, and fetal well-being.

Maternal status. Observe the patient's spontaneous verbal and nonverbal expressions to assess discomfort. Keep in mind that excessive anxiety may impede cervical dilation; a small dose of an analgesic agent may relax an anxious patient sufficiently to allow cervical dilation and shorten labor.

Labor status. Certain factors, such as epidural anesthesia, may slow labor. Also consider contraction intensity, frequency, and duration to help determine the need for pain relief.

Assess cervical dilation to ensure that pharmacologic agents are given at the safest times during labor. Timing is essential to achieve appropriate pain relief without adversely affecting the fetus.

Fetal status. Carefully consider fetal age and development before administering prescribed pain-relief agents. An immature fetus has a diminished ability to metabolize analgesic or anesthetic agents used to reduce labor pain; the physician or nurse-midwife must carefully consider fetal status before drug administration. Obtain and document baseline fetal heart rate and pattern before pharmacologic measures are instituted.

Follow-up assessment

To determine the effectiveness and safety of comfort promotion and pain-relief measures, continue to assess the patient and fetus throughout labor. Observe maternal and fetal vital signs frequently (especially respirations), assess the patient's cardiovascular response, and watch for such adverse drug reactions as vomiting, itching, and drowsiness. Also assess the primary support person's feelings and actions to determine their effect on the patient.

Nursing diagnoses

After assessing the patient, fetus, and support persons, review the findings and formulate nursing diagnoses related to comfort promotion and support. (For a partial list of applicable diagnoses, see Nursing Diagnoses: *Comfort promotion and support.*)

Planning and implementation

The nurse provides or assists with comfort promotion and pain-reduction measures when caring for a patient in labor. The nurse also assists the support person to ensure adequate and appropriate support for the patient and to balance patient and family needs.

Comfort measures

Intervene to decrease anxiety, promote hygiene, and help the patient find comfortable positions that reduce labor pain and facilitate childbirth. Some patients find these actions adequate to maintain comfort throughout labor.

Decrease anxiety. Anxiety leads to tension, which may cause additional pain. Nursing measures seek to reduce anxiety, thus decreasing blood pressure and heart rate, allowing greater energy production for

NURSING DIAGNOSES

Comfort promotion and support

The following list of potential nursing diagnoses gives examples of the problems and etiologies that the nurse may encounter when caring for a patient in labor:
- Anxiety related to labor pain
- Decreased cardiac output related to epidural anesthesia
- Ineffective breathing pattern, related to labor progress and pain
- Knowledge deficit related to analgesia and anesthesia options
- Pain related to the frequency and intensity of uterine contractions
- Urine retention related to spinal anesthesia

---

effective uterine contractions, and reducing muscle tension and the heightened pain perception caused by tension.

The nurse's presence, confidence, attention, and concern help control the patient's anxiety. As labor progresses, keep the patient informed, teach and reinforce coping strategies, and assure the patient that labor is progressing normally. Reassure, encourage, and praise the patient throughout labor.

A support person provides comfort, reassurance, and assistance with such pain control techniques as breathing exercises, imagery, and distraction.

Promote hygiene. Nursing interventions to maintain hygiene can increase the patient's comfort level by boosting self-esteem, providing distraction, removing an additional source of discomfort (such as wet sheets), and blocking pain perception. Simple nursing measures that promote hygiene and the patient's comfort include showers and bathing during active labor; frequent perineal care; oral hygiene, as needed; and frequent linen and clothing changes.

Position the patient for comfort. During the latent and early active stages, encourage the patient to move about. A patient in an upright position will have stronger, more regular, and more frequent contractions because gravity helps align the fetus with the pelvic angle as the uterus tilts forward with each contraction. Maintaining this position may shorten labor and reduce pain and medication requirements.

As labor progresses and an upright position becomes uncomfortable, the patient might alternate walking with sitting, side-lying, or kneeling to provide rest and vary the intensity and frequency of contractions. If she must remain in bed during labor because of potential obstetric complications or fetal conditions, advise her to assume a side-lying position as often as possible to minimize fetal stress and enhance circulation.

Relaxation techniques
The goal of relaxation techniques is to reduce anxiety and muscle tension, thus quieting or calming the mind and muscles. Relaxation de-

creases oxygen consumption, heart rate, respiratory rate, arterial blood lactate concentration, and sympathetic nervous system activity.

Techniques used to promote relaxation include distraction, progressive muscle relaxation, yawning, controlled breathing, imagery, touch, and music therapy. Ensure that the environment is conducive to relaxation. Minimize unnecessary interruptions.

Pharmacologic pain control

Analgesic and anesthetic agents are the two types of pharmacologic pain relief used during labor (for a summary, see *Drugs used to relieve labor pain*).

Analgesia refers to pain reduction without loss of consciousness. Although the patient may continue to perceive pain, an analgesic agent can make it more tolerable by affecting the peripheral nervous system (by relaxing muscles and increasing blood flow) and the central nervous system (CNS).

Anesthesia refers to partial or complete loss of sensation, sometimes with loss of consciousness. Affecting the entire body or only a region of the body, an anesthetic agent blocks conduction of impulses along pain pathways to the brain.

Regional anesthetic agents are injected into areas surrounding nerves. Types used for labor pain include pudendal block, epidural block, spinal block, saddle block, or paracervical block.

General anesthetic agents render the patient unconscious and thus unable to feel pain. These agents may be inhaled or administered I.V. or I.M. Typically, they are used only for emergency cesarean delivery or other surgical interventions because they greatly increase the risk of aspiration, the leading cause of anesthesia-related maternal death.

Ideally, the patient should receive information and make choices about pharmacologic options before labor begins. The patient's obstetrician and anesthesiologist are responsible for describing obstetric analgesia and anesthesia and obtaining written consent to administer these therapies.

Provide additional information as needed, including the route of administration, degree and timing of pain relief, impact on labor and the fetus, potential adverse drug reactions, and the effectiveness of the technique selected. Describe the immediate and prolonged effects of pharmacologic agents on the neonate. Take steps to ensure that the patient's caregivers will support her decision.

Analgesia. The patient usually receives an analgesic agent when active labor is established and the cervix begins to dilate. Administration usually takes place via an intravenous or intramuscular injection.

Analgesic agents may cause drowsiness, euphoria, orthostatic hypotension, and dizziness. Use side rails on the bed to ensure patient safety if a member of the health care team or a support person cannot be in constant attendance. Caution the patient and support person that the patient should not get out of bed without a nurse's help.

Drugs used to relieve labor pain

The following drugs provide analgesia or anesthesia for labor.

DRUG AND INDICATION	POSSIBLE ADVERSE REACTIONS	NURSING CONSIDERATIONS
Narcotic agonists		
meperidine, morphine *Indication:* Alter pain perception	*Maternal:* decreased respirations, orthostatic hypotension, nausea and vomiting, itching, drowsiness, urine retention *Fetal:* moderate central nervous system (CNS) depression, decreased beat-to-beat variability *Neonatal:* moderate CNS depression, mild behavioral depression	• Review maternal history for drug allergy, substance abuse, chronic respiratory disease, and renal and liver disease. • Frequently assess maternal vital signs, respirations, and level of consciousness. • Assess labor stage and progress. • Use continuous electronic fetal heart rate (FHR) monitoring, if possible. • A degree of neonatal respiratory depression can be anticipated if administered 1 to 2 hours prior to birth. Inject naloxone (0.01 mg/kg) into umbilical cord vein or neonate's thigh, as prescribed.
Narcotic antagonists		
naloxone *Indication:* Reverse respiratory depression caused by narcotic toxicity in patient or neonate	*Maternal:* may reverse analgesia if given 5 to 10 minutes before delivery, increasing pain perception *Fetal:* none *Neonatal:* may induce withdrawal symptoms in a narcotic-dependent neonate	• Keep resuscitation equipment nearby during administration. • Do not administer to patient with known drug dependency. • Develop a plan for alternative pain relief. • Narcotic antagonists will not reverse respiratory depression caused by sedatives, hypnotics, anesthetics, or non-narcotic CNS depressants.
Narcotic agonist-antagonists		
butorphanol tartrate, nalbuphine *Indication:* Alter pain perception	*Maternal:* may induce withdrawal symptoms in a narcotic-dependent patient; may cause decreased respirations, orthostatic hypotension, nausea and vomiting, itching, drowsiness *Fetal:* moderate CNS depression, decreased beat-to-beat variability *Neonatal:* moderate CNS depression, mild behavioral depression	• Review the patient's history for drug allergy, substance abuse, chronic respiratory disease, and renal and liver disease. • Frequently assess maternal vital signs, respirations, and level of consciousness. • Assess labor stage and progress. • Use continuous electronic FHR monitoring, if possible.
Sedative-hypnotics (tranquilizers)		
phenothiazines (promethazine, propiomazine), piperazine (hydroxyzine) *Indication:* Promote rest and sleep; may reduce anxiety and reduce narcotic requirements	*Maternal:* may cause dizziness, lassitude, incoordination, fatigue, euphoria, or excitation *Fetal:* decreased beat-to-beat variability; moderate CNS depression, especially with larger doses *Neonatal:* possible hypotonia, decreased feeding, lethargy, and hypothermia	• Review the patient's history for drug allergies before administration. • These drugs usually are given only during the early first stage of labor; they may have antiemetic effects. *(continued)*

Drugs used to relieve labor pain (continued)

DRUG AND INDICATION	POSSIBLE ADVERSE REACTIONS	NURSING CONSIDERATIONS
Sedative-hypnotics (tranquilizers) (continued)		
barbiturates (secobarbital) *Indication:* Decrease anxiety during the prodromal or early latent phase of labor	*Maternal:* possible paradoxically increased pain and excitability *Fetal:* none *Neonatal:* possible CNS depression that can persist for several days	• Barbiturates are administered less commonly than other tranquilizers because of their prolonged depressant effects on the neonate. • Barbiturates should be administered only if delivery is not expected for 12 to 24 hours.
Regional anesthetic agents		
bupivacaine, lidocaine, chloroprocaine, mepivacaine *Indication:* Preferred regional method for analgesia and anesthesia during first and second stages of labor; provide anesthesia for vaginal or cesarean delivery; relieve uterine pain (pudendal block relieves perineal pain)	*Maternal:* hypotension (epidural and spinal); delayed analgesia (10 to 20 minutes); one-sided block or ineffective pain relief (spinal); prolonged labor if epidural block given too early; urine retention (epidural and spinal); increased toxicity from vascularity of region (pudendal); hematoma (pudendal); diminished bearing-down efforts (epidural) *Fetal:* transient decreased beat-to-beat variability with lidocaine and mepivacaine; late decelerations; fetal distress secondary to maternal hypotension; about 30% incidence of bradycardia (paracervical) *Neonatal:* CNS depression in presence of severe hypotension; neonatal bradycardia, hypotonia, and decreased responsiveness with accidental fetal intracranial injection (pudendal block)	• Determine baseline maternal vital signs and FHR; assess throughout labor as needed. • Explain procedure and expected feelings as anesthesia is initiated. • Pudendal: Assess for diminished bearing-down reflex and fetal symptoms associated with accidental scalp injection. • Epidural: Ensure adequate patient hydration by administering 500 to 1,000 ml I.V. fluid before injection. Take vital signs every 5 minutes for 30 minutes after injection and report hypotension. Monitor vital signs every 15 minutes throughout continuous epidural infusion. Catheterize if patient retains urine. Labor may be augmented with oxytocin if uterine contractions diminish. Assist with positioning and maintain safety. • Spinal: Ensure adequate patient hydration by administering 500 to 1,000 ml I.V. fluid before injection. Take vital signs every 5 minutes until delivery and treat as prescribed. Observe for signs of total spinal block (apnea, unconsciousness, absent blood pressure, absent pulse, pupil dilation). Encourage the patient to lie flat for 8 to 10 hours after administration.
General anesthetic agents		
halothane, enflurane, thiopental sodium *Indication:* Anesthesia for cesarean delivery; surgical intervention for obstetric complications, version, extraction, or uterine manipulation	*Maternal:* increased risk of regurgitation and aspiration; increased risk of uterine atony; decreased risk of hypovolemia compared to regional anesthesia *Fetal:* increased risk of fetal CNS depression *Neonatal:* short-term behavioral changes	• Assess for risk of aspiration. Maintain nothing by mouth (NPO) status. • Administer antacid or H_2 blocking agent, as prescribed. • Continuously monitor FHR, especially during induction of anesthesia and in response to anesthesia. • Maintain respiratory support, I.V. fluids, and uterine fundal massage, as necessary, during recovery from anesthesia. • Drowsiness may persist after recovery. Assist with positioning and maintain safety.

Categories of systemic analgesic agents used during labor include sedatives, narcotic agonists, mixed narcotic agonist-antagonists, anti-anxiety agents, and inhalation analgesics (see *Drugs used to relieve labor pain,* pages 143 and 144).

Regional anesthesia. By blocking pain transmission without altering consciousness, regional anesthesia allows the patient to participate in labor and childbirth while decreasing pain perception and the amount of drug that crosses to the fetus. Many physicians advocate regional anesthesia. Its disadvantages include potential CNS toxicity, hypotension, diminished bearing-down efforts, pruritus, urine retention, nausea, and vomiting.

The physician or anesthesiologist administers the anesthetic. Drugs used most commonly include ester-type agents (chloroprocaine hydrochloride, procaine hydrochloride, and tetracaine hydrochloride) and amide-type agents (bupivacaine hydrochloride, etidocaine hydrochloride, lidocaine hydrochloride, and mepivacaine hydrochloride). The choice of agent will differ with the type of anesthetic block used.

Regional anesthesia techniques include local infiltration (including pudendal and paracervical blocks), epidural block, and spinal block. Epidural and spinal blocks carry an increased risk of hypotension and must be monitored closely. (For descriptions of administration techniques, see *Types of regional anesthesia,* page 146.)

General anesthesia. Because it requires intubation and increases the risk of aspiration, general anesthesia usually is used only when the patient undergoes emergency cesarean delivery, intrauterine manipulation, or other surgical intervention. General anesthesia may be attained through inhalation or I.V. drug administration. Inhalation involves high concentrations of the same agents used for inhalant analgesia (nitrous oxide, halothane, and enflurane). The intravenous agent thiopental sodium (Pentothal) produces deep anesthesia and may cause depression in the neonate.

Evaluation

Evaluation findings should be stated in terms of actions performed or outcomes achieved for each goal. The following examples illustrate appropriate evaluation statements for the patient experiencing labor pain.

• The patient and her support person demonstrated knowledge of such comfort promotion techniques as controlled breathing and progressive muscle relaxation.

• The patient expressed understanding of pain-relief measures available to her.

• The patient reported relief from pain after administration of regional anesthesia.

• Fetal heart rate remained stable after anesthesia administration.

Types of regional anesthesia

This chart explains the administration techniques for five types of regional anesthesia.

Local infiltration

Used to numb perineal tissue for episiotomy or laceration repair, this technique involves injection of anesthetic through a 22G needle into the fascia of the perineum. The patient may feel a burning sensation. This technique poses no threat to the patient, fetus, or neonate.

Pudendal block

Used to block perineal and vaginal pain but not uterine contractions during the second stage of labor, this technique involves injection of 3 to 5 ml of anesthetic into the pudendal nerve on each side of the sacrum. The needle crosses the sacrosciatic notch and passes the tip of the ischial spine. Accidental injection into the fetus's scalp or cranium may cause neonatal bradycardia and decreased responsiveness.

Paracervical block

Used to anesthetize the uterus and cervix during the first stage of labor, this technique involves insertion of an Iowa trumpet into the lateral fornix of the vagina and injection of 5 to 10 ml of anesthetic. The block provides anesthesia through the second stage of labor. This rarely used technique is associated with a high incidence of fetal adverse reactions.

Epidural block

Used to anesthetize the lower half of the body, this technique involves insertion of an 18G stylet into lumbar interspace 3, 4, or 5. Then the tip of the needle is advanced into the epidural space to administer the anesthetic. An epidural block may prolong labor and cause hypotension.

Spinal block

Performed in a similar manner to the epidural block, this technique is used to anesthetize the lower half of the body. However, the needle is advanced somewhat farther, into the subarachnoid space. Thus, the anesthetic is injected directly into spinal fluid. The patient loses perception of contractions and ability to bear down. A spinal block to the level of T10 is used for vaginal delivery, to T8 for cesarean delivery.

Documentation

The nurse must document all findings and actions taken using the nursing process. Documentation applicable to the patient experiencing labor pain includes:
• comfort measures taken and their effectiveness
• analgesic agents administered and their effectiveness
• anesthetic agents administered and their effectiveness
• vital signs
• changes in uterine contractions after drug administration
• changes in fetal heart rate after drug administration
• actions taken by the support person, such as applying a cool cloth to the patient's forehead
• patient reactions to the support person's assistance.

STUDY ACTIVITIES   **Short answer**   .

1. During her childbirth education class, Chandra Thompson asks the nurse-educator where the pain of labor actually comes from. Ms. Thompson also wonders whether all labor pain feels basically the same in intensity. How could the nurse-educator respond?

_____

_____

2. Carolyn Andrews, a 19-year-old multigravida, asks the nurse if her mother can be permitted to be with her in labor. She explains that having a support person with her was a big help during the birth of her first baby. Identify the benefits of including Ms. Andrews's mother during labor for her continuous support.

_____

_____

3. What follow-up assessment should the nurse do to determine the effectiveness and safety of the Meperidine (Demerol) that was administered to Ms. Andrews 30 minutes ago?

_____

_____

4. Identify at least six relaxation techniques that a nurse could employ to promote a patient's comfort during labor.

_____

5. What must the nurse include in an informed consent regarding analgesia prior to its administration?

_____

_____

6. When documenting the administration of analgesia or anesthesia, what should the nurse include?

_____

_____

7. Identify five techniques used to provide regional anesthesia or analgesia.

_____

Multiple choice

8. A narcotic antagonist, such as naloxone, is indicated for:
   A. Altering pain perception
   B. Reversing respiratory depression caused by analgesic administration
   C. Promoting rest and sleep
   D. Decreasing anxiety

9. One essential nursing measure to ensure patient safety after administering Meperidine is:
   A. Use side rails on the bed if the patient is to be unattended
   B. Insert a Foley catheter to prevent urine retention
   C. Advise the patient of possible adverse reactions, such as dizziness
   D. Apply internal fetal monitoring equipment to assess fetal response closely

10. An expected fetal adverse reaction to Meperidine is:
    A. Decreased beat-to-beat variability
    B. Bradycardia
    C. Late decelerations
    D. None known

11. When administering an epidural block during the first stage of labor, the nurse must anticipate which of the following adverse reactions:
    A. Nausea and vomiting
    B. Prolonged labor
    C. Decreased respirations
    D. Drowsiness
    E. Urinary retention
    F. Diminished bearing-down efforts
    G. Increased toxicity from vascularity of region
    H. Hypotension
    I. Transient decreased beat-to-beat variability
    J. Euphoria

ANSWERS   **Short answer**

1. During the first stage of labor, pain results primarily from cervical effacement and dilation. This pain is perceived differently by each woman, yet there is a progressive intensity to the pain experienced in the first stage. At 0 to 3 cm of cervical dilation, the pain is often described as an ache or discomfort; at 4 to 7 cm, as moderately sharp; at 7 to 10 cm, as severe, sharp, and cramping. During the second stage of labor, pain results from friction between the fetus and birth canal and from pressure on the perineum, bladder, bowel, and uterine ligaments; during the third stage, pain results from ischemia caused by contraction of uterine blood vessels. Uterine contractions may perpetuate pain after the placenta has been expelled.

2. Support from trusted family members can help an individual gain, regain, and use personal strength during difficult or challenging periods that demand extra energy and resources. Patients who have a continuous support during labor can benefit physically and psychologically. Women with a constant companion during labor have shorter labors, fewer obstetric complications, reduced feelings of pain and anxiety, less use of labor-inducing drugs and anesthesia, more positive feelings about the birth experience, and better coping behaviors than those without a support person.

3. To determine the effectiveness and safety of the analgesia that Ms. Andrews received, the nurse should continue to assess the patient and her fetus throughout labor. Maternal and fetal vital signs (especially maternal respirations) should be checked frequently and cardiovascular response assessed. A continuous electronic fetal monitor also should be applied. Side rails should be up on the patient's bed if she is unattended. Adverse drug reactions such as vomiting, itching, and drowsiness also should be evaluated.

4. Techniques used to promote relaxation include distraction, progressive muscle relaxation, yawning, controlled breathing, imagery, touch, and music therapy.

5. The patient's obstetrician and anesthesiologist are responsible for describing obstetric analgesia and anesthesia and obtaining written consent to administer these therapies. The nurse would provide additional information as needed, including the route of administration, degree and timing of pain relief, impact on labor and the fetus, potential adverse drug reactions, and the effectiveness of the technique selected. In addition, the nurse should describe the immediate and prolonged effects of pharmacologic agents on the neonate.

6. The nurse must document all findings and actions taken, using the nursing process. For the patient experiencing labor pain, the following must be documented: comfort measures taken and their effectiveness, analgesic and anesthetic agents administered and their effectiveness, vital signs, changes in uterine contractions and fetal heart rate after drug administration, actions taken by the support person, and patient reactions to the support person's assistance.

7. Five different types of regional anesthesia are local infiltration, pudendal block, paracervical block, epidural block, and spinal block.

Multiple choice

8. B. Naloxone reverses respiratory depression caused by narcotic toxicity in the patient or neonate.

9. A. Side rails on the bed ensure patient safety when she is unattended because Meperidine can cause drowsiness and dizziness.

10. A. Possible fetal adverse reactions include both moderate CNS depression and decreased beat-to-beat variability.

11. B, E, F, H, I

CHAPTER 10

The first stage of labor

OBJECTIVES

After studying this chapter, the reader should be able to:

1. Differentiate between true labor and false labor.

2. Obtain pertinent health history information during the patient's admission to the labor and delivery area.

3. Describe the physical assessment during admission to the labor and delivery area.

4. Describe how to assess the patient and fetus during the first stage of labor.

5. Implement comfort and support measures for the patient and her family.

OVERVIEW OF CONCEPTS

The first stage of labor begins with the onset of regular, rhythmic uterine contractions that cause progressive cervical changes. It ends with complete cervical dilation of approximately 10 cm. Labor, however, is more than the physiologic process of birth. It also is a significant life event that represents a pivotal point in the lives of each member of this new family. Labor is a psychological and developmental task that demands adaptation. During the first stage of labor, nursing care must meet the patient's physical, psychosocial, and cultural needs.

Nursing care before admission

Before any patient can be admitted for care in the labor and delivery area, she must be in true labor or show signs of a medical or obstetrical complication, such as hypertension, that could affect her or the fetus. To make this determination, the nurse performs an initial assessment that focuses on the imminence of the birth and on fetal stability. This assessment, which includes a brief history and physical examination, should provide sufficient data to distinguish true labor from other conditions that mimic it, such as false labor, urinary tract infection (UTI), "terminal pregnancy blues" (generalized physical discomfort and emotional distress near the end of pregnancy), and abruptio placentae (see *Characteristics of true and false labor*). However, if delivery appears imminent, omit the preadmission assessment and admit the patient immediately.

Characteristics of true and false labor

The information in this chart helps the nurse determine whether the patient is in true labor.

CHARACTERISTIC	TRUE LABOR	FALSE LABOR
Contractions	Regular and rhythmic	Irregular
Pain	Discomfort that moves from the back to the front of the abdomen	Mild discomfort or pressure in the abdomen and groin; may be relieved by walking
Fetal movement	Unchanged	May intensify
Fetal descent	Progressing	Unchanged
Show	Pinkish mucus, possibly with the mucus plug from the cervix	None
Cervix	Progressing effacement and dilation	Unchanged after 1 to 2 hours

Initial assessment

During the introductory period, observe the patient closely to identify clues to her labor status. Postures, facial expressions, or gestures that connote tension, anxiety, or pain may accurately reflect a patient's labor progress. To help form an accurate initial impression, be sure to relate the patient's behavior to her cultural background and its influences on her pain response.

If the patient is in active labor, shorten the initial assessment and prioritize the questions. Focus on collecting data about her current labor status. (For more information, see *Intrapartal preadmission health history,* page 152.) Refer to prenatal records, if available, and use the previously documented information.

Perform a brief physical examination to determine labor progress and fetal well-being. The patient needs to be in a comfortable position for the assessment, especially if she is in active labor. Calmly conduct both the history and the physical assessment between contractions.

Physical assessment

The initial physical assessment includes evaluation of vital signs; fetal heart tones; uterine contractions; fetal lie, presentation, and position; estimated fetal weight; edema and deep tendon reflexes; status of amniotic membranes; and cervical changes, fetal descent, and other factors determined by vaginal examination.

Vital signs. For a patient in labor, vital signs provide necessary information about maternal and fetal health. They also provide baseline data for future comparisons.

Check the patient's blood pressure, which should range from 90 to 140 mm Hg systolic and from 60 to 90 mm Hg diastolic. A rise of 30

Intrapartal preadmission health history

During the initial intrapartal nursing assessment, the nurse collects data to determine the patient's health status, health promotion, and health protection behaviors as well as her significant roles and relationships. The following order is suggested to prioritize the collection of this information:

BIOGRAPHICAL DATA

	Record name, address, and other biographical information required by the facility. Age may affect labor progress and outcome.

HEALTH STATUS

Expected delivery date	"Due date" will help in assessing for preterm or post-term neonate, determining gestational age, and evaluating fetal size.
Previous pregnancies and outcomes	Gravidity (number of pregnancies) and parity (number of births) can affect duration of—and potential for complications in—successive labors. Determine if any pregnancies ended in spontaneous or induced abortions as well as status of living children.
Previous labor and delivery experiences	Ask dates and lengths of previous labors. Ask about any complications requiring forceps or cesarean sections. Ask about birth weights, which can be important to predicting current labor progress.
Contraction pattern	Onset, frequency, and duration of contractions, and their perceived intensity, can help predict phase and stage of labor, distinguish between true and false labor, and differentiate labor from urinary tract infections (UTIs) and abruptio placentae.
Status of amniotic membranes	Ask if amniotic membranes have ruptured and if they broke with a gush or in a trickle. Inquire about fluid color or odor. Time of occurrence also is significant.
Presence of bloody show or vaginal bleeding	Increasing show may signal onset of second stage. Vaginal bleeding may signal placenta previa or abruptio placentae, with subsequent fetal distress.
Prenatal complications or concerns	Any prenatal problems such as anemia, UTI, infections, or increased blood pressure are significant to labor. Tests such as ultrasonography or amniocentesis can provide additional data about potential outcomes.
Prior medical problems	Any medical problems such as diabetes, heart disease, high blood pressure, or kidney disease must be documented and incorporated into care.
Current fetal movements	Ask about current fetal activity and whether frequency of movements has changed from usual daily rate. A fetus usually moves at least 10 times a day.

HEALTH PROMOTION AND PROTECTION

Prenatal care	Initiation of prenatal care and frequency of visits indicate constancy and vigilance of care. Lack of prenatal care or recently initiated care increases risk of complications. A copy of prenatal records can guide completion of health history and physical assessment.

ROLES AND RELATIONSHIPS

Labor support	Identify the labor coach or support person. Childbirth education or preparation may ease labor pain and facilitate labor progress.
Family involvement	Determine family support and participation, and encourage it as permitted by the facility.

mm Hg systolic and 15 mm Hg diastolic above the patient's usual blood pressure may signal pregnancy-induced hypertension (PIH).

The temperature normally should range from 98° to 99.6° F (36.2° to 37.6° C). A temperature elevation may signal dehydration; a serious obstetric infection, such as chorioamnionitis (fetal membrane inflammation); or another type of infection, such as a UTI. Pulse rate typically should range from 60 to 90 beats/minute. An elevated pulse rate may be caused by anxiety, pain, infection, dehydration, or drug use.

Respirations normally should range from 16 to 24 breaths/minute. Increased respirations may indicate hyperventilation, anxiety, pain, or infection. Decreased temperature, pulse, and respirations do not commonly occur during labor.

Fetal heart tones. Evaluate fetal heart tones to determine fetal well-being. An electronic fetal heart monitor may be used for this part of the assessment (see Chapter 8, Fetal assessment in labor). Otherwise, assess the heart tones via auscultation. A variation from the normal fetal heart rate of 120 to 160 beats/minute may indicate fetal distress.

Uterine contractions. Distinguish true labor from Braxton Hicks contractions by using an external fetal monitor or palpating the patient's abdomen. Note the frequency, duration, and intensity of the uterine contractions (see *Palpating uterine contractions,* page 154). Also observe the patient during and between contractions to estimate her level of discomfort.

Fetal lie, presentation, and position. Perform Leopold's maneuvers to determine the fetal lie, presentation, and position. (For an illustrated procedure, see *Performing Leopold's maneuvers,* page 155.) Leopold's maneuvers also help anticipate the course of labor.

Estimated fetal weight. Assess the fetal weight by evaluating the fundal height. Then correlate the estimated weight with the gestational age to identify a fetus that is large or small for gestational age.

Edema and deep tendon reflexes. Slight localized edema of the feet and ankles is normal late in pregnancy. However, edema of the face (especially in the periorbital area and bridge of the nose), hands, or pretibial area may signal generalized edema and PIH, especially if accompanied by brisk deep tendon reflexes or clonus. If these signs are present, notify the physician.

Vaginal examination. The vaginal examination determines the patient's labor progress by assessing cervical changes, confirming amniotic membrane status, and evaluating fetal position and descent. If specially educated in this skill and if the facility permits, the nurse conducts the vaginal examination. Otherwise, the nurse assists a physician or nurse-midwife. The nurse immediately documents the vaginal examination findings. Note the date, time, findings, examiner's name, and any procedures that were performed, such as an amniotomy or placement of fetal scalp electrode or intrauterine pressure catheter.

Palpating uterine contractions

Assessment of uterine contractions by palpation requires no special equipment. It does, however, demand nursing skill and sensitivity to touch. Uterine tightening and abdominal lifting occur with contractions that can be lightly palpated on the uterine fundus. Each contraction has three phases: the increment (building up) phase, the acme (peak) phase, and the decrement (letting down) phase.

The nurse determines the frequency, duration, and intensity of several contractions. The frequency is assessed by the time period between the beginning of one contraction and the beginning of the next. Duration is evaluated by the time period from the onset of uterine tightening to its relaxation. While the uterus is tightened, the intensity of the contraction is determined by pressing the fingertips into the fundus. During mild contractions, the fundus indents easily and feels like a chin. In moderate contractions, the fundus indents less easily and feels more rigid, like the tip of a nose. With strong contractions, the fundus is firm, resists indenting, and feels like a forehead.

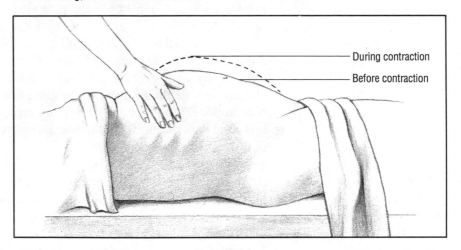

During contraction

Before contraction

Preparation for admission or discharge

After reviewing the health history and physical assessment findings to develop a complete clinical picture of the patient, consider the health care facility's policy for admission. If the patient is in true labor or meets the standards for admission, continue to prepare her for delivery. If she is in false labor and she and the fetus are in stable condition, call the physician or nurse-midwife for discharge orders and instructions for the patient's return.

For a patient who must be discharged, be sure to instruct her to return to the health care facility if her membranes rupture, if she develops bleeding, if her contractions become more intense, or if she shows signs of infection, such as fever. Advise her to return if normal fetal movements decrease significantly. Instruct her to keep her next prenatal appointment with her physician or nurse-midwife.

Performing Leopold's maneuvers

Leopold's maneuvers allow the nurse's systematic evaluation of the patient's abdomen to determine fetal position. Before Leopold's maneuvers are performed, the patient should void and lie supine with her abdomen uncovered. Abdominal muscle tension can be reduced by placing a pillow under her shoulders and drawing her knees up slightly.

1. The first maneuver is used to determine which part of the fetus lies in the upper uterus.

2. The second maneuver is performed to locate the back.

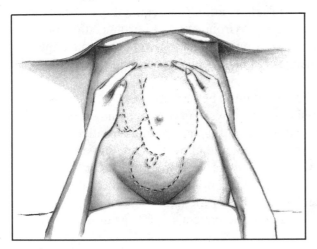

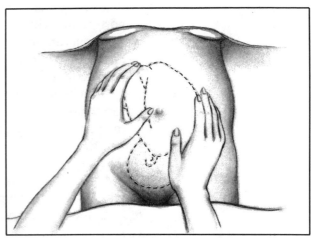

3. The third maneuver is carried out to identify the presenting part (the part of the fetus above the pelvic inlet).

4. The fourth maneuver determines the descent of the presenting part.

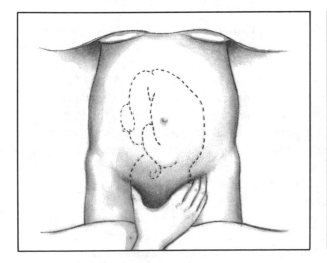

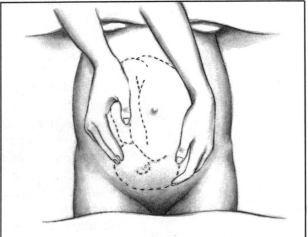

Document the patient's discharge. Record the initial assessment findings and recommendations that the patient received, including follow-up with the health care provider.

Nursing care after admission

Patients and their support persons enter the labor and delivery area in widely varying emotional states and degrees of preparedness. The nurse should make every effort to create a calm, welcoming environment. This helps decrease their apprehension and stress and promote a more positive childbirth experience.

Orientation

After the patient has been officially admitted, acquaint her and her support person with their physical environment and introduce the nurse who will care for them. A thorough orientation will help reduce their anxiety and convey openness to their needs, encouraging them to participate fully.

An informed consent is obtained before any procedure is performed on a patient in labor. The physician or nurse-midwife informs the patient of each procedure's benefits, risks, and alternatives and obtain the consent. Then the nurse should allow time to answer the patient's questions and discuss her concerns. If medications or the stress of labor compromises the patient's ability to make rational decisions, include her support person or a family member in discussions about care and procedures. Document the patient's—or her family's—consent in her records.

Ongoing assessment

After the patient is admitted, complete her health history, perform a detailed physical assessment, and collect laboratory data. The assessment data will serve as the basis for developing a care plan for the patient and her family.

Health history. This interview supplements the initial health history, which emphasized the patient's current labor status, with questions that review body systems and assess her psychosocial status. If the patient's prenatal record includes this information, do not collect it again. Vary the length of the ongoing health history based on the patient's condition. If the patient's labor is progressing rapidly, shorten the interview.

Family history. Ask the patient if anyone in her family has a disorder that may affect her labor and delivery, such as pregnancy-induced hypertension. A patient with a family history of this disorder may develop similar complications during the stress of labor.

Medical and surgical history. Document allergies to any medications, anesthetics, foods, or other substances. If the patient had ever had a blood transfusion, note any history of transfusion reactions. Record any surgery she has had, whether she received an anesthetic during surgery, the type, and how well she tolerated it.

Personal habits and activities of daily living. Determine personal habits and the patient's use of alcohol, cigarettes, or any prescription, over-the-counter, or street drugs. Use of alcohol or drugs may endanger maternal and fetal health. Cigarettes reduce fetal weight and produce maternal respiratory congestion, causing difficulty if the patient receives a general anesthetic.

Ask the patient about her prenatal weight gain, her last meal, and how well rested she is entering labor.

Psychosocial status. A psychosocial assessment is an important part of the total nursing evaluation. Key factors that influence a patient's response to labor include her personality, previously established reaction patterns, and other childbirth experiences. Other influential factors include her relationship with her support person and various social, cultural, and economic adjustments required during childbearing.

Observe the patient carefully to obtain a full picture of her current psychosocial status. Note how she presents herself for care by considering her general appearance, facial expression, posture, and body language. Study her verbal and nonverbal cues to determine how she is coping with labor and impending parenthood.

Cultural or ethnic background. Culture and ethnicity can affect expectations and perceptions of childbirth. A culturally sensitive, nonjudgmental nurse can find out what the patient expects and try to meet her needs.

Child care considerations. Ask about the patient's plans for breastfeeding or bottle-feeding the neonate. If she has not made a decision about feeding, discuss the options with her. If she has made a decision, support it.

Knowledge and concerns about labor and delivery. If the patient had attended childbirth education classes, this information provides an estimate of her knowledge of labor and delivery and allows proper nursing support for her chosen childbirth method.

Assess the patient's understanding of—and worries about—her impending labor and delivery. Lack of knowledge can lead to nonproductive efforts and stress.

Goals for labor and delivery. Assess the patient's goals to see if they are realistic and flexible, and aid in planning for the support person's participation. Conclude the assessment by finding out what kind of support the patient prefers during labor and delivery. Note the patient's preferences and help her support person and family understand them.

Physical assessment

A physical assessment is performed by the physician or nurse-midwife to evaluate findings that could affect labor, delivery, and maternal or fetal well-being. Be alert to some of the following significant clinical findings that would alter nursing care planning:

• Skin rash or lesions, especially on the genitals. These signs may indicate a sexually transmitted disease, such as herpes, that could be transmitted to the fetus.

- Jaundice. This sign may signal liver disease, which could reduce the patient's ability to clear anesthetics and medications from her body.
- Signs and symptoms of dehydration, such as thirst or dry mucous membranes. A dehydrated patient will need fluids to maintain her blood volume and prevent further problems.
- Edema. A patient with generalized or excessive edema may have PIH or a kidney disorder that may cause labor complications.
- Vulvar varicosities or hemorrhoids. A patient with these swollen, tortuous veins should be monitored for pain or thrombosis during labor.
- Problems with back, pelvis, or abduction of legs that involve stiffness, difficulty in moving, or pain. Any of these problems may make the patient uncomfortable when in the lithotomy position. Back problems may worsen during labor.

Laboratory studies
Review all of the patient's laboratory data, including the results of routine antepartal studies, special antepartal tests (if the patient has a chronic disease, such as diabetes, or an obstetric concern, such as a genetic disorder), and the routine studies performed on admission to the labor and delivery area.

Nursing diagnoses
Review all health history, physical assessment, and laboratory test findings. Based on these, formulate nursing diagnoses for the patient, fetus, support person, or other family members, as needed. (For a partial list of applicable diagnoses, see Nursing Diagnoses: *First stage of labor.*)

Initial planning and implementation
After assessing the patient and fetus, plan and implement routine admission procedures, such as I.V. fluid infusion and skin preparation. Prioritize these procedures based on the labor progress, the ease of implementation, and the patient's comfort, safety, preference, and need to move about.

I.V. fluid infusion. Due to delayed gastric emptying time, the patient's intake may be limited to minimum oral fluids and ice chips. However, a patient in labor may perspire heavily, breathe rapidly, and urinate frequently, creating the potential for a fluid volume deficit. Therefore, the physician or nurse-midwife may order continuous I.V. fluid infusion.

Skin preparation. In most health care facilities, complete pubic skin preparation, or "prep," has been omitted or replaced by removal of hair from the lower third of the labia or from around the part of the perineum where an episiotomy or laceration would be repaired. Perform the procedure according to the health care facility's policy and medical orders.

Enema administration. For a patient in labor, enema administration is no longer a routine procedure. However, if an enema is ordered, administer it according to the health care facility's policy.

NURSING DIAGNOSES

First stage of labor

The following potential nursing diagnoses are examples of the problems and etiologies that a nurse may encounter when caring for a patient in the first stage of labor.
- Altered placental tissue perfusion; related to maternal position
- Anxiety related to hospital environment
- High risk for fluid volume deficit related to restricted oral intake and increased fluid output
- Impaired physical mobility related to electronic fetal monitoring equipment
- Ineffective family coping: compromised, related to patient's pain
- Ineffective individual coping related to lack of family support
- Knowledge deficit related to appropriate relaxation techniques
- Knowledge deficit related to the labor process
- Pain related to uterine contractions

Ongoing planning and implementation

During the first stage of labor, continually monitor the status of the patient and the fetus as well as the labor progress. Also provide comfort and support to the patient and her family.

Monitor vital signs. To provide safe care, evaluate vital signs as often as required by health care facility policy. During the early phase of labor (0 to 3 cm of cervical dilation), assess the patient's blood pressure, pulse, and respirations hourly, if no problems are anticipated or discovered. Monitor her temperature every 4 hours throughout labor, unless she has ruptured membranes or a temperature above 99.6° F (37.5° C). In these instances, monitor her temperature every 2 hours while checking her pulse. Record all findings.

During the active phase of labor (4 to 10 cm of cervical dilation), check blood pressure, pulse, and respirations every hour (if normal). When the patient reaches transition, the final part of the active phase of labor, evaluate her at least every 30 minutes.

Monitor uterine contractions. The policy of the health care facility— and the physician's or nurse-midwife's orders—will determine exactly how often uterine contractions must be monitored. Unless a deviation occurs, assess contractions every hour during the early phase and every 30 minutes during the active phase of the first stage of labor.

The facility's policy and physician's or nurse-midwife's orders also will determine whether uterine contractions are monitored by abdominal palpation or electronic fetal monitoring (EFM). Monitor the intensity, frequency, and duration of the contractions.

Monitor fetal response to labor. Frequently evaluate the fetus to maintain well-being (see *Fetal evaluations during labor,* page 160). Depending on the health care facility's policies and orders written by the physician and nurse-midwife, assess the fetus by auscultating fetal heart tones or using EFM.

Fetal evaluations during labor

During labor, the nurse must frequently monitor the fetus as well as the patient to help maintain their health.

- For the low-risk patient, assess the fetal heart rate every 60 minutes in the latent phase, every 30 minutes in the active phase, and every 15 minutes in the second stage.
- For the high-risk patient, evaluate the fetal heart rate, rhythm, and response to contractions at least every 30 minutes in the early phase of labor, every 15 minutes during active labor, and every 5 minutes in the second stage as ordered, with either auscultation or electronic fetal monitoring.
- Note the amniotic fluid color when the membranes rupture. Meconium-stained fluid indicates fetal stress.
- Document the results of fetal scalp sampling and cord blood pH testing, if obtained.

Monitor labor progress. Monitor cervical dilation, effacement, station, and other indicators of labor progress through vaginal exams.

Monitor urinary function. Regularly assess the patient's urine output and presence of proteinuria and ketonuria. The patient should urinate at least every 2 hours, and her urine should contain no protein or ketones. If ketonuria or proteinuria are present, notify the physician or nurse-midwife and monitor the patient and fetus more closely.

During active labor, the patient may develop bladder distention with decreased urine output. This increases her discomfort, impedes labor progress by preventing fetal descent, and can lead to postpartal UTIs. An order for straight catheterization to empty the bladder may become necessary.

Provide comfort and support. During childbirth, the patient needs not only physical care but also a supportive human presence, pain relief, acceptance, information, and reassurance. By constantly providing for the patient's physical comfort and emotional support, the nurse can meet most or all of these needs. (For more information, see *Nursing measures for comfort and labor support.*)

When caring for a patient in the first stage of labor, individualize her care by selecting comfort and support measures that are most effective for her. These measures include creating a supportive atmosphere, promoting good positioning and walking, maintaining hygiene, conserving energy, promoting rest and effective breathing, integrating cultural beliefs and practices, educating the patient and advocating on her behalf, and relieving pain. (See also Chapter 9, Comfort promotion during labor and childbirth.)

Care for the family

Throughout labor, provide care not only for the patient and fetus but also for the family. Each family requires individualized interventions

Nursing measures for comfort and labor support

PHASE	MATERNAL BEHAVIOR	COMFORT MEASURES
Latent	• May be excited or apprehensive • Usually talkative and sociable • Receptive to diversional activities	• Suggest distractions such as watching television or reading. • Encourage walking or upright posture in rocker. • Promote rest and relaxation depending on time of day.
Active	• More serious and preoccupied with contractions • May become quiet and withdrawn, or panicked and verbal • May begin to doubt ability to cope	• Encourage companionship with partner or family member. • Promote quiet, relaxed atmosphere. • Promote rest between contractions. • Encourage breathing techniques to help maintain her self-control.
Transition	• Self-absorbed, restless • Irritable and hypersensitive • May develop nausea and vomiting, hiccups, or belching • May experience maternal amnesia between contractions • Increased perspiration with intermittent chills and hot flashes common • May feel discouraged or panicky	• Never leave patient alone. • Provide constant reassurance. • Offer firm guidance in using modified breathing techniques. • Offer steadfast physical care and emotional support and comfort. • Employ analgesics with caution—this phase is intense but brief.

based on needs and childbirth goals. Suggest ways to provide comfort for the patient.

Keep in mind that some people choose not to participate in a family member's childbirth experience. The partner may prefer not to be involved; the patient may not want her partner to see her during labor. Respect each person's preferences and avoid imposing personal values.

Evaluation

To complete the nursing process, evaluate the effectiveness of nursing care by reviewing the goals attained and the family's involvement and satisfaction with the care. Remember that evaluation stimulates continued reassessment—and improvement—of the effectiveness of nursing care throughout the intrapartal period.

Documentation

Document assessment findings and nursing activities as thoroughly and objectively as possible. Thorough documentation not only allows evaluation of the effectiveness of the nursing care plan, but also helps ensure consistent care from others on the health care team. The entries should describe events exactly, completely, and in chronological order to be accurate.

Although each health care facility may require documentation of slightly different information, most require the nurse to record the following information on the continuing labor record after initial assessment is completed:

- patient's vital signs
- fetal heart rate pattern (variability, baseline, periodic changes, and use of external or internal monitor)
- uterine contraction pattern (intensity, frequency, and duration)
- vaginal examination findings (cervical dilation, effacement, station, position, and status of membranes)
- spontaneous or artificial rupture of membranes and description of amniotic fluid
- application of internal fetal scalp electrode or intrauterine pressure catheter
- patient's position changes or behaviors, such as crouching or vomiting
- fluid intake and output
- administration of medications, oxygen, I.V. fluids, and epidural anesthesia
- patient's response to treatments received
- presence of family members
- physician or nurse-midwife visits with the patient.

STUDY ACTIVITIES

Short answer

1. LeVonne Foster, a 28-year-old gravida 3 para 2002, arrives with her husband in the labor and delivery area to be admitted. She is at full-term gestation, after a healthy, uneventful pregnancy. During the nursing assessment, Ms. Foster's contractions appear irregular. They come every 4 to 7 minutes, last about 30 to 40 seconds, and are of mild intensity, feeling more like "pressure." She denies any bloody show or rupture of membranes. Fetal heart tones are stable, and she reports active fetal movement. Her pelvic examination reveals cervical dilation of 2 cm, 50% effaced, with an unengaged vertex presentation.

After walking for 2 hours, Ms. Foster is reexamined. Her contractions are less frequent, coming every 12 to 15 minutes and lasting 20 to 30 seconds, and her pelvic exam remains unchanged. Maternal and fetal status are stable. What is most likely occurring? Explain your answer.

_____

2. After obtaining a discharge order, what instructions would the nurse give to Ms. Foster and her husband? What, then, would the nurse document?

_____

3. Betty Smith, a graduate nurse, is being oriented to the labor and delivery unit. The charge nurse explains the guidelines for fetal evaluations during labor. How frequently should Ms. Smith expect to assess the fetal heart rate?

_____

_____

4. List ten comfort measures that the nurse can provide for the woman in labor.

_____

_____

5. Why is it important for the nurse to encourage the patient to urinate at least every 2 hours during labor?

_____

6. Briefly describe a patient going through the transitional phase of her labor and at least four comfort measures that the nurse could employ at this time.

_____

_____

True or false

7. The first stage of labor begins with the onset of regular, rhythmic uterine contractions and ends with the birth of the neonate.
☐ True ☐ False

8. It is important for the nurse to auscultate fetal heart tones throughout several contractions and for at least 60 seconds afterward to establish the well-being of the fetus.
☐ True ☐ False

9. Contraction duration is evaluated by the time period from the onset of uterine tightening to the beginning of the next contraction.
☐ True ☐ False

10. Leopold's maneuvers allow the nurse's systematic evaluation of the patient's abdomen to determine fetal position.
☐ True ☐ False

11. Nursing responsibilities include the immediate documentation of vaginal examination findings as well as any procedures that were performed, such as amniotomy.
☐ True ☐ False

ANSWERS **Short answer**

1. Based on her contraction pattern, experience of pain as pressure, and her lack of show, cervical dilation, or descent, Ms. Foster is most likely in false labor.

2. Ms. Foster would be instructed to return to the health care facility if her membranes rupture, if she develops bleeding, if her contractions become more intense, or if she shows signs of infection, such as fever. She also would be advised to return if normal fetal movements changed. The nurse then would document Ms. Foster's discharge, including the initial assessment findings and recommendations that the nurse had given Ms. Foster, such as follow-up with her physician.

3. For the low-risk patient, Ms. Smith would expect to assess the fetal heart rate every 60 minutes in latent labor, every 30 minutes in the active phase, and every 15 minutes in the second stage. For the high-risk patient, she would expect to evaluate the fetal heart rate, rhythm, and response to contractions at least every 30 minutes in the early phase of labor, every 15 minutes during active labor, and every 5 minutes in the second stage, as ordered with either auscultation or EFM.

4. The nurse can individualize care for a patient in the first stage of labor by selecting comfort and support measures that are most effective for her. These measures include creating a supportive atmosphere, promoting good positioning and walking, maintaining hygiene, conserving energy, promoting rest and effective breathing, educating the patient and advocating on her behalf, integrating her cultural beliefs and practices, and relieving pain.

5. During active labor, the patient may develop bladder distention with decreased urine output. This increases discomfort, impedes labor progress by preventing fetal descent, and can lead to postpartal UTIs.

6. A patient in the transitional phase of the first stage of labor might be self-absorbed, restless, irritable, and hypersensitive; she may develop nausea and vomiting, hiccups, or belching; she may experience a natural amnesia between contractions and increased perspiration with intermittent chills or hot flashes. The patient may feel discouraged or panicky. Nursing comfort and support measures would include never leaving the patient alone at this time, providing constant reassurance, offering firm guidance in using modified breathing techniques, offering steadfast physical care as well as emotional support and comfort, and employing analgesics with caution (because this phase is intense but brief, so neonatal considerations must be kept in mind).

True or false

7. False. The first stage of labor begins with the onset of regular, rhythmic contractions and ends with complete cervical dilation of approximately 10 cm.

8. True.

9. False. The duration is evaluated by the time period from the onset of uterine tightening to its relaxation.

10. True.

11. True.

CHAPTER 11

The second stage of labor

OBJECTIVES

After studying this chapter, the reader should be able to:

1. List characteristics of the onset and progression of the second stage of labor and compare its typical length for primiparous versus multiparous patients.

2. Describe assessment of a patient in the second stage of labor.

3. Outline the nurse's responsibilities during childbirth for both the patient and neonate.

OVERVIEW OF CONCEPTS

The second stage of labor begins with complete cervical dilation and ends with delivery of the neonate. It requires tiring maternal efforts coupled with strong, effective uterine contractions. The patient will need much emotional support and encouragement. During this highly emotional and stressful period, the nurse must also meet the needs of the family and fetus as well as monitor the progress of labor, prepare the environment and equipment needed for delivery, and evaluate the neonate's status after delivery.

The transition from the first to the second stage of labor signals impending birth. The nurse should be aware of the characteristics that indicate the onset of the second stage and its expected duration. After assessing the patient's progress into the second stage, the nurse must notify the physician or nurse-midwife to prepare for the delivery.

Onset

Several characteristics indicate a transition from the first to the second stage of labor, including some or all of the following:
- an increasing urge to push
- an increase in bloody show
- increased facial perspiration
- involuntary shaking of extremities
- grunting
- gaping of the anus, involuntary defecation
- bulging of the vaginal introitus
- spontaneous rupture of membranes, if this has not already occurred

• abrupt onset of early decelerations (beginning early in the contraction) in fetal heart rate (FHR); such FHR changes, although common, should be reported to the physician or nurse-midwife.

Duration

For primiparous patients, the second stage of labor averages 66 minutes, ranging from 48 to 174 minutes. For multiparous patients, the second stage averages 24 minutes, ranging from 6 to 66 minutes. The duration depends on the combined effects of fetal, maternal, psychological, and environmental factors.

Although a prolonged second stage (over 2 hours in a primigravida or over 1 hour in a multigravida) may indicate a disorder, the physician or nurse-midwife may allow the labor to continue if all is stable and progressing.

As the patient reaches the threshold for a prolonged second stage, the nurse must notify the physician or nurse-midwife of the patient's labor status, fetal condition, and need for further evaluation. Thereafter, the nurse must carefully monitor both the patient and the fetus for continuing evidence of labor progress and signs of distress (see *Factors affecting the duration of the second stage of labor*). Thorough documentation at frequent intervals is especially important at this time.

Nursing care

Assessment

During the second stage of labor, assessment occurs more frequently than during the first stage.

Vital signs

Take vital signs at least every 15 minutes or more often, especially if the patient has continuous epidural anesthesia, is hypertensive, or has other complicating conditions. Bearing-down efforts may increase patient blood pressure, pulse, and respirations. Take blood pressure as necessary between contractions, but use discretion if pressure has been stable and birth is imminent. A temperature rise of one degree may occur even in the absence of infection, but a temperature over 100° F (37.8° C) should be reported to the physician or nurse-midwife. Dehydration may play a role in temperature elevation.

Cervical dilation

When characteristics of the onset of the second stage appear, expect a vaginal examination to be performed to confirm complete dilation and assess the presenting part, fetal station, status of the fetal membranes, and color of the amniotic fluid.

Some patients have a strong urge to bear down before the cervix dilates completely. Premature pushing can cause cervical edema, and it may slow cervical dilation and fetal descent. If examination reveals incomplete dilation and the patient has a strong urge, help the patient avoid bearing down by repositioning and encouraging deep-breathing techniques, such as panting and blowing during contractions.

Factors affecting the duration of the second stage of labor

When working with a patient during the second stage of labor, the nurse must be aware of the various factors that may affect the duration of labor in order to provide support, encouragement, and any necessary interventions.

FETAL FACTORS
- Physical condition
- Size, station, and position
- Molding
- Method of internal rotation
- Rate of descent

MATERNAL FACTORS
Age and parity
- Size and shape of the bony pelvis
- Strength of uterine contractions
- Resistance or relaxation of soft tissues
- Labor positioning
- Fatigue level

- Degree of expulsive efforts
- Obstetric interventions, such as anesthesia or episiotomy

Psychological factors
- Emotional readiness
- Degree of relaxation
- Level of trust in care providers
- Previous preparation for childbirth

Environmental factors
- Bright lights
- Noise
- Hectic activity

Contractions

Assess the strength, frequency, and duration of uterine contractions every 15 minutes during the second stage. Contractions that have occurred every 2 or 3 minutes may extend to every 5 minutes during this stage, allowing the patient to rest between contractions. Some patients have more frequent contractions and report unceasing pain. This pain may relate to increasing pressure from the presenting part and difficulty relaxing between contractions.

When the second stage lasts longer than 2 hours, uterine contractions may decrease in strength and frequency. The physician or nurse-midwife then evaluates the need for oxytocin (to stimulate labor) and assesses for cephalopelvic disproportion or other abnormalities.

Bearing-down efforts

Assess the effectiveness of the patient's bearing-down efforts and her energy resources as the second stage progresses.

Although epidural anesthesia can be useful in the first stage of labor, it may create problems for a patient in the second stage; the amount of sensory and motor block necessary to relieve pain may reduce, delay, or eliminate bearing-down efforts. Moreover, epidural anesthesia may lengthen the second stage and increase the need for forceps or vacuum assistance.

Fetal heart rate

Assess the FHR more frequently during the second stage of labor than during the first, based on the patient's risk status, underlying medical conditions, medications and anesthetic agent used, and any alterations in FHR patterns that arose during the first stage. For a low-risk patient, auscultate FHR every 15 minutes or use an electronic fetal monitor, depending on the patient's wishes, the physician's or nurse-midwife's preference, and facility policy. If the patient finds repeated FHR auscultation disruptive, consider switching to electronic monitoring. A patient with complications placing her at risk may require electronic monitoring, possibly with an internal scalp electrode to detect fetal distress or beat-to-beat variability and must have FHR recorded at 5-minute intervals.

Descent
The fetus normally begins descent during active labor; if descent has not begun by 7 cm of cervical dilation, an abnormality may exist. Failure to descend occurs in a small percentage of patients due to such causes as the largeness of the fetus (over 4,000 g), cephalopelvic disproportion, or fetal malposition (primarily persistent occiput transverse or occiput posterior positions).

During a pelvic examination, descent is assessed during the first stage of labor by measuring the relationship between the fetus's head and the patient's ischial spines.

Amniotic fluid
Note any change in the color of the amniotic fluid during the second stage of labor because it may indicate fetal distress. When stained with meconium, amniotic fluid becomes green and may range in consistency from thin to thick. An increase in bloody show, which commonly occurs early in the second stage, may cause pink-tinged amniotic fluid. Port wine–colored fluid may indicate abruptio placentae. Notify the physician or nurse-midwife of any change in amniotic fluid color.

Nursing diagnoses
The following diagnoses address representative problems and etiologies that the nurse may encounter when caring for a patient during the second stage of labor.
• Anxiety related to duration of labor
• Fatigue related to duration of labor, energy expenditure, and possible lack of sleep
• Fluid volume deficit related to restricted fluid intake and fluid loss during labor efforts
• Hopelessness related to prolonged bearing-down efforts that produce little progress
• Ineffective breathing pattern related to painful uterine contractions and inefficient bearing-down efforts
• Ineffective individual coping related to exhaustion
• Knowledge deficit related to typical duration of labor
• Pain related to rapid delivery or fetal malposition
• Pain related to stretching of vaginal and perineal tissues during birth

Planning and implementation

During the second stage of labor, the nurse must plan and act almost simultaneously to comfort the patient and assist with delivery of the neonate.

Provide emotional support

Provide general emotional support to the patient by assuring her that labor is progressing normally, that she will not be left alone, and that the physician or nurse-midwife will be summoned. Depending on the support person's participation, the nurse's role can range from reassuring to active coaching during the second stage. If the support person participates actively and responds appropriately to the patient's efforts, the nurse will need only to supply positive feedback and encouragement.

Coordinate bearing-down efforts

Coordinate the patient's bearing-down efforts to minimize discomfort and maximize her energy and efficiency. Encourage her to push at the peak of contractions and to rest between contractions.

Assist with positioning

Position changes may be especially helpful to maximize the patient's efficiency during bearing down. The side-lying position helps slow a rapid delivery and may reduce perineal tension. The forearms-and-knees position can reduce back pain related to labor. When the fetus descends slowly, the patient may benefit from a squatting position. Be sure to consider the advantages and disadvantages of a position before suggesting a change to the patient.

Monitor hydration

A patient who shows decreased bearing-down efforts after a period of effective efforts may be dehydrated. To avoid this, frequently offer her juice, water, or tea, as ordered. If bearing down lasts more than 2 hours, start an I.V. line to deliver fluids, as prescribed.

Facilitate delivery

As delivery approaches, nursing responsibilities include making a judgment about when to transfer the patient to the delivery room (or when to summon the physician or nurse-midwife), preparing the delivery area, preparing the patient, and assisting with delivery.

Transfer to the delivery room. Judging when to transfer a patient to the delivery room and when to summon the physician or nurse-midwife is a learned skill. The goal is to allow sufficient time for the patient to reach the delivery room before giving birth, but not to allow so much time that the patient and staff have an extended wait. Always consider the patient's labor history, current progress, and rate of descent.

Prepare the delivery area. Make all necessary physical preparations for the impending birth. This includes gathering and setting up needed equipment and reviewing the patient's and physician's or nurse-midwife's wishes for the delivery.

Plan ahead for emergencies. Know how to operate all delivery room equipment, including stirrups, infant resuscitation equipment, and the bed.

Prepare the patient. Once the patient is positioned in the delivery room bed, prepare the perineum by swabbing with an antiseptic solution.

Assist with delivery. Although the nurse does perform or repair an episiotomy (small incision in perineum to assist delivery of the fetus), the nurse should communicate the patient's wishes to the physician or nurse-midwife. Further, the nurse should provide care and support during and after an episiotomy. The nurse is responsible for providing the necessary suture equipment and proper lighting for repair by the physician or nurse-midwife.

Care for the neonate

Immediately after delivery of the head (before delivery of the body), the physician or nurse-midwife suctions the neonate to ensure an adequate airway. After the neonate's delivery, nursing care shifts from the patient to the neonate.

Perform an initial physical assessment after drying and positioning the neonate. Continue to suction the upper airway as needed, complete the clamping of the cord, and initiate bonding between the neonate and parents within the first few minutes after delivery.

Note the time of birth and the condition of the neonate's airway, amount of mucus, and respiratory efforts. Continue the physical assessment, noting the neonate's heart rate, reflex irritability, color, and muscle tone in addition to evaluating the umbilical cord. Assign an Apgar score at 1 minute and 5 minutes after delivery (for instructions, see *Assigning an Apgar score*); explain the Apgar score's meaning to the patient and her partner. Also note any obvious congenital anomalies, birthmarks, or bruises associated with delivery. Record the passage of neonatal meconium or urine in the delivery room.

Initiate parent-infant bonding as soon as the neonate's condition is stable. Place the neonate on the patient's abdomen, and cover both the neonate and the patient with a warm blanket. Assess the patient's and partner's response to the neonate, and facilitate their interaction.

Evaluation

Evaluate the effectiveness of nursing care by reviewing the goals attained and the outcome of the second stage of labor for the patient, support person, and neonate. The following are examples of appropriate evaluation statements.

• The patient bore down productively during the final phase of the second stage of labor.

• The patient and her partner expressed appropriate bonding behavior with the neonate immediately after delivery.

Assigning an Apgar score

The Apgar score, a method of indicating neonatal vigor, combines the results of individual assessments: heart rate, respirations, muscle tone, reflex irritability, and color. Typically assigned by the nurse at 1 minute and 5 minutes after the neonate is delivered, the score may reveal the need for resuscitation, confirm trauma during delivery, and indicate congenital anomaly, among other findings. If the heart rate is less than 100 beats/minute or respirations are absent, request help and initiate resuscitation immediately.

ASSESSMENT STEPS
Use the guidelines below to assign a score from 1 to 2 in each assessment category. Be sure to follow the appropriate assessment procedures.

Heart rate
Using a stethoscope, count heartbeats for 30 seconds and multiply by 2. Alternatively, feel for a pulse at the base of the umbilical cord or over the heart. If the heart rate exceeds 100 beats/minute, give a score of 2. A heart rate under 100 beats/minute warrants a 1, and no detectable heart rate should receive a 0.

Respirations
After counting and observing, assign a score of 2 for vigorous crying or regular respirations. Irregular, shallow, or gasping respirations score a 1, and absent respiratory effort gets a 0.

Muscle tone
Normally, the neonate's elbows are flexed and thighs and knees drawn up. If the limbs return to this position quickly after being extended, assign a score of 2. If muscles have some tone but do not respond briskly, give a 1. Assign a 0 for flaccid muscles.

Reflex irritability
Insert a bulb syringe into one of the neonate's nostrils or lightly flick the sole of one foot. If the response is a vigorous cry, assign a score of 2. Some motion or weak crying warrants a 1; no response rates a 0.

Color
Observe the skin or mucous membranes for pallor or cyanosis. If the neonate appears completely pink, assign a score of 2 (few neonates receive this score). Acrocyanosis, which refers to bluish hands and feet and applies to most neonates, receives a score of 1. A completely pale or blue neonate receives a score of 0. (In a dark-skinned neonate, check the palms of the hands and soles of the feet to determine pallor or cyanosis.)

Add the scores assigned in each assessment category to arrive at a total Apgar score. The highest score possible is 10; the lowest is 0. Interventions, if necessary, are based on the score.

INTERVENTIONS
A neonate with a score of 8 to 10 is normal and needs only routine interventions. Aspirate the mouth and nose with a bulb syringe. Dry and wrap the neonate in warm blankets. Perform a brief physical examination.

A score of 5 to 7 indicates mild respiratory, metabolic, or neurologic depression. Stimulate breathing by gently but firmly slapping the soles of the feet or rubbing the spine or back. Administer 100% oxygen via bag and face mask. If the neonate shows no improvement and the mother received a narcotic analgesic, expect to administer 0.01 mg/kg of naloxone I.M.

A score of 3 or 4 requires interventions as described above; also, the neonate may require a feeding tube to decompress the stomach. Expect to maintain oxygen administration until the neonate's heart rate exceeds 100 beats/minute and skin is completely pink.

A score of 0 to 2 indicates severe depression and requires immediate intubation and bag ventilation at 40 to 60 breaths/minute with pressures high enough to move the upper chest. Closed chest cardiac massage is performed for bradycardia under 60 beats/minute (or between 60 and 80 beats/minute but not increasing) or cardiac arrest. Resuscitation drugs also are needed.

Documentation
The nurse documents initial and ongoing assessment findings, pertinent characteristics of the patient and support person, and all nursing activities and interventions as completely as possible. Although documentation records vary among health care facilities, most require the nurse to document at least the following whenever appropriate:
• vital signs (blood pressure, pulse, temperature)

- fetal heart rate (variability, baseline, periodic changes, use of external or internal fetal monitor)
- vaginal examination findings (document time of complete cervical dilation, ongoing fetal station, fetal position, and crowning)
- uterine contractions (duration, frequency, intensity)
- bearing-down efforts
- amniotic fluid (color and amount)
- fluid intake and output
- emotional responses
- presence of support person or others
- transfer to delivery room or birthing chair
- time of birth (full expulsion of neonate)
- names of all people in the room at the time of birth
- episiotomy or lacerations and description of repairs
- Apgar scores
- neonatal resuscitation, if necessary
- passage of meconium or urine
- any neonatal abnormalities or umbilical cord variations
- initial parent-infant bonding.

STUDY ACTIVITIES

1. Sara Jones, a 19-year-old multigravida, has been pushing ineffectively for over 30 minutes. She has been uncomfortable since her epidural anesthetic was allowed to wear off as she entered the second stage of labor. List at least eight maternal or neonatal factors that may affect the duration of second-stage labor and that the nurse will need to assess to provide appropriate support or interventions.

_____

_____

2. At 38 weeks' gestation, Drew James is born by normal spontaneous vaginal delivery over an intact perineum after an unmedicated labor. After positioning him under a radiant warmer, the nurse conducts an assessment that reveals a heart rate of 120 beats/minute, a somewhat shallow and irregular respiratory effort, some flexion of the extremities, grimacing after stimulation with a bulb syringe, and a completely pale complexion. Based on these findings, which Apgar score would the nurse assign him, and what nursing actions (if any) should be taken?

_____

_____

3. After pushing for 45 minutes in the second stage, Bernadette Gregory, a 27-year-old primigravida, is showing evidence of progressive fetal descent, although delivery is not imminent. Noting decreased FHR variability and increasing decelerations, the nurse notifies the physician. Which nursing actions are then appropriate until a medical evaluation is made?

_____

4. Identify at least five characteristic signs of the onset of the second stage of labor.

_____

5. Identify the major nursing responsibilities when facilitating a delivery and caring for the patient and neonate immediately afterward.

_____

True or false

6. The second stage of labor begins with complete cervical dilation and culminates in the delivery of the placenta.
□ True   □ False

7. The nurse should suspect an abnormality and notify the physician or nurse-midwife if no fetal descent occurs after a primigravid patient effectively bears down for over 2 hours.
□ True   □ False

8. Meconium staining of the amniotic fluid during the second stage typically indicates fetal distress.
□ True   □ False

9. The average duration of the second stage for multiparous patients is 1 hour.
□ True   □ False

ANSWERS **Short answer**

1. Maternal factors that may affect the duration of Ms. Jones's second stage include her age and parity, the size and shape of her bony pelvis, the strength of her uterine contractions, the resistance or relaxation of her soft tissues, her labor position and fatigue level, the degree of her expulsive efforts, and the effect of her epidural anesthesia. Fetal factors may include the fetus's physical condition, size, station, and position; the presence of molding; the method of the fetus's internal rotation; and the rate of descent.

2. The nurse would assign Drew an Apgar score of 5: 2 points for heart rate; 1 point each for respiratory effort, muscle tone, and reflex irritability; and 0 points for color. Because this score can indicate mild respiratory, metabolic, or neurologic depression, the nurse would stimulate Drew's breathing by gently but firmly slapping the soles of his feet or rubbing his spine or back. The nurse also would administer 100% oxygen via bag and face mask. The neonate would be observed continuously for improvement in his respirations, heart rate, color, tone, and reflexes and assigned another Apgar score at 5 minutes.

3. Decreased FHR variability, especially when accompanied by pronounced or prolonged decelerations, is cause for concern and reflects fetal distress. If delivery is not imminent, while awaiting further medical evaluation the nurse should try to raise the FHR by repositioning the patient, offering oxygen by mask, increasing I.V. fluids, and encouraging the patient to breathe through contractions rather than push.

4. Signs of the second stage of labor include an increasing urge to push, an increase in bloody show, increased facial perspiration, involuntary shaking of the extremities, decreased restlessness, grunting, involuntary defecation, gaping of the anus, bulging of the vaginal introitus, spontaneous rupture of membranes, and abrupt onset of early decelerations.

5. As delivery approaches, nursing responsibilities include making a judgment about when to transfer the patient to the delivery room (and when to summon the physician or nurse-midwife), preparing the delivery area, preparing the patient, and assisting with delivery. Immediately after delivery, nursing care shifts from the patient (now cared for by the physician or nurse-midwife) to the neonate. Nursing responsibilities for the neonate include drying and positioning the neonate, suctioning the upper airway as needed, performing an initial physical assessment, completing the clamping of the umbilical cord, and initiating bonding between the neonate and parents within the first few minutes after delivery.

True or false

6. False. The second stage of labor begins with complete cervical dilation and ends with delivery of the neonate.

7. True.

8. True.

9. False. The average duration of the second stage for multiparous patients is 24 minutes, ranging from 6 to 66 minutes.

CHAPTER 12

The third and fourth stages of labor

OBJECTIVES

After studying this chapter, the reader should be able to:

1. Describe maternal assessment and care during the third stage of labor.

2. Describe placental separation and delivery.

3. Discuss nursing interventions for a patient with a postpartum hemorrhage.

4. Explain neonatal assessment and care during the third and fourth stages of labor.

5. Discuss normal assessment findings during the fourth stage of labor.

6. Describe abnormal fourth-stage findings and possible nursing interventions.

OVERVIEW OF CONCEPTS

The third stage of labor begins with delivery of the neonate and ends with delivery of the placenta. It may last from a few minutes to 30 minutes. For most patients, this stage occurs without incident and produces a blood loss of less than 500 ml. However, postpartal hemorrhage may occur, signaling a common obstetric emergency.

In this stage, the nurse assesses the patient for homeostasis, placental status, and delivery and assists with perineal repair. The nurse also evaluates the neonate's adaptation to the extrauterine environment and assesses the family's response to the patient and neonate. The nurse must respond quickly to changing circumstances, resetting priorities as needed.

The fourth stage of labor begins after delivery of the placenta and lasts about 1 hour. It marks the beginning of the "fourth trimester" (the first 3 postpartal months), during which the patient recovers from the stresses of labor and physiologically returns to a nonpregnant state. During this stage, the patient, her partner, and the neonate experience heightened awareness and sensitivity as they further their bonding.

During the third and fourth stages of labor, the patient's cultural beliefs can influence her self-care and health promotion measures, interactions with health care professionals, and care of and bonding with the neonate. To provide adequate care, the nurse should become acquainted with the patient's cultural beliefs and exercise care to avoid stereotyping her.

In most facilities, the patient, her partner or support person, and the neonate remain together during the fourth stage of labor. In others, the neonate may be moved to the nursery while the patient remains in the postpartum recovery area. Therefore, the type of nursing care needed will depend on facility policy.

Nursing care during the third stage of labor

During this stage, the nurse may care for the mother and neonate simultaneously. To provide the best possible care, the nurse should apply the nursing process.

Assessment

Because the third stage of labor is brief, rapidly assess maternal vital signs and the status of the placenta, perineum, fundus, and neonate.

Maternal vital signs. Assess vital signs frequently, reporting changes or abnormal findings to the physician or nurse-midwife immediately. An increasing pulse rate followed by increased respirations and decreased blood pressure may be the first signs of postpartal hemorrhage and hypovolemic shock, which can occur rapidly. These complications are relatively common and typically result from uterine atony and excessive blood loss during placental separation and delivery or from perineal lacerations.

Placenta. After delivery of the neonate, watch for these normal signs of placental separation:
- a sudden gush or trickle of blood from the vagina
- increased umbilical cord length at the vaginal introitus
- change in the shape of the uterus from discoid (disk-shaped) to globular (globe-shaped)
- change in the position of the uterus to a location at or above the patient's umbilicus.

When these signs occur, expect placental delivery shortly. After the placenta separates completely, it descends to the lower uterine segment. Myometrial contractions, which may have subsided temporarily, return at 4- to 5-minute intervals and propel the placenta into the vagina. At this point, the patient may be asked to gently bear down to help expel the placenta.

Note the mechanism of placental expulsion (refer to "Placental delivery" in Chapter 7, Physiology of labor and childbirth).

Examination of the placenta determines whether fragments remain in the uterus and provides additional information about the neonate's status. Calcifications, discolorations, malformations, or other abnormalities may indicate poor placental function, explain fetal distress in labor or low birth weight, and indicate the need to evaluate the neonate more thoroughly.

Note the umbilical cord and its insertion into the placenta. Some cord variations pose potential hazards to the neonate. For example, the normal umbilical cord contains three vessels: two arteries and one vein. Fewer than three vessels correlates with various congenital anomalies.

Perineum. If the patient underwent an episiotomy or sustained lacerations, assist with surgical repair of the tissue by providing adequate light, suture material, a local anesthesia kit (if necessary), and patient support. Assess for an intact suture line, and note the degree of swelling, oozing, or discoloration caused by bruising or hematoma formation.

If the physician or nurse-midwife did not perform an episiotomy, assist with inspection of the perineum for lacerations or edema. Also assist with inspection of the vagina and cervix for lacerations or retained placental fragments, as necessary.

Fundus. Palpate the fundus to determine its location and consistency. After the placenta is delivered, the fundus normally is midline, 1 to 2 cm below the umbilicus, and firmly contracted. A boggy (soft and poorly contracted) fundus is a sign of uterine atony (lack of muscle tone). (See *Factors associated with postpartum hemorrhage,* page 178, and *Uterine palpation and massage,* page 179.)

Neonate. Depending on facility policy, the physician, nurse-midwife, or nurse assesses the neonate immediately after delivery. (For more information, see *Assigning an Apgar score* in Chapter 11, The second stage of labor.) Continue to assess the neonate throughout the third stage of labor, focusing on evaluation of respiratory and cardiovascular status and thermoregulatory functions.

Nursing diagnoses

Based on assessment findings, formulate nursing diagnoses for the patient (for a partial list of applicable diagnoses, see Nursing Diagnoses: *Third and fourth stages of labor,* page 180). Then use the assessment findings and diagnoses to define care priorities during the postpartal period.

Planning and implementation

Routine care includes hygienic care, repositioning the patient and transferring her to the recovery area (or assisting recovery in the labor-delivery-recovery area), providing neonatal care, and promoting bonding.

Provide hygienic care

Immediately after the physician or nurse-midwife has finished inspecting or repairing the perineum, help prevent infection by cleaning the patient. Dislodge and remove dried blood or fecal material, leaving the perineal area free of bacterial contamination. Help the patient change from her soiled delivery gown into a clean gown, and cover her with a clean, warm bath blanket.

Factors associated with postpartum hemorrhage

The following factors commonly are associated with uterine atony and the potential for postpartal hemorrhage. If uterine atony is not identified and corrected, postpartal hemorrhage can occur.

- History of postpartal hemorrhage with previous delivery
- Delivery of a macrosomic neonate
- Precipitous labor and delivery
- Hydramnios
- Multiple fetuses
- Extended stimulation of labor with oxytocin (Pitocin)
- Bladder distention
- Traumatic delivery
- Grand multiparity (more than 5 deliveries)
- Anesthesia or excessive analgesia

Reposition and transfer the patient

Pay close attention to body dynamics and homeostasis when repositioning the patient. When helping her lower her legs from stirrups or from the flexed position, advise her to flex her legs together and assist her to lower them simultaneously. After the patient has been repositioned, transfer her to the recovery area or allow her to remain in the labor and delivery area, depending on facility policy.

Care for the neonate

While the neonate remains with the mother or parents, provide appropriate care (for specific nursing care, see *Neonatal status: Third and fourth stages of labor,* page 181). Be especially alert for signs of cold stress, which may include an accelerated respiratory rate; labored respirations; and an increased metabolic rate accompanied by hypoglycemia, which indicates greater use of glucose stores. (For more information about cold stress and heat loss in the neonate, see Chapter 17, Physiology of neonatal adaptation, and Chapter 19, Care of the healthy neonate.)

Promote bonding

The neonate's introduction to the parents is paramount. While necessary assessments and procedures are performed, keep the mother and neonate together. Bonding commonly begins at this time, unless the patient is distracted by pain or her environment.

Encourage both parents to touch and talk to the neonate immediately. Upon hearing the parents' voices, the neonate should gaze in their direction and may open the eyes fully if they are shaded from the light.

Immediately after delivery, try promoting mother-infant bonding by encouraging breast-feeding. During breast-feeding, the mother and

Uterine palpation and massage

Through uterine palpation, the nurse can assess the location and firmness of the fundus. Uterine massage can help stimulate uterine contractions, which promote involution and prevent hemorrhage. Also, blood clots may be expelled during uterine massage. To perform uterine palpation and massage, expose the patient's lower abdomen and follow these steps.

1. Place one hand at the level of the symphysis pubis, cupping it against the abdomen to support the fundus and prevent downward displacement. Keep in mind that the elasticity of the ligaments supporting the uterus and the stretching experienced at term place the postpartal uterus at risk for inversion if the uterus is not fixed in place during palpation and massage.

2. Place the other hand at the top of the fundus, cupping it against the abdomen.

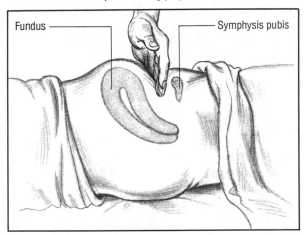

Fundus — Symphysis pubis

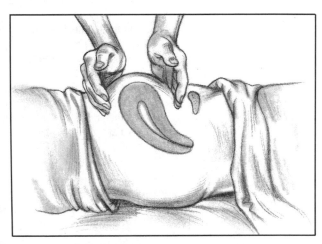

3. Gently compress the uterus between both hands. Note the level of the fundus above or below the umbilicus in finger-breadths or centimeters. (One fingerbreadth measures about 1 cm.) Also note the firmness of the fundus.

4. To massage the fundus, use the side of the hand above the fundus. Without digging into the abdomen, gently compress and release the uterus, always supporting the lower uterine segment with the other hand. Lochia flow during massage is observed.

5. Massage the uterus long enough to produce firmness. Because the fundus is tender, use only enough pressure to produce desired results without causing discomfort.

infant face each other, have skin-to-skin contact, and interact as the mother responds to the feel, smell, and movement of her infant.

While the patient is being repositioned or transferred to another bed, encourage the father or support person to hold the neonate. When the neonate is transferred to a crib, warmer, or the nursery, encourage the father or support person to remain with the neonate and report weight and activity to the mother. This helps parents and neonate maintain contact and continue bonding.

NURSING DIAGNOSES

Third and fourth stages of labor

The following nursing diagnoses address representative problems and etiologies that a nurse may encounter when caring for a patient during the third and fourth stages of labor.

Third stage of labor
- Decreased cardiac output related to postpartal hemorrhage
- High risk for injury related to neonatal birth trauma
- Impaired gas exchange related to excess secretions in the neonate
- Ineffective individual coping related to the birth experience
- Ineffective thermoregulation related to neonate's adaptation to extrauterine life
- Pain related to perineal trauma
- Pain related to uterine contractions

Fourth stage of labor
- Altered parenting related to unmet expectations about the neonate's capabilities
- Fluid volume deficit related to fluid restriction during labor and delivery
- High risk for infection related to perineal trauma
- High risk for infection related to episiotomy
- Pain related to episiotomy
- Pain related to maternal positioning
- Pain related to uterine contractions

Evaluation

Before the fourth stage of labor begins, evaluate nursing care provided during the third stage. In many facilities, the delivery nurse continues to care for the mother; in others, another nurse assumes care for the mother after transfer to the recovery area. In either case, evaluate maternal status by reviewing and comparing assessment data and considering the effectiveness of nursing interventions. The following examples illustrate appropriate evaluation statements:
- The patient's fundus was firm.
- The patient lost less than 500 ml of blood.
- The neonate adapted appropriately to the extrauterine environment.
- The patient held and gazed at the neonate immediately after delivery.

Documentation

The nurse usually documents assessments and activities of the third stage on the delivery record.

Although each health care facility may require documentation of slightly different information, most expect the nurse to record the following on the delivery record:
- episiotomy or laceration repair
- drugs or fluids administered
- time, mechanism, and completeness of delivery of the placenta
- maternal and neonatal vital signs
- interaction between parents and neonate

Neonatal status: Third and fourth stages of labor

When caring for the mother during the third and fourth stages of labor, the nurse also must assess and provide care for the neonate.

Assessment

To assess the neonate's respiratory status, count respirations and note skin color. Respirations should range from 40 to 60 breaths/minute. Except for the hands and feet, which may have a blue tinge, the neonate's skin color should be similar to that of the parents.

To assess cardiovascular status, palpate the heart rate or auscultate it. The rate should range from 120 to 160 beats/minute, increasing with crying and activity. Palpate the femoral pulse for presence and quality. Lack of a femoral pulse may indicate coarctation of the aorta, a congenital cardiovascular condition.

Assess respiratory and cardiovascular status, muscle tone, reflex irritability, and color at 1 and 5 minutes, then at 5-minute intervals unless the situation warrants more frequent assessment. Evaluate the neonate each time the mother is assessed routinely.

Nursing care

An important aspect of care during this time is maintenance of the neonate's temperature. Dry the neonate thoroughly immediately after delivery. Skin-to-skin contact with the mother provides the warmest environment for the neonate because heat from her body conducts to the neonate. If the mother holds the neonate, cover both with a warm blanket. If she does not, keep the neonate wrapped in warm blankets under a radiant warmer.

The neonate's largest surface area and area of greatest potential heat loss is the head. After drying the scalp, cover it with a stockinet cap or other head covering.

Other routine neonatal care includes applying identification bands and footprinting, as facility practice dictates.

In many facilities, the neonate is weighed and measured in the delivery area and receives vitamin K and eye prophylaxis (ophthalmic anti-infective treatment) there as well.

• maternal status at the time of transfer to the recovery area
• neonatal status at the time of transfer to the recovery area or nursery.

Nursing care during the fourth stage of labor

The nurse uses the nursing process to care for a patient during the fourth stage of labor. To interpret assessment data properly and make decisions about care, the nurse must understand the physiology of the recovery period, including changes in the cardiovascular, respiratory, urinary, reproductive, gastrointestinal, and musculoskeletal systems.

Assessment

Maternal status can change rapidly during the fourth stage of labor, and such life-threatening complications as postpartal hemorrhage can occur. Therefore, frequent assessments are necessary. Begin the assessment by reviewing subjective and objective data obtained during the previous stages of labor. Continue the assessment by collecting current data.

If the neonate stays with the mother during this period, continue to maintain the neonate's warmth and monitor cardiovascular and respiratory status.

Health history

First, review all data obtained on admission and throughout labor and delivery. The following elements of the patient's history help interpret fourth-stage assessment findings.

Vital signs. Postpartal deviations from the patient's baseline blood pressure, pulse, respirations, or temperature can indicate hemorrhage, pregnancy-induced hypertension (PIH), dehydration, or infection.

Obstetric history. The patient's gravidity and parity help predict her uterine contractility and response to oxytocic medication. The patient's obstetric history can predict her probable postpartal recovery. For example, a patient who experienced postpartal hemorrhage after a previous childbirth has greater risk for hemorrhage after this one.

Labor duration and progress. Prolonged labor can lead to uterine atony, particularly if accompanied by many hours of oxytocic stimulation. It also may cause dehydration and exhaustion. Precipitous labor and delivery can cause uterine atony, predispose the patient to hemorrhage, and produce lacerations or cervical tears that may increase blood loss.

Physical assessment

Begin patient assessment after the neonate is stabilized and during or immediately after perineal repair. Assess the patient's vital signs and level of consciousness.

After any perineal repair is complete and the patient has been helped into a more comfortable position, assess postpartal parameters and evaluate her discomfort, recovery from analgesia and anesthesia, and fatigue, hunger, and thirst. Also observe the family's response to the neonate's birth.

Postpartal parameters. During this assessment, evaluate vital signs, fundus, lochia, perineum, leg pain, and edema as well as the presence of any tremors (for more information, see *Parameters of postpartal assessment*). Assess these parameters at least every 15 minutes during the fourth stage. In situations that deviate from the norm, such as a sudden drop in blood pressure or a large increase in bright red lochia, alert the physician or nurse-midwife.

Discomfort. With each assessment during the fourth stage, determine the patient's discomfort. Determine the character, intensity, and source of discomfort, such as uterine contractions, ("after pains"), laceration repair, or perineal hematoma. Sources of discomfort during the fourth stage of labor directly relate to the length and intensity of labor, the conduct of the delivery, the presence of perineal trauma, and uterine muscle contractility (which affects hemorrhage control). A report of discomfort coupled with physical assessment findings may indicate a problem, such as hematoma formation.

Parameters of postpartal assessment

For each postpartal assessment parameter, this chart describes assessment techniques, normal and abnormal findings, and related nursing interventions. During the fourth stage of labor, the nurse must assess these parameters at least every 15 minutes.

PARAMETER ASSESSMENT TECHNIQUE	FINDINGS	NURSING INTERVENTIONS
Vital signs Palpation of the pulse for a full minute, observation of respiratory rate and rhythm, and blood pressure auscultation; temperature usually taken 1 hour after birth	*Normal findings* • Pulse within 4 to 17 beats/minute of predelivery rate • Respiratory rate within 2 to 4 breaths of predelivery rate • Systolic and diastolic blood pressure within 10 mm Hg of predelivery pressure	*For a patient with normal findings* • Repeat assessments every 15 minutes until stable; then repeat according to facility policy or as prescribed. • Assess for orthostatic changes in blood pressure and increase in pulse if the patient reports light-headedness when rising or walking.
	Abnormal findings • Rapid pulse rate, characteristic of hemorrhage • Pulse rate more than 17 beats/minute slower than predelivery rate, which may indicate heart block or other postpartal cardiac anomaly • Depressed respiratory rate, which can result from medications or anesthesia • Tachypnea, which indicates oxygen need from hemorrhage or shock • Hypotension (less than 10 mm Hg between systolic and diastolic measurements), which may suggest extensive blood loss and impending shock • Hypertension (15 mm Hg increase in diastolic, 30 mm Hg systolic), which may occur with pregnancy-induced hypertension (PIH) • Elevated temperature, which may be caused by dehydration, fatigue, or infection	*For a patient with abnormal findings* • Notify the physician or nurse-midwife. • Repeat vital sign assessments at least every 5 minutes along with other assessments. • Maintain fluid balance, as needed. • Be prepared to administer oxygen and medications, as prescribed. • If hypertension is present, check the patient's reflexes. A patient with pregnancy-induced hypertension (PIH) who develops symptoms will show brisk reflexes with ankle clonus.
Fundus Palpation	*Normal findings* • Fundal height between the umbilicus and 1 to 2 cm below the umbilicus • Fundus at midline, firm, and about the size of an average cantaloupe	*For a patient with normal findings* • Repeat fundal palpation every 15 minutes with other assessments. • Teach the patient the significance of a well-contracted uterus. Teach her to palpate her fundus and practice fundal massage. *(continued)*

Parameters of postpartal assessment *(continued)*

PARAMETER ASSESSMENT TECHNIQUE	FINDINGS	NURSING INTERVENTIONS
Fundus *(continued)*	*Abnormal findings* • Boggy (soft, poorly contracted) uterus, deviated from midline and above the umbilicus, which suggests atony, clot retention, or a full bladder	*For a patient with abnormal findings* • Massage the fundus until it becomes firm and clots are expressed. • Reassess the fundus at least every 5 minutes. • Encourage the patient to void. • Encourage the patient who has chosen to breast-feed to begin because nipple stimulation causes the pituitary gland to release oxytocin. • Notify the physician or nurse-midwife, who may need to evaluate patient further. • Administer oxytocic medications, as prescribed.
Lochia Inspection of lochia flow and observation for clots at the perineum while assessing the fundus. Check to ensure that blood is not pooling under the patient	*Normal findings* • Serous fluid with no clots • Scant (1″ stain on perineal pad), light (1″ to 4″ stain), or moderate (4″ to 6″ stain) flow within 15 minutes	*For a patient with normal findings* • Repeat the assessment in 15 minutes.
	Abnormal findings • Heavy flow (saturation of one or more perineal pads) in 15 minutes or less, which indicates excessive bleeding and possible uterine atony • A steady trickle of bleeding in a patient with a well-contracted uterus, which may indicate cervical, vaginal, or perineal laceration	*For a patient with abnormal findings* • Evaluate for uterine atony. • Massage the fundus. • Notify the physician or nurse-midwife, who may need to evaluate the patient's condition further.
Perineum Inspection. Remove the perineal pad, position the legs so that the perineum can be observed, and use an adequate light source. Alternatively, position the patient in the left or right lateral position with the upper leg flexed. Raise the upper buttock slightly to observe the perineum. Ask the patient to contract and relax the perineal muscles to assess muscle function. Place a clean pad on the perineum and help the patient into a comfortable position.	*Normal findings* • Intact perineum, possibly with slight edema (depending on the duration of the second stage of labor) • Incision with approximated edges (straight edges meeting without separations), minimal swelling, no discoloration or bleeding from the incision, and possible burning sensation in the incision area when voiding (if episiotomy or laceration repair was performed)	*For a patient with normal findings* • Maintain cleanliness and comfort if the perineum is intact. • Assess the perineum every 15 minutes in a patient with an episiotomy. Place an ice pack on the perineum to increase comfort and decrease edema. Initiate perineal care after assessing the area.

Parameters of postpartal assessment (continued)

PARAMETER ASSESSMENT TECHNIQUE	FINDINGS	NURSING INTERVENTIONS
Perineum (continued)	*Abnormal findings* • Swelling and discoloration, which may indicate hematoma development • Bleeding, which may indicate unligated blood vessels • Dehiscence (separation of the suture line) • Increasing, throbbing perineal pain • Visible fluctuant mass at introitus	*For a patient with abnormal findings* • Report edema, discoloration, or dehiscence immediately, which may indicate hematoma formation. • If signs of hematoma exist, monitor for signs of impending shock, such as restlessness, increased respirations, increased pulse, and decreased blood pressure.
Leg pain and tremors Dorsiflexion of the foot. Support the patient's thigh with one hand and her foot with the other. Then bend her leg slightly at the knee, and firmly and abruptly dorsiflex the foot.	*Normal findings* • No discomfort in the calf or popliteal space • No ankle clonus	*For a patient with normal findings* • Encourage patient activity. • Repeat this assessment every 15 minutes.
	Abnormal findings • Pain in the calf or popliteal space, which may result from a thrombus • Ankle clonus, which may result from PIH	*For a patient with abnormal findings* • Report findings. • Obtain elastic stockings and advise the patient to wear them as prescribed. • Instruct the patient not to massage her legs. • Monitor for signs of embolism, such as shortness of breath, rapid drop in blood pressure, elevated heart rate, ashen coloring, and sweating.

Dull aching or burning constitute normal episiotomy pain. Pain that throbs, increases, or does not respond to comfort measures may indicate an abnormality, such as perineal, vulvar, or vaginal hematoma.

A hematoma can form when blood seeps into the tissue because open blood vessels are not closed adequately during episiotomy repair. Characteristically, it swells gradually and reddens or becomes purple. Symptoms may include increasing and throbbing perineal pain, tachycardia, restlessness, and, in severe cases, hypotension.

During the fourth stage, the patient may experience other discomforts related to second-stage occurrences, such as the exertion and method of pushing, use of regional anesthesia, or positioning during delivery.

Recovery from anesthesia and analgesia. If the patient received an anesthetic or other medications during labor and delivery, evaluate her recovery with each assessment during the fourth stage. (For more information, see *Selected major drugs in the fourth stage of labor,* page 186.) As the effects of the drugs begin to dissipate, evaluate the patient's con-

Selected major drugs in the fourth stage of labor

This chart summarizes the drugs commonly used during the fourth stage of labor.

DRUG	MAJOR INDICATIONS	USUAL ADULT DOSAGES	NURSING IMPLICATIONS
oxytocin (Pitocin)	Ineffective uterine contractions after delivery of the placenta; heavy amount of lochia	1 to 4 ml (10 to 40 units) in 1,000 ml D$_5$W or normal saline solution I.V., infused at a rate to control bleeding, usually 20 to 40 mU/minute; many clinicians follow with ergonovine maleate or methylergonovine maleate I.M.	• Administer drug I.M. or by I.V. infusion, never by bolus injection. If possible, use an infusion pump or a drip regulator to ensure accurate delivery. • Monitor the patient's heart rate, central nervous system (CNS) status, blood pressure, uterine contractions, and blood loss every 15 minutes. • Watch for signs of hypersensitivity, such as blood pressure elevation. In a patient who had a long labor accompanied by infusion of oxytocin and large volumes of parenteral fluid, watch for signs of water intoxication, such as edema; oxytocin has an antidiuretic effect. • Use appropriate comfort measures to control pain caused by uterine contractions.
ergonovine maleate (Ergotrate) and methyl-ergonovine maleate (Methergine)	Prevent or control postpartal hemorrhage	For both drugs, 0.2 mg I.M. every 2 to 4 hours to a maximum of five doses.	• Be aware that these drugs may be given if oxytocin does not control postpartal bleeding. • Assess the patient's vital signs (especially blood pressure) before administration. • Do not administer this drug before delivery of the neonate because it can cause tetanic contractions. • Do not administer this drug if the patient is hypertensive. • Watch for adverse reactions, which may include severe hypertension and signs of cerebral hemorrhage (such as loss of consciousness), myocardial infarction (such as chest pain), and retinal detachment (such as blurred vision). • Monitor the patient's blood pressure, pulse rate, uterine contractions, and vaginal bleeding. Report sudden changes in vital signs, frequent periods of uterine relaxation, and any change in lochia character or amount. • Use appropriate comfort measures to control pain caused by uterine contractions.
acetamino-phen (Tylenol)	Relief of mild to moderate pain caused by episiotomy or uterine contractions	325 to 650 mg by mouth every 3 to 4 hours as needed	• Assess the patient's need for analgesia. Her discomfort may increase with oxytocin administration and development of vaginal or perineal hematoma. • Monitor the patient's response to the drug; hypersensitivity (very rare) may cause general malaise, rash, sweating, or anaphylaxis.

Selected major drugs in the fourth stage of labor *(continued)*

DRUG	MAJOR INDICATIONS	USUAL ADULT DOSAGES	NURSING IMPLICATIONS
meperidine hydrochloride (Demerol)	Relief of moderate to severe pain caused by uterine contractions	25 to 100 mg I.M., depending on the patient's weight and degree of pain	• Drug should be used only for short-term management of pain. • Assess the patient's need for analgesia. Evaluate the drug's appropriateness in relation to the patient's vital signs, history of drug sensitivity, and degree of discomfort. • Obtain the patient's baseline blood pressure and pulse and respiratory rates before administering this drug. Assess vital signs regularly to determine the patient's response to the drug. • Observe for adverse reactions, such as dry mouth, dizziness, and respiratory depression. • Keep naloxone hydrochloride (Narcan) readily available to reverse respiratory depression.
promethazine hydrochloride (Phenergan)	Adjunct to narcotic administration to sedate patient and control nausea related to narcotic administration	12.5 to 25 mg by mouth, I.M., or rectally every 4 to 6 hours	• Use with caution in a patient with hypersensitivity to this drug or with CNS depression. • Assess the patient's need for analgesia and nausea control. Evaluate the drug's appropriateness in relation to the patient's vital signs, history of drug sensitivity, and degree of discomfort. • Monitor the patient's vital signs and CNS status regularly. • Observe for adverse effects, such as transient hypotension, drowsiness, tinnitus, nervousness, hysteria, blurred vision, and seizures. • Advise the patient to rise slowly, and assist with ambulation.

dition and response to pain. Assess the character, intensity, and location of pain, and monitor response to measures such as repositioning and applying ice. These assessments will help distinguish between normal discomfort and pain that signals a problem.

If the patient had continuous regional anesthesia, assess the return of motor function to her legs. During each postpartal assessment, note the color and temperature of her legs and toes and her abiity to move them.

Fatigue, hunger, and thirst. Depending on the duration of labor and the second stage, the patient may experience extreme fatigue or exhaustion immediately after delivery. Shaking or tremors may indicate muscle exhaustion or PIH. To differentiate normal postpartal tremors from those caused by PIH, evaluate the patient's blood pressure, assess for ankle clonus by dorsiflexing the foot, and assess deep tendon reflexes.

After the neonate is born, the patient may feel extremely hungry and thirsty, especially if she was restricted to ice chips or clear fluids during labor and if her labor was long. Keep in mind that labor and delivery consume a great amount of energy and may have been preceded by a period of restricted food and fluid intake.

Response to birth. Assess the parents' response to the neonate's birth at least once during the fourth stage of labor. Sensitive postpartal assessment of family interaction can provide valuable information that predicts future family interactions.

Nursing diagnoses

Carefully review assessment findings and use them to develop appropriate nursing diagnoses. (For a partial list of applicable diagnoses, see Nursing Diagnoses: *Third and fourth stages of labor,* page 180.)

Planning and implementation

Although the fourth stage of labor is brief and focuses on assessment, planning is necessary and may occur during assessment. During this stage, interventions may include maintaining appropriate maternal positioning and activity, preventing hemorrhage, maintaining hygiene and comfort, maintaining fluid balance, meeting nutritional needs, and promoting bonding. (See *Planning and implementing nursing care during the fourth stage of labor.*)

Evaluation

At the end of the fourth stage of labor, evaluate the effectiveness of nursing care while making a final assessment of the patient's stability. The following examples illustrate some appropriate evaluation statements:

• The patient's fundus is firm and located 1 cm below the umbilicus.
• The patient's perineum is intact.
• The father and other family members held the neonate.
• The patient began breast-feeding her neonate.

Documentation

As part of the nursing plan of care, document all nursing care provided as well as the patient's response to the care. In addition to a verbal report, a written record will help the postpartal nurse meet the patient's individual needs.

Although each health care facility may require documentation of slightly different information, most require the nurse to record the following information:

• the patient's vital signs
• location and consistency of the uterus
• amount and quality of lochia
• condition of perineum
• the parents' response to the neonate's birth
• patient discomfort

Planning and implementing nursing care during the fourth stage of labor

Maintain positioning and activity
- Encourage supine positioning for fundal and perineal assessments.
- Suggest semi-Fowler's, high Fowler's, or lateral positioning to promote comfort and provide better position to view or breast-feed neonate.
- Assist with ambulation when out of bed for the first time after delivery. Be alert to orthostatic hypertension. Encourage slow, purposeful movement.
- Promote bed rest for those with a long or difficult labor and delivery, regional anesthesia, heavy analgesia during or after delivery, or a postpartum hemorrhage. Take special care with these patients when up for the first time.

Prevent hemorrhage
- Massage uterus gently during each nursing assessment and encourage the patient to do so at regular intervals.
- Administer oxytocin, as prescribed.
- Encourage breast-feeding.
- Encourage voiding to prevent bladder distention, which causes uterine atony.
- Promote adequate hydration through fluid intake.

Maintain hygiene and comfort
- Remove collected secretion, such as lochia and perspiration, with modified bed bath.
- Teach the patient self-care activities such as perineal care—wiping front to back after eliminating, perineal rinsing—as well as frequent showers for increased perspiration in early postpartum period.
- Provide clean, warm clothing and a blanket.
- Change perineal pads and underpads after each assessment or more frequently, if appropriate.

Prevent discomfort from uterine contractions
- Administer analgesic agents, as prescribed.
- Reduce the rate of continuous oxytocin infusion, as prescribed.
- Teach abdominal effleurage (light, fingertip massage over the abdomen) to ease the pain of contractions.

- Place a pillow over the patient's lower abdomen and help her assume a prone position, if her condition allows. The uterus should contract strongly several times and the pain should subside for a while. When the pain subsides, help the patient assume a comfortable position.
- Offer a modified bed bath to remove perspiration and relax sore muscles.
- Offer a back and neck massage to relieve tension and stiffness caused by labor, pushing, or positioning.

Relieve perineal pain
- Apply an ice pack to the area.
- Apply witch hazel compresses to the area.
- Encourage the patient to contract and relax the perineal muscles (Kegel exercises).
- Administer analgesic agents, as prescribed.

Alleviate discomfort from initial chills
- Wrap warm blankets around the patient's feet or head.
- Provide warm oral fluids if the patient's condition warrants.
- Adjust the room temperature.

Maintain fluid balance and nutritional needs
- Monitor temperature, pulse rate, and blood pressure and compare them to baseline measurements to estimate the extent of the deficit.
- Provide oral fluids.
- Regulate I.V. fluids as directed by the physician or nurse-midwife.
- Provide nourishment according to the patient's preference, if not contraindicated by complications. Assess the appropriateness of her food choices and recommend easily digestible alternatives, if necessary.

Promote bonding
- Encourage immediate, continuous mother-infant contact.
- Offer anticipatory guidance regarding the neonate's needs and abilities.
- Help establish an emotionally warm and sensitive environment.

• reports of fatigue, hunger, or thirst
• urinary status (whether the patient has voided)
• drugs, fluids, and food given to the patient.

STUDY ACTIVITIES

Short answer

1. Karen Christopher, a 32-year-old gravida 8 para 6107, has just delivered her seventh child by normal spontaneous vaginal delivery after a precipitous labor. Ms. Christopher and her husband had been worried during this pregnancy after hydramnios was detected while she was being followed for gestational diabetes. Their vigorous new son weighs in at 9 lb, 7 oz, during the initial neonatal assessment in the delivery room. Once the placenta is delivered, the physician begins to suture a perineal laceration. During a nursing assessment at this time, the nurse notes a boggy uterus on palpation. Efforts to control the ensuing postpartum hemorrhage are initiated immediately. What are the factors in Ms. Christopher's history that predispose her to a postpartum hemorrhage?

_____

2. After an uneventful labor, Xiaoming Han has given birth to her first child, a healthy daughter. Her husband has been present throughout and very supportive of his wife. How can the nurse promote bonding for this couple, who are in a birthing room?

_____

_____

3. During a nursing assessment on Ruth Richmond, a 27-year-old gravida 1 para 1001, the nurse notes that Ms. Richmond's lochia is slowly but consistently saturating a perineal pad every 10 minutes or so, despite a well-contracted uterus. What should the nurse suspect and what nursing intervention is indicated?

_____

4. Identify four sources of early postpartal discomfort that the nurse would evaluate during a postpartum assessment.

_____

5. Describe nursing measures to relieve discomfort caused by uterine contractions.

_____

6. What are the common causes of an elevated maternal temperature during the fourth stage?

_____

Multiple choice

7. During Francie Pitts's recovery from her uneventful vaginal birth 1 hour ago, she begins to complain of increasing, throbbing perineal pain. The nurse notes that Ms. Pitts is increasingly restless and has tachycardia. On perineal evaluation, the nurse observes a large, purple, swollen area at the vaginal introitus. What is most likely occurring?

    A. An engorged hemorrhoid
    B. A dehiscence of the episiotomy
    C. A vaginal hematoma
    D. A uterine prolapse

8. When estimating a normal blood loss after a spontaneous vaginal delivery, the nurse would expect:

    A. More than 500 ml
    B. Less than 500 ml
    C. More than 750 ml
    D. Less than 250 ml

9. Nursing interventions to prevent a postpartum hemorrhage in the fourth stage would include all but which of the following:

    A. Encouraging voiding to prevent bladder distention
    B. Repositioning the patient on her left side
    C. Performing fundal massage at regular intervals
    D. Administering oxytocin, as ordered

True or false

10. The normal umbilical cord contains two arteries and one vein.
    ☐ True   ☐ False

11. The neonate's largest surface area, hence the area of greatest potential heat loss, is the body.
    ☐ True   ☐ False

12. A contraindication to the use of ergonovine maleate (Ergotrate) or methylergonovine (Methergine) is hypotension.
    ☐ True   ☐ False

13. A boggy uterus can suggest atony, clot retention, or a full bladder.
    ☐ True   ☐ False

ANSWERS   ### Short answer

1. The factors commonly associated with uterine atony and the risk of postpartum hemorrhage that are in Ms. Christopher's history include grand multiparity, prenatal history of hydramnios, a precipitous labor, and the delivery of a macrosomic neonate.

2. The nurse can begin by introducing the neonate to the parents as soon as possible. The mother and neonate should be kept together while any further assessments or procedures are being done during the third and fourth stage. The parents should be encouraged to touch and talk to their daughter immediately. The nurse can point out that the neonate will gaze in their direction and may open her eyes fully if they are shaded from the light. The father can be encouraged to hold her while the mother is being settled after the delivery of the placenta and perineal repair. If the neonate needs to be transferred to the nursery, the nurse should encourage the father to go with his daughter to maintain contact and continue bonding.

3. A heavy lochial flow saturating a perineal pad in 15 minutes or less indicates excessive bleeding. In a patient with a well-contracted uterus, such as Ms. Richmond, the nurse should suspect a cervical, vaginal, or perineal laceration. The nurse would intervene by notifying the physician or nurse-midwife, who would need to evaluate the patient's condition further.

4. Sources of discomfort during the fourth stage of labor directly relate to the length and intensity of labor, the conduct of the delivery, the presence of perineal trauma, and uterine muscle contractility.

5. To relieve discomfort caused by uterine contractions, the nurse might administer analgesic agents, as prescribed; reduce the rate of continuous oxytocin infusion, as prescribed; teach abdominal effleurage; position the patient in a prone position with a pillow supporting her lower abdomen; offer a modified bed bath; and offer a back and neck massage.

6. Common causes of an elevated maternal temperature during the early postpartum period are dehydration, fatigue, and infection.

Multiple choice

7. C. The nurse should suspect a possible perineal or vaginal hematoma.

8. B. The normal blood loss expected with a spontaneous vaginal delivery is less than 500 ml.

9. B. Positioning the patient on her left side would hinder a complete nursing assessment of the uterus to prevent uterine atony.

True or false

10. True.

11. False. The neonate's largest surface area and area of greatest potential heat loss is the head.

12. False. Ergonovine maleate (Ergotrate) and methylergonovine (Methergine) should not be administered if the patient is hypertensive.

13. True.

CHAPTER 13

Intrapartal complications and related obstetrical interventions

OBJECTIVES   After studying this chapter, the reader should be able to:

1. Identify factors or conditions that place a patient, fetus, or neonate at risk for complications during labor and delivery.

2. Assess for signs and symptoms that indicate the potential for or presence of an intrapartal complication.

3. Recognize the emotional and psychological needs of a patient and her family during an intrapartal complication.

4. Discuss specific nursing interventions for a patient experiencing selected intrapartal complications as well as for her fetus or neonate, based on her condition.

5. Identify emergencies that may arise when caring for a patient with an intrapartal complication and describe appropriate nursing interventions.

OVERVIEW OF CONCEPTS   Certain physiologic problems that affect the reproductive system during childbirth place any intrapartal patient at risk and require obstetrical interventions to achieve optimal outcomes for the mother and the neonate. These include reproductive system disorders related to uterine, membrane and amniotic fluid, umbilical cord, placental, and pelvic factors; systemic disorders of the pregnant patient; and fetal complications.

In addition, some medical or obstetrical conditions identified either prior to or during the intrapartal period also require specialized care to achieve the health and well-being of both patient and neonate. These encompass medical disorders, such as cardiac disease, diabetes mellitus, infection, and substance abuse; and pregnancy-related conditions, such as pregnancy-induced hypertension (PIH) and Rh isoimmunization.

A pregnancy with complications has a much higher chance of perinatal complications. Many conditions create an unfavorable intrauterine environment that does not support normal fetal growth or oxygenation. This fetus is especially sensitive to hypoxia, stress, and trauma.

Signs of fetal distress, such as fetal heart rate (FHR) abnormalities and meconium-stained amniotic fluid, may develop more quickly during labor.

For a neonate of a patient with complications, perinatal concerns involve the significant increase in the morbidity and mortality associated with prematurity, postmaturity, or low birth weight. These conditions predispose the neonate to birth trauma, perinatal asphyxia, meconium aspiration, hypoglycemia, heat loss, polycythemia, and death.

Although the goal of care is a safe, satisfying delivery that produces a normal, healthy neonate, this goal may not be achieved. If a neonate is born seriously ill, disabled, or without hope for survival, the parents' worst fears are confirmed. If perinatal death or disability occurs, the family will need assistance with coping and grieving. The nurse plays a vital role in detecting intrapartal complications, assisting in their resolution, and providing the patient with appropriate care.

Nursing responsibilities

For the high-risk patient and her family, the nurse must provide basic intrapartal care. (See Chapters 9, 10, 11, and 12, on the four stages of labor.) In addition, an experienced nurse who understands the complexities of labor and delivery for a patient at risk for or experiencing an intrapartal complication provides specialized care at a critical-care level of specialized practice. These responsibilities should not be undertaken by the beginning nurse.

To manage the nursing care of the high-risk intrapartal patient, the nurse must perform specialized maternal and fetal monitoring (which demands advanced knowledge and skills), be familiar with the technology used to improve perinatal outcomes, and be ready to provide nursing care as an important part of a specialized perinatal team.

Assessment

As with any patient who seeks admission for labor and delivery, the nurse obtains the intrapartal patient's health history, conducts an abbreviated physical assessment, and assists in collecting specimens for appropriate laboratory tests.

With an intrapartal patient with or at risk for complications, however, the nurse must make additional assessments, be aware of maternal and fetal risks, be prepared to notify the physician of significant findings, and plan care accordingly. (For more information, see *Selected intrapartal conditions and risks.*)

Health history

When taking a history, keep in mind that a patient may perceive a common, normal variation as a problem. Depending on the intrapartal patient's condition, adjust the approach to the health history, augmenting the basic interview with appropriate questions. These questions depend on the patient's age, disorder, and labor status.

Selected intrapartal conditions and risks

During the intrapartal period, the nurse should be alert to certain conditions that may pose risks for the patient and her fetus or neonate, as shown in the chart below.

MATERNAL RISKS	FETAL OR NEONATAL RISKS	NURSING CONSIDERATIONS
Cardiac disease		
• Cardiac decompensation • Pulmonary edema • Congestive heart failure • Maternal death • Preterm labor, if certain cardiac drugs were used	• Increased risk of congenital heart defects • IUGR • Fetal hypoxia or asphyxia	• Management in labor requires coordination of obstetrician, cardiologist, anesthesiologist, and critical-care obstetrical nurse. • Carefully monitor vital signs frequently. • Maintain strict fluid intake and output records. • Provide continuous, internal EFM and continuous maternal electrocardiogram hemodynamic monitoring with an arterial line, central venous pressure, or indwelling pulmonary artery catheter. • Keep resuscitation equipment near the patient at all times. • Promote proper positioning; avoid supine position and encourage lateral recumbent position; avoid lithotomy position for delivery. • Provide adequate analgesia or anesthesia; prepare for epidural anesthesia and possibility of forceps or vacuum extraction delivery. • Alert the neonatal team to be present when birth is imminent. • Plan to assess continuously for at least 24 hours postpartum.
Diabetes mellitus		
• Hypoglycemia • Hydramnios • Hyperglycemia • Diabetic ketoacidosis • Preterm labor • Excessive postpartal bleeding from uterine atony or birth trauma	• Hydramnios • Congenital malformations • Fetal distress • Fetal death, especially in a patient with diabetic ketoacidosis • Macrosomia, which can lead to birth trauma • Neonatal hyperinsulinism leading to hypoglycemia • Respiratory distress syndrome • Polycythemia • Hyperbilirubinemia • Hypocalcemia	• On admission, determine the patient's last meal and insulin dose; screen for insulin deficiency leading to ketoacidosis. • Assess for signs and symptoms of maternal hypoglycemia or hyperglycemia. • Prepare for elective induction or cesarean delivery, as ordered. • Provide continuous EFM to screen for fetal distress. • Monitor maternal blood glucose levels; provide proper I.V. insulin and glucose infusions, as ordered; follow closely in postpartum period for adjustments in dosages. • Screen closely for evidence of diabetic ketoacidosis—hyperglycemia and ketonuria, signs of dehydration, hypotension, deep and rapid respirations, decreased level of consciousness, fruity or acetone-like breath, nausea and vomiting. • Assess vital signs, fluid intake and output, and evidence of PIH. • If hydramnios is present, be alert to ruptured membranes and increased chance of umbilical cord prolapse. • At birth, monitor neonate closely for hypoglycemia; if macrosomic, for evidence of birth trauma.

(continued)

Selected intrapartal conditions and risks *(continued)*

MATERNAL RISKS	FETAL OR NEONATAL RISKS	NURSING CONSIDERATIONS
Infection		
• PROM • Premature labor • Fever	• Premature neonate • Neonatal infection or sepsis • Respiratory distress syndrome • Fetal death	• Assess history or physical examination for evidence of infections. • Be vigilant about following infection control guidelines and observe universal precautions for all patients. • Administer I.V. fluids immediately to improve hydration, reduce fever, and prevent maternal exhaustion. • Utilize external EFM to avoid further contamination of the fetus. • Once an infection is identified, anticipate labor induction or oxytocin augmentation to shorten diagnosis-to-delivery time; cesarean delivery typically is avoided. • Limit vaginal exams; avoid amniotomy; provide meticulous perineal care. • When anticipating the delivery, summon neonatal team. • Coordinate family care and communication between postpartum and nursery staff. • Provide emotional support, especially if isolation precautions are indicated. • Expect to collect various laboratory specimens to determine the type and degree of infection.
Pregnancy-induced hypertension		
• Insufficient perfusion of vital organs, including fetal-placental unit • Seizures, hypertonic uterine activity, and abruptio placentae, if patient develops eclampsia • Preterm labor	• Premature neonate • Magnesium sulfate toxicity in neonate, if magnesium sulfate was administered to patient • IUGR	• Monitor vital signs closely, to determine evidence of impending eclampsia. • Cardiovascular monitoring with an indwelling pulmonary artery or central venous pressure catheter for a patient with severe PIH may be prescribed as well as strict fluid intake and output measures. • Assess the patient's level of consciousness, especially if receiving medications to treat PIH. • Anticipate continuous, internal EFM to detect signs of placental insufficiency and fetal distress as well as uterine contraction pattern for evidence of hypertonicity and increased risk of abruptio placenta. • Prepare to assist with emergencies; employ seizure precautions. • Assist with prevention or treatment of seizures with magnesium sulfate ($MgSO_4$) treatment. • Assess maternal and fetal response to treatment; monitor lab values for $MgSO_4$ and maternal respirations. • Provide calcium gluconate at bedside for $MgSO_4$ overdose. • Expect $MgSO_4$ therapy for at least 24 hours postpartum. • Anticipate vaginal delivery, be prepared for precipitous delivery, especially if oxytocin induction is employed. • Summon neonatal team for delivery, especially if neonate is preterm; be prepared for $MgSO_4$ toxicity in neonate, which produces respiratory depression, hypotonia, and hypotension.

Selected intrapartal conditions and risks *(continued)*

MATERNAL RISKS	FETAL OR NEONATAL RISKS	NURSING CONSIDERATIONS
Rh isoimmunization		
• Placental hypertrophy with uteroplacental insufficiency • Chorioamnionitis • Abruptio placentae • Hydramnios (may cause inefficient contractions) • Preterm labor and delivery	• Fetal hypoxia and distress • Anemia • Jaundice • Liver, spleen, and heart enlargement • Anasarca (severe, generalized edema) • Myocardial failure	• Assess for signs of chorioamnionitis (maternal or fetal tachycardia, fever, uterine or abdominal tenderness, and purulent secretions with rupture of membranes), which may occur due to contamination during intrauterine blood transfusions or amniocentesis. • Carefully observe for signs and symptoms of abruptio placentae, such as vaginal bleeding or uterine tetany. • Continuous internal EFM may be indicated, depending on fetal gestational age and delivery options. Typically, patient is preterm. • Anticipate fetal blood scalp sampling to estimate fetal tolerance for labor and to determine need for cesarean delivery. • Monitor uterine contraction pattern for hypotonic dysfunction, common in this patient. • Promote comfort and support; limited analgesia or anesthesia may be available because of fetal prematurity and instability. Be sensitive to anxieties regarding fetal status and prognosis. Provide reassurance and information, as available. • Alert neonatal team of maternal status during labor and coordinate their efforts at the time of delivery.
Substance abuse		
• Preterm labor • Precipitous birth • Abruptio placentae • Maternal infection • Psychosocial problems, such as isolation • Interactions between abused substance and drugs administered during delivery	• LBW or SGA neonate caused by IUGR • Premature neonate • Neonatal infection • Congenital malformations • Neonatal withdrawal symptoms	• Due to lack of prenatal care, thorough history, physical, and laboratory data may need to be collected during intrapartal admission. • Monitor vital signs for evidence of maternal or fetal tachycardia, depressed maternal respirations, or elevated blood pressure. • Carefully assess the patient's labor progress; be prepared for precipitous labor or delivery. • Anticipate external EFM; prepare for amniotomy to determine presence of meconium-stained fluid and evidence of fetal distress. • Promote comfort measures; observe for interactions between analgesics and illicit drugs. • Work with the neonatal team to anticipate potential problems. • Provide emotional support; express acceptance and patience. • Encourage maternal-neonatal bonding; explain any state laws or social service interventions affecting discharge.

Physical assessment

During the physical assessment, modify the standard examination to meet the high-risk intrapartal patient's needs, and note significant findings that are related to her condition.

Laboratory tests

Expect to collect all standard admission laboratory tests as well as those ordered for specific high-risk intrapartal conditions. (For details, see Chapter 10, The first stage of labor.) Consider the patient's condition when reviewing the results.

Nursing diagnoses

The nurse reviews all health history, physical assessment, and laboratory test findings and then formulates nursing diagnoses appropriate for the intrapartal patient. (For a partial list of applicable diagnoses, see Nursing Diagnoses: *Intrapartal complications.*)

Planning and implementation

Some nursing interventions for the patient at risk for or with an intrapartal complication are the same as those for any other intrapartal patient. For example, the nurse must assess the patient and fetus, assist in labor management, promote comfort, assist with delivery, provide emotional support, promote bonding, perform patient teaching, and care for the patient's family. However, the nurse also must be prepared to respond to intrapartal emergencies and may need to approach the usual tasks differently, modifying or augmenting normal intrapartal care.

Nursing care in this situation requires advanced knowledge and skills. The nurse must participate as an integral perinatal team member and work closely with the physician to achieve optimal outcomes.

The family of the intrapartal patient at risk is likely to be very concerned about the patient and her fetus or neonate. The nurse must provide sensitive nursing care adapted to the family's needs.

Evaluation

During the final step of the nursing process, the nurse evaluates the effectiveness of nursing care. State all evaluations in terms of actions performed or outcomes achieved for each goal. (See *Selected high-risk evaluation statements,* page 200, for examples.)

Documentation

Document assessment findings and nursing activities as thoroughly and objectively as possible. Thorough documentation not only allows evaluation of the effectiveness of the care but also makes data available to other members of the health care team, which helps to ensure consistent care. To document as accurately as possible, ensure that the entries describe events exactly, completely, and in chronological order.

Record physician management decisions and how nursing care was accomplished. Make sure to record all information required. Examples of appropriate documentation topics include:
- maternal vital signs
- FHR patterns
- continuous labor progress and outcome
- physical examination findings (edema, deep tendon reflexes, evidence of bleeding, infection)
- laboratory studies and their values
- medications given, time of administration, and effectiveness

NURSING DIAGNOSES

Intrapartal complications

The following nursing diagnoses address problems and etiologies the nurse may encounter when caring for the patient with intrapartal complications. Specific nursing interventions for many of these diagnoses are provided in the "Planning and implementation" section of this chapter.

Intrapartal complications and special procedures
- Altered role performance related to unmet expectations for childbirth
- Anxiety related to fear of death during childbirth
- Anxiety related to uncertain maternal or perinatal outcome
- Ineffective family coping: compromised, related to unexpected need for obstetric procedure
- Ineffective individual coping related to lack of family support
- Knowledge deficit about obstetric procedure or condition
- Pain related to required obstetric or special procedure

Age-related concerns
- Body image disturbance related to labor and delivery
- Decisional conflict related to offering the neonate for adoption
- Fear related to labor and delivery
- Knowledge deficit related to labor and delivery
- Self-esteem disturbance related to unexpected cesarean delivery

Cardiac disease
- Altered cardiopulmonary tissue perfusion related to stress of labor or an abnormal heart
- Pain related to labor and delivery

Diabetes mellitus
- Altered nutrition: less than body requirements, related to increased glucose needs
- Anxiety related to labor and delivery
- Fear related to possible congenital malformations from uncontrolled diabetes
- Powerlessness related to condition that threatens maternal and fetal health

Infection
- Anxiety related to unexpected fetal outcome
- Fatigue related to maternal dehydration and exhaustion
- Ineffective denial related to socially unacceptable infection
- Ineffective individual coping related to disruption of bonding
- Social isolation related to isolation precautions

Substance abuse
- Altered nutrition: less than body requirements, related to substance abuse
- Fear related to removal and loss of neonate by statute

- Ineffective individual coping related to lack of family support
- Knowledge deficit related to infant care
- Social isolation related to substance abuse

Pregnancy-induced hypertension (PIH)
- Altered cardiopulmonary tissue perfusion related to elevated blood pressure
- Altered renal tissue perfusion related to elevated blood pressure
- Anxiety related to perinatal outcome
- High risk for injury related to seizures
- Ineffective family coping: compromised, related to perinatal outcome
- Knowledge deficit related to PIH treatments

Rh isoimmunization
- Altered parenting related to the neonate's transfer to the neonatal intensive care unit
- Ineffective family coping: compromised, related to lack of opportunity for bonding

Reproductive system disorders
- Anxiety related to abnormally prolonged labor
- Fatigue related to prolonged labor
- High risk for fetal injury related to alteration in the fetal placental unit
- High risk for fetal injury related to premature delivery
- High risk for fetal injury secondary to fetal hypoxia and traumatic delivery
- Ineffective individual coping related to exhaustion and anxiety
- Pain related to strong uterine contractions

Systemic disorders
- Anxiety related to uncertain perinatal outcome
- Decreased cardiac output related to hemorrhage
- High risk for injuary related to alteration in maternal hemodynamic status caused by hemorrhage

Fetal complications
- Anticipatory grieving related to death of the fetus
- Ineffective family coping: compromised, related to grieving
- Ineffective individual coping related to grieving
- Powerlessness related to having to carry a dead fetus to full gestation

Selected high-risk evaluation statements

The following examples illustrate appropriate evaluation statements for a variety of intrapartal complications.

Unexpected intrapartal complications
- The patient expressed decreased anxiety when discussing the usual outcomes of cesarean delivery or forceps delivery.
- The patient and support person expressed acceptance and understanding of the need for the procedure.
- The patient and her fetus completed labor and delivery safely with few or no additional complications.

Reproductive system disorders
- After initial oxytocin infusion, the patient gave birth vaginally.
- The patient exhibited no signs of infection after amniotomy.
- The patient and her fetus completed labor and delivery safely with little or no additional complications.

Cardiac disease
- The patient assumed labor positions that supported cardiac function.
- The patient delivered successfully without further maternal or neonatal complications.

Diabetes
- The patient's blood glucose levels remained within acceptable limits.
- The patient displayed no signs of hypoglycemia or hyperglycemia.

- The patient delivered a stable neonate.

Infection
- The patient verbalized an understanding of the need for infection control techniques.
- The patient's family expressed support and concern for the patient.

Pregnancy-induced hypertension
- The patient's blood pressure was stabilized.
- The patient's fluid intake and output were balanced.
- The patient did not develop seizures.

Rh isoimmunization
- The patient expressed an accurate understanding of her condition and that of her fetus.
- The patient delivered a stable neonate.

Substance abuse
- The patient received sufficient analgesia to relieve labor pain.
- The patient demonstrated appropriate signs of bonding after birth by holding and gazing at the neonate.

- patient's physiologic response to necessary treatments
- fluid intake and output
- coping responses
- interactions among patient and family
- interactions with physician.

Unexpected intrapartal complications

Complications that arise during labor may raise the patient's fears as well as threaten the health and well-being of both the mother and her fetus. The nurse plays a vital role in detecting intrapartal complications, assisting in their resolution, and providing the patient with appropriate clinical and emotional care.

Occasionally the patient requires obstetrical interventions to ensure a healthy intrapartal outcome. These interventions may be aimed, for example, at initiating or enhancing uterine contractions, assisting the fetus in moving through the birth canal, or delivering the neonate surgically. In order to provide optimal care, the nurse must be familiar with these special procedures and be able to explain them to the patient and her family as well as assisting, as needed.

Reproductive system disorders related to uterine factors

Many uterine factors can affect the progress of labor. Uterine contractions, the primary power of labor, play a critical role in determining whether labor is normal or dysfunctional. (For more information, see *Dysfunctional labor,* page 202.) Other, more commonly encountered intrapartal complications related to the uterus include precipitate labor, uterine rupture, and uterine inversion.

Dysfunction

Uterine dysfunction may be classified as hypotonic or hypertonic. In hypotonic dysfunction, the more common of the two, contractions grow less frequent and less powerful as labor continues. Eventually, they become too weak to produce adequate cervical dilation. Hypotonic dysfunction typically occurs during the active phase of labor.

Such a patient may receive an amniotomy followed by oxytocin to augment her contractions. Although labor augmentation differs from labor induction with oxytocin, take similar precautions and care for the patient as if labor were being induced.

Hypertonic dysfunction, which typically occurs during the latent phase of labor, is characterized by intense, painful contractions unaccompanied by normal cervical dilation. Continuous, careful monitoring of labor progress and fetal status is essential because fetal hypoxia may occur. The nurse must bc aware of any signs of fetal distress and be prepared to intervene appropriately.

The patient may be given narcotic analgesia to produce sleep for several hours. Upon awakening, she may have a normal, progressive labor pattern. This intervention is used only if the membranes are intact and no evidence of fetal distress is detected because this treatment delays delivery.

Precipitate labor

Characterized by rapid progression, precipitate labor typically lasts 3 hours or less. It may result from decreased resistance of soft tissue in the birth canal or from abnormally strong uterine contractions. Although research suggests that precipitate labor poses no greater risk to the patient and fetus than does normal labor, some experts believe that precipitate labor increases the risk of maternal lacerations and fetal intracranial hemorrhage and asphyxia. Additional risks include unattended delivery, fetal hypoxia from intense uterine contractions, and decreased uterine tone after delivery.

A patient with a history of precipitous labor will need careful and constant monitoring of fetal and maternal status. Prolonged periods of uterine contractions with decreased periods of uterine relaxation may lead to periods of fetal hypoxia.

Dysfunctional labor

When a fetus fails to move out of the uterus and through the birth canal, or when this progression takes an abnormally long time, the patient is in dysfunctional labor. (Other terms used to describe dysfunctional labor include dystocia, prolonged labor, and failure to progress.) Experts estimate that dysfunctional labor has a 1% to 7% incidence. Depending on the circumstances involved, it may threaten the health or life of the patient and fetus.

Dysfunctional labor has several causes. Altered uterine muscle contractility can prevent cervical dilation and effacement, thus blocking fetal descent. Altered muscle contractility may result from abnormalities of the uterus or bony pelvis or fetal position and presentation. Administration of narcotic or anesthetic agents, primiparity, and maternal exhaustion are other causes. In many cases, the cause cannot be identified with certainty.

Progression of labor can be depicted by plotting cervical dilation in centimeters against elapsed time. In normal labor, the resulting graph will form an S-shaped curve. In dysfunctional labor, the dilation curve will become flattened or strung out.

Effects of prolonged labor on the fetus may include hypoxia, asphyxia, and physical injuries during descent. In many cases, dysfunctional labor is an indication for cesarean delivery.

Uterine rupture

A serious medical emergency, rupture of the uterus may occur before or during labor. A complete rupture tears all layers of the uterus, establishing direct communication between the uterine and abdominal cavities. In an incomplete rupture, the myometrium tears, but the peritoneal covering of the uterus remains intact.

Uterine rupture occurs more frequently after previous cesarean delivery and during prolonged labor, difficult forceps delivery, and oxytocin administration. Although signs and symptoms of uterine rupture vary widely with location and severity, they typically include abdominal pain, vaginal bleeding, hypovolemic shock, and fetal distress. If rupture occurs during labor, contractions may cease.

If a patient experiences uterine rupture, surgical intervention must take place immediately to save the fetus's life and, at times, the patient's life. After cesarean delivery, the surgeon will repair the ruptured uterus if it can sustain a future pregnancy or remove it if it cannot.

Uterine inversion

In this rare, potentially life-threatening emergency, the uterus turns inside out so that its internal surface protrudes into or beyond the vagina. Uterine inversion may occur during or after delivery of the placenta. Although the cause may not be apparent, excessive traction on the umbilical cord and attempts to deliver the placenta while the uterus is relaxed may be contributing factors. The patient may experience significant blood loss and shock. The clearest sign of uterine inversion is the craterlike depression that forms in the abdomen during the third or fourth stage of labor.

If uterine inversion occurs, immediate interventions must be taken to save the patient's life, including blood transfusions and surgical reinversion of the uterus. This emergency situation requires the nurse's assistance.

Induction of labor

Uterine contractions may be induced through hormone infusion or through amniotomy. Induction may be necessitated by an emergency when medical or obstetric problems threaten the health of the patient or fetus. The physician also can use labor induction methods to strengthen natural contractions. Occasionally, labor may be induced by choice if the patient has a term pregnancy and is free of complications.

The two most common induction methods are amniotomy and intravenous synthetic oxytocin (Pitocin or Syntocinon) infusion. A more recent development is a procedure that involves the intra-vaginal or intracervical administration of prostaglandin (PGE_2) gel.

Amniotomy. To accomplish an amniotomy, a physician or nurse-midwife artificially ruptures the amniotic membranes to augment or induce labor. Some call the procedure artificial rupture of the membranes, or AROM.

The physician or nurse-midwife performs the procedure under sterile conditions with the patient in the lithotomy position. During and immediately after the procedure, the obstetric team monitors the fetus to ensure that the umbilical cord has not prolapsed.

Amniotomy improves the efficiency of uterine contractions by releasing prostaglandins, which naturally stimulate labor progress. If amniotomy fails to induce labor, the physician may initiate oxytocin infusion. If this fails, cesarean delivery may be required.

Intravenous oxytocin. During natural labor, the posterior lobe of the pituitary gland releases the hormone oxytocin. This hormone stimulates strong, rhythmic contractions of the uterine muscle. Because oxytocin stimulates such a powerful response, the physician can induce labor by infusing minute amounts of it.

Oxytocin infusion may cause excessive or tetanic uterine contractions that last longer than 70 seconds each, occur more often than once every 3 minutes, and increase intrauterine pressure to more than 75 mm Hg. These excessive contractions may rupture the uterus. They also may reduce oxygen to the fetus, reducing or disrupting heartbeat.

Excessive contractions or reduced FHR warrants an immediate halt to oxytocin infusion. The oxytocin level will drop by half within about 3 minutes, and the tetanic contractions usually will return to a normal level.

Reproductive system disorders related to membrane and amniotic fluid factors

Several complications may arise during labor that are linked to the membranes and amniotic fluid. They include hydramnios, oligohydramnios, and amniotic fluid embolism.

Hydramnios

Normally, amniotic fluid volume equals approximately 1,000 ml at term. In hydramnios, volume reaches or exceeds 2,000 ml and is associated with fetal anomalies, the most common being congenital anomalies of the central nervous and gastrointestinal systems.

Hydramnios occurs in about 0.9% of all pregnant patients; the risk increases in patients with diabetes. In 90% of mild cases, the cause of hydramnios cannot be determined. Ultrasonography and physical assessment are used to diagnose this condition.

During labor, the primary risk is the potential for a sudden rupture of membranes (ROM) with a resultant prolapse of the umbilical cord caused by the force behind the release of this large volume of fluid. Fetal assessment is critical upon ROM, especially in this case.

Oligohydramnios

The counterpart of hydramnios, oligohydramnios refers to an abnormally small amount of amniotic fluid. Its cause is unknown, but a normal reduction in amniotic fluid after week 36 may create or aggravate the condition in post-term pregnancies. Reduced amniotic fluid is associated with maternal hypertension, fetal congenital anomalies, intrauterine growth retardation (IUGR), and risk to the fetus's life.

When oligohydramnios has been diagnosed before delivery through ultrasonography, cord accidents due to an occult prolapse or cord occlusion are a concern. Thus, vigilant fetal monitoring during labor is important.

Amniotic fluid embolism

A rare obstetric disorder, amniotic fluid embolism has a maternal mortality rate approaching 80%. The fetal mortality rate also is high. In this syndrome, amniotic fluid enters the maternal circulation and causes respiratory distress and shock. Classic symptoms include sudden onset of dyspnea and hypotension, possibly followed by cardiopulmonary arrest. Other significant signs include chest pain; cyanosis; frothy, pink-tinged sputum; tachycardia; and hemorrhage. Coagulopathy affects approximately 40% of patients with this syndrome and may be the cause of death in those who survive the initial hemodynamic insult.

The treatment of a patient with amniotic fluid embolism includes maintaining oxygenation and cardiac output as well as managing any coagulation problems, recognizing the symptoms of respiratory distress and shock, and knowing emergency procedures for respiratory and cardiac arrest.

Reproductive system disorders related to placental factors

Placental abnormalities may become apparent during pregnancy, or they may remain undetected until labor or just after delivery (the puerperium). During any stage, they present a major risk to the patient and fetus. The most common placental complications include placenta previa, abruptio placentae, and failure of placental separation.

Placenta previa

When the placenta forms near or over the cervical os instead of taking a position higher in the body of the uterus, the patient risks mild to potentially life-threatening hemorrhage, depending on the location of the placenta.

Placenta previa occurs in 0.4% to 0.6% of pregnancies. Incidence increases with multiparity, previous cesarean delivery, advanced maternal age, twin fetuses, and abnormal fetal lie.

The main symptom of placenta previa is painless vaginal bleeding after week 20. In some patients, bleeding may not occur until labor begins. When bleeding begins before the onset of labor, it tends to be episodic, beginning without warning, stopping spontaneously, and beginning again later. The patient may experience slow, steady bleeding that could affect blood count. Typically, the uterus is soft and nontender.

To avoid potentially severe hemorrhage, the patient should not have a manual pelvic examination until results of the ultrasound examination are available, especially if the fetus is premature. Severe hemorrhage warrants immediate emergency delivery. (See "Cesarean delivery" later in this chapter.)

Abruptio placentae

In approximately 1% of pregnancies, some or all of the placenta separates from the uterine wall after week 20 of gestation and before delivery. Called abruptio placentae, this condition may threaten the life of the patient and fetus. (For more information, see *Comparing placenta previa and abruptio placentae,* page 206.)

Although the primary cause of abruptio placentae is unknown, the following conditions may contribute to it: maternal hypertension, a short umbilical cord that places traction on the placenta, trauma, a uterine anomaly or tumor, sudden decompression of the uterus, pressure on the vena cava from the enlarged uterus, and dietary deficiency.

Whether an abruption involves a small area of the placenta or total separation, vaginal bleeding after week 20 of pregnancy and constant abdominal pain are its classic signs. Additional signs also may include uterine tenderness or back pain, fetal distress, frequent contractions, hypertonic uterus, preterm labor, and fetal demise.

Diagnosis of abruptio placentae should be based on the patient's history, physical assessment, and ultrasound examination. Most often, a patient will report an episode of vaginal bleeding, typically accompanied by continuous abdominal pain. In some cases, she may report uter-

Comparing placenta previa and abruptio placentae

By distinguishing between similar placental abnormalities, the nurse can anticipate care measures that the health care team must take.

PLACENTA PREVIA	ABRUPTIO PLACENTAE
Description	
Development of the placenta in the lower uterine segment. Classified according to the degree that it obstructs the cervical os.	Premature separation of some or all of the normally implanted placenta from the uterine wall. Classified according to the type of hemorrhage and degree of separation.
Signs and symptoms	
Abdomen appears normal; painless bleeding; uterus soft, except during contractions; fetus palpable; fetal heart tones almost always present; fetal movement not affected.	Abdomen distended, tense, and painful (boardlike); possible concealed hemorrhage; fetus nonpalpable; possible signs of fetal distress; if fetus has died, fetal heart tones absent, no fetal movement.
Management	
Bed rest; vaginal or cesarean delivery; vaginal examinations are contraindicated; Trendelenburg position to prevent shock.	Immediate cesarean or vaginal delivery to preserve the life of a live fetus or prevent further bleeding with a dead fetus.
Complications	
Hemorrhage; shock; infection; maternal or fetal death.	Hemorrhagic shock; hypofibrinogenemia; disseminated intravascular coagulation; hemorrhage into the myometrium; renal failure (acute tubular necrosis); maternal or fetal death.

ine contractions. Preparations must be made for immediate delivery, usually by cesarean delivery.

Failure of placental separation

The placenta normally separates from the uterine wall within 10 to 20 minutes after fetal delivery. Occasionally, however, placental separation may be delayed—a condition known as retained placenta. Separation may not occur at all—a condition known as abnormal adherence that takes one of three forms: placenta accreta, placenta increta, or placenta percreta.

Retained placenta. When spontaneous placental separation does not occur within 30 minutes after fetal delivery, the nurse-midwife or physician may attempt to remove the retained placenta manually. The patient may require a dilatation and curettage (D&C) procedure afterward to ensure that all fragments have been removed. She also may receive an oxytocic drug to promote uterine contractions and reduce bleeding.

Abnormal adherence. In some patients, absence of the decidua basalis allows the placenta to adhere too firmly to the uterine wall. Known as placenta accreta, this condition may occur over the entire placenta or only in a portion of it.

Although the etiology of these conditions is unknown, predisposing factors may include placenta previa, previous cesarean delivery, previous curettage, and multiparity. Incidence of these abnormalities is unknown as well, but placenta accreta is the most commonly reported of the three conditions.

The treatment of a patient with placenta accreta depends on the amount of placenta adhering to the uterine wall and subsequent hemorrhage. A small accreta may be managed by D&C; an oxytocic drug may be used to control bleeding. Total accreta, increta, or percreta requires hysterectomy. Nursing care also depends on the amount of adhering placenta, the severity of blood loss, and whether hysterectomy was performed.

Reproductive system disorders related to umbilical cord factors

Anomalies involving the umbilical cord typically are not detected until delivery. Some may threaten the fetus's life. Complications that may arise during labor include abnormal cord implantation, abnormal cord length, and cord prolapse.

Abnormal cord implantation

Normally, the umbilical cord inserts in the center of the placenta. In a velamentous (membranous) insertion, the cord vessels separate into branches before reaching the placenta and the cord inserts into the membranes rather than the placental disk. Occasionally with a velamentous insertion, fetal vessels in the membranes cross the internal os and take up a position ahead of the fetal presenting part. This potentially serious condition, known as vasa previa, may be discovered during a pelvic examination when the examiner feels vessels through the cervical os.

Abnormal cord length

On average, an umbilical cord measures 55 cm (22″). An excessively long cord raises the risk of knots and prolapse or a nuchal cord. A short cord may contribute to abruptio placentae.

Cord prolapse

Displacement of the umbilical cord to a position at or below the fetus's presenting part most commonly occurs when amniotic membranes rupture before fetal descent. The sudden gush of fluid carries the long, loose cord ahead of the fetus toward and possibly through the patient's cervix and into the vagina. Serious asphyxia may occur when the fetus compresses the cord, interrupting blood flow from the placenta. Factors that increase the risk of cord prolapse include hydramnios, more than one fetus, ruptured membranes, a transverse or breech lie, a small

Umbilical cord prolapse

If not corrected within minutes, umbilical cord prolapse may cause fetal hypoxia, central nervous system damage, and possible death. Fortunately, rapid assessment and intervention by the health care team can help the patient and fetus survive this traumatic event. Discussed below are the signs and symptoms of cord prolapse and appropriate interventions until emergency cesarean or forceps delivery can take place.

Signs and symptoms
- Patient reports feeling the cord "slither" down after membrane rupture
- Visible or palpable umbilical cord in the birth canal
- Violent fetal activity
- Fetal bradycardia with variable deceleration during contractions

Nursing actions
- Immediately summon another member of the health care team who can notify the physician and prepare the team for a prompt delivery or emergency surgery.
- Place the patient in a Trendelenburg or knee-chest position with her hips elevated. Either position will shift the fetus's weight off the cord. (Two gloved fingers also can assist in pushing the fetus's presenting part off the cord while the operating room is being prepared.)
- Do not attempt to press or push the cord back into the uterus. This may traumatize the cord, stop blood flow to the fetus, or start an intrauterine infection.
- Expect to assist in giving the patient supplemental oxygen by face mask at 10 liters/minute, initiating or increasing I.V. fluids with 5% dextrose in lactated Ringer's solution (to enhance fluid volume and circulation), and sending blood for type and crossmatch (if this was not done on admission).
- Expect to assist in monitoring fetal heart tones with an internal fetal scalp electrode on the presenting part.
- It is dangerous to try to reinsert the cord if it protrudes from the vagina. Instead, lift it with gloved hands and gently wrap it in loose, sterile towels saturated with sterile saline solution.
- Keep the patient informed throughout this emergency. Calmly convey the seriousness of the situation and emphasize the importance of cooperation. Reassure the patient and her family that the medical and nursing staff will do everything possible to ensure a safe and successful delivery.
- Accompany the patient to the operating room, continuing to keep pressure off the cord and monitoring for signs of maternal and fetal distress.

fetus, a long umbilical cord, a low-lying placenta, premature delivery, and an unengaged fetal presenting part.

Umbilical cord prolapse incurs a high infant mortality rate if not detected and treated immediately. Diagnosis of cord prolapse is based on observation of the cord outside the vulva, feeling the cord during a vaginal examination, or observation of fetal distress. (For more information, see *Umbilical cord prolapse*.)

Preparing for a cesarean delivery

To prepare the patient and her family for surgery, the nurse begins by explaining all the steps in the procedure and by ensuring that the patient has given her written consent. Steps in physical preparation for the patient undergoing a cesarean include:
- Abdominal preparation or shaving
- Bladder catheterization with indwelling urinary catheter
- Collecting laboratory tests, as ordered, including a complete blood count, as well as a type and crossmatch for blood replacement
- Establishing an intravenous infusion, as prescribed
- Antacid administration, as prescribed
- Positioning on surgical table to prevent the gravid uterus from occluding placental perfusion through compression of the vena cava while awaiting surgery to commence
- Preparation of the operating room and equipment, surgical team
- Coordination of obstetrician, anesthesiologist, and pediatrician as well as nursing staffs
- Documentation

Related obstetrical interventions

Upon the identification of a serious intrapartal complication which threatens the health of the mother, fetus, or both, the nurse must be prepared to assist with related obstetrical interventions and coordinate efforts with other members of the health care team.

Cesarean delivery

In some cases, the nurse may need to assist with a cesarean delivery, which involves surgical incision of the abdominal and uterine walls (see *Preparing for a cesarean delivery*). The most common reasons for cesarean delivery encompass five general categories:
- Dystocia (difficult or abnormal delivery) accounts for about 29% of all cesarean deliveries. The most common cause of dystocia is cephalopelvic disproportion, which results from a large fetus, malpresentation, a contracted pelvis, or—in rare cases—a tumor that blocks the birth canal.
- Previous cesarean delivery is the cause in 35% of all cesarean deliveries.
- Breech presentation prompts 10% of cesarean deliveries. This indication is becoming more common, particularly in nulliparous patients. Many practitioners now consider cesarean delivery safer for breech fetuses.
- Fetal distress is the indication in 8% of all cases.
- Other indications account for the remaining 18% of cesarean deliveries. These include active herpes genitalis or condylomata acuminata lesions in the birth canal. Both are potentially dangerous if transmitted to the fetus during delivery. Condylomatous lesions also may obstruct the birth canal.

All methods of obstetric anesthesia pose some risks for the patient and fetus that must be weighed against benefits when choosing an anesthetic agent. Choice of an agent should reflect the circumstances and the patient's desires. If the patient wishes to witness the delivery, the choice typically is spinal or epidural anesthesia. In an emergency requiring immediate cesarean delivery, a rapid-induction general anesthesia may be the type of choice.

If time is adequate and the patient and fetus are normal, the physician makes a transverse incision at or just below the pubic hairline. Much less common today is the classical incision, in which the physician cuts vertically through the body of the uterus. This type of incision increases the possibility of rupture during subsequent pregnancies.

Forceps delivery

In this procedure, the physician uses two curved, articulated, blunt metal blades to extract the fetus from the birth canal or to rotate the fetus.

Fetal station determines the type of forceps used. Low or outlet forceps may be appropriate when the head has reached the perineum and is visibly separating the labia. Forceps can help the patient push the fetus out, shortening the second stage of labor. Use of low forceps is relatively safe; complications usually are limited to bruising of the fetus's head and minor perineal, vaginal, or cervical trauma. Today, most physicians will perform a cesarean delivery rather than using mid or high forceps.

Vacuum extraction

To accomplish vacuum extraction, the physician uses a suction-cup device known as a ventouse. The ventouse is attached by tubing to a suction pump. After positioning the ventouse on the fetus's scalp, air is pumped out of the space between the cup and the scalp, creating a vacuum. By pulling a chain or cord attached to the ventouse, the physician draws the fetus through the birth canal.

Those who favor vacuum extraction believe that it decreases delivery time. They also point out that the procedure does not require additional space inside the vaginal canal, as forceps do.

Vaginal birth after cesarean delivery

In vaginal birth after cesarean delivery (VBAC), a patient who has had a cesarean delivery attempts to deliver vaginally. This approach offers several advantages over repeated cesarean deliveries:
• reduced risk of infection and death
• less discomfort than cesarean delivery
• less recovery time than cesarean delivery
• less cost than cesarean delivery.

The American College of Obstetricians and Gynecologists has established specific criteria and guidelines for the patient attempting VBAC. Acceptable criteria for attempting a VBAC include:
• previous uterine incision made in the low transverse position
• patient desire to try vaginal delivery
• available blood for transfusion
• an obstetric team prepared to perform cesarean delivery if necessary
• no patient medical or obstetric problems that contraindicate VBAC.

Reproductive system disorders related to pelvic factors

Critical to normal fetal descent is the relationship between the size of the pelvis and the size and presentation of the fetus. Complications develop when the pelvis is too small (contracted) to allow normal fetal descent. Additional complications involving obstructed fetal descent include lacerations of the vaginal canal and surrounding soft tissues. For this reason, the physician or nurse-midwife may elect an episiotomy.

Structural contractures

The pelvis may be contracted at the inlet, midpelvis, or outlet, or it may be generally small. This may not be a problem with a small fetus. With a fetus of normal or above-normal size, however, contracture may prevent passage.

The patient has a contracted pelvic inlet when the anteroposterior diameter measures less than 10 cm or when the diagonal conjugate measures less than 11.5 cm. The patient has a contracted midpelvis when the interspinous diameter measures less than 10 cm and a contracted outlet when the interischial tuberous diameter measures 8 cm or less. A contracted outlet rarely occurs without a contracted midpelvis.

With a normal fetopelvic relationship, uterine contractions gradually rotate the fetus's head to an anterior position that provides the most favorable adaptation between the head and the pelvis. A contracted pelvis may prevent this internal rotation, thus placing the fetus's head in the transverse position. This would lead to a cesarean delivery after a diagnosis of arrest of cervical dilation is made.

Lacerations

During delivery, the soft tissues of the birth canal commonly sustain trauma and lacerations of the cervix, vagina, or perineum. If the patient is bleeding heavily after expelling the placenta and her fundus is firm, suspect a cervical laceration. Small cervical lacerations occur commonly during delivery and may not need repair. Severe lacerations, possibly affecting the upper vagina, will require surgical attention. Expect the cervix to be examined after a difficult vaginal delivery.

Lacerations of the lower portion of the birth canal may be classified by severity:
• First-degree lacerations involve the fourchette, perineal skin, and vaginal mucous membranes.

• Second-degree lacerations extend to the fascia and muscles of the perineal body.
• Third-degree lacerations extend to the anal sphincter.
• Fourth-degree lacerations extend to the anal canal.

Episiotomy

Lacerations of the birth canal may be prevented or minimized by episiotomy. Episiotomy may be accomplished by two methods. The most common in the United States is a median episiotomy. Using round-tipped scissors, the physician or nurse-midwife cuts straight downward from the vaginal orifice. In the alternative method—mediolateral episiotomy—the cut is oblique, angling away from the anus.

Systemic disorders

Complications involving hemorrhage, shock, and disseminated intravascular coagulation can occur at any time during labor and delivery.

Hemorrhage and shock

Many factors predispose the patient to hemorrhage and subsequent shock, including placenta previa, abruptio placentae, uterine rupture, and lacerations during delivery. (See Chapter 16, Selected postpartal complications, for a more detailed description.)

Disseminated intravascular coagulation (DIC)

A pathological form of diffuse rather than localized clotting, DIC leads to massive internal and external hemorrhage as clotting factors (such as fibrinogen) are consumed. Intrauterine fetal death, abruptio placentae, septic shock, or amniotic fluid embolism can initiate normal clotting mechanisms. If these clotting factors are depleted, DIC may occur.

Treatment of a patient with DIC must include treatment of the causative factor as well as aggressive support of blood volume and pressure. The patient may require replacement of blood components, such as platelets or fresh frozen plasma.

Fetal complications

Many fetal factors can affect the progress of labor, including malpresentation, malposition, macrosomia, shoulder dystocia, and intrauterine fetal death. (For more information, see *Signs of fetal distress*.)

Malpresentation

When the fetal presenting part is not the head, the condition is known as a malpresentation. Examples of malpresentations include breech, shoulder, and face.

The most common malpresentation is breech, which occurs in 3% to 4% of births and more frequently in twins. Currently in the United States, approximately 80% of breech fetuses that reach term are delivered by cesarean. Breech presentation is associated with increased incidence of preterm labor, congenital anomalies, and birth trauma.

Signs of fetal distress

Signs of fetal distress indicate that the health—and possibly the life—of the fetus is in jeopardy. For example, meconium-stained or yellow amniotic fluid signals fetal hypoxia, which can lead to anoxia, central nervous system damage, or death. The nurse can use the following chart to identify signs of fetal distress and appropriate interventions.

Signs
- Abnormal fetal heart rate pattern, including a heart rate below 120 or above 160 beats/minute, decreased or increased variability, or periodic changes, such as late decelerations or deep, wide, variable decelerations
- Increased or decreased fetal activity
- Meconium-stained or yellow amniotic fluid after membrane rupture

Nursing actions
- Help the patient into the lateral or knee-chest position to relieve fetal pressure on the vena cava, aorta, or umbilical cord and improve maternal and fetal circulation.
- Supply oxygen to improve oxygenation of the patient and the fetus. Administer by face mask at 8 to 10 liters/minute.
- Notify the physician and the surgical team.
- Expect to assist with initiating or increasing I.V. fluids, such as lactated Ringer's solution, to manage hypotension or hypovolemia.
- Expect to discontinue oxytocin immediately (if it is being administered) to improve uteroplacental perfusion.
- Be calm and purposeful when caring for the patient. This will help prevent undue fear and anxiety, which could adversely affect uteroplacental perfusion.
- Explain what is happening, and reassure the patient to help her gain control and cooperate fully. Keep her family informed and encourage their support.

A transverse lie occurs when the long axis of the mother is perpendicular to that of the fetus and includes shoulder and arm presentations. Either one requires cesarean delivery.

Malposition

Malposition occurs when the fetus's presenting part enters the birth canal in an abnormal position that makes delivery difficult. An example is the persistent occiput posterior position where the occiput of the fetus's head is in one of the posterior quadrants of the maternal pelvis. If the occiput fails to rotate spontaneously to the anterior position, the physician may use forceps to complete the rotation and facilitate delivery.

Macrosomia

The classic definition of macrosomia is a fetus that weighs more than 4,500 g. This occurs in approximately 1% of births. A large fetus does not necessarily preclude vaginal delivery; in fact, many are delivered vaginally or with low forceps. The fetopelvic relationship must be assessed for each patient.

A risk of shoulder dystocia must be considered. Predisposing factors for macrosomia include maternal diabetes, multiparity, maternal age over 34, previous macrosomia, maternal height over 67″ (170 cm), and maternal weight over 154 lb (70 kg).

Shoulder dystocia

In shoulder dystocia, the fetus's head emerges but the anterior shoulder catches on the pubic arch—a rare and usually unexpected condition. Typically in shoulder dystocia, the head emerges and is immediately pulled back tightly against the vulva. Predisposing factors include macrosomia, a prolonged second stage of labor, multiparity, prolonged pregnancy, and previous delivery of a neonate weighing more than 4,000 g. Because this condition has the potential to cause fetal trauma or death, interventions must be immediate. For these reasons, cesarean sections may be elected if shoulder dystocia is anticipated.

Intrauterine fetal death

If fetal activity fails to begin or if it ceases after 20 weeks' gestation, the patient should be monitored for fetal heart tones. Absence of fetal heart tones warrants a real-time ultrasound examination to detect heart wall motion. Absence of such motion offers reliable evidence of fetal death.

In more than half the cases of fetal death, the cause cannot be determined. Where the cause is known, however, it may be associated with severe maternal disease, diabetes mellitus, hypertension, abruptio placentae, erythroblastosis fetalis, and umbilical cord accidents.

Anticipated high-risk intrapartal complications

High-risk intrapartal patients may have chronic medical disorders that predispose them to obstetric complications such as cardiac disease, diabetes, infection, or substance abuse. They may have pregnancy-related conditions that require special care, such as PIH or Rh isoimmunization. (For details, see *Selected intrapartal conditions and risks,* pages 195 to 197.)

Cardiac disease

Maternal cardiac disease complicates nearly 1% of all pregnancies and is a major cause of maternal death in the United States. The intrapartal period poses the greatest risk for the patient with cardiac disease because the hemodynamic changes of pregnancy peak at this time.

Labor can produce sudden, profound changes in the cardiovascular system. During each contraction, pain and increased venous blood return from the uterus raise cardiac output 20%. Mean arterial pressure rises and is followed by a reflex bradycardia.

Intrapartal management of the patient with a cardiac disease requires the expertise of an obstetrician, cardiologist, anesthesiologist, and obstetric nurse with critical-care skills. The patient needs intensive obstetric and cardiac monitoring. Interventions are based on the patient's degree of cardiac decompensation (inability of the heart to compensate for impaired functioning). Even a patient with minimal activity limitation during pregnancy can experience sudden worsening of the disease during labor. The nurse should be familiar with the normal changes of pregnancy and with the maternal and fetal consequences of cardiac disease. (For more information, see Chapter 6, Selected antepartal complications.)

Diabetes mellitus

During pregnancy, a patient with diabetes mellitus requires close monitoring and management to prevent intrapartal problems. Prevention of hyperglycemia before conception and during pregnancy improves perinatal outcomes but does not remove all risks. Uncontrolled diabetes is associated with increased maternal, fetal, and neonatal morbidity and mortality. (For more information about the maternal, fetal, and neonatal effects of diabetes, see Chapter 6, Selected antepartal complications.)

Uncontrolled diabetes can cause hydramnios. It also is associated with hypertensive disorders, such as chronic hypertension and PIH, which affect 15% to 30% of all pregnant patients with diabetes. Women with diabetes also are at risk for preterm labor and, if associated with vascular changes, placental abnormalities.

Neonates of diabetic mothers whose diabetes has not been well controlled have a higher morbidity and mortality rate than those born to nondiabetic mothers. They also are at risk for neonatal hypoglycemia at birth and for macrosomia, which can lead to birth trauma. A neonate of a pregestational diabetic patient is at increased risk for congenital malformations, especially if the patient's glucose levels were uncontrolled during fetal organ development.

Infection

Infections are a major cause of maternal, fetal, and neonatal death. During the intrapartal period, they are more common in patients with premature labor, PROM (especially before 36 weeks' gestation), fever, or fetal death.

The primary perinatal infections are bacterial or viral and are caused by such organisms as group B beta-hemolytic streptococcus, herpes simplex virus, hepatitis B virus or human immunodeficiency virus (HIV). They may be transmitted to the fetus through an infected uterus or birth canal and can lead to morbidity or mortality because the fetus's immature immune system cannot fight off these life-threatening organisms. Fungal (candidiasis) or protozoal (trichomoniasis) infections are not potentially fatal.

Many factors can predispose a patient to infection, including obesity, severe anemia, poor hygiene, uncontrolled diabetes, chronic renal or respiratory disease, and a depressed immune response.

During labor, predisposing factors to intrapartal infection may include preterm labor, prolonged labor, prolonged PROM (rupture that occurs more than 24 hours before labor), use of such invasive equipment as internal fetal scalp electrodes or intrauterine pressure catheters, and multiple vaginal examinations.

Pregnancy-induced hypertension (PIH)

A hypertensive syndrome that occurs during pregnancy, PIH has two forms: preeclampsia (causing hypertension, proteinuria, and edema, leading to oliguria, headache, blurred vision, and increased deep tendon reflexes) and eclampsia (causing convulsions along with the signs of preeclampsia). Affecting about 5% of all pregnancies, preeclampsia may progress to eclampsia suddenly or gradually. The patient with PIH may be very ill. Failure to recognize and appropriately manage PIH accounts for about 1% of maternal deaths in the United States.

PIH is characterized by insufficient perfusion of many vital organs, including the fetal-placental unit (all fetal and maternal systems that work together to exchange nutrients, excrete toxins, and perform other functions); it is completely reversible with pregnancy termination, but symptoms may remain for 24 to 48 hours after delivery. The patient may report sudden weight gain, varying degrees of edema, numbness in her hands or feet, headache, or vision problems—warning signs of increasing preeclampsia.

The major goal of intrapartal preeclampsia management is to deliver the patient efficiently through aggressive medical management while preventing eclampsia. To achieve this goal, the nurse must understand the pathophysiology, progression, and prognosis of the disorder, and must recognize and immediately report to the physician the classic signs of preeclampsia. (For more information on PIH, see Chapter 6, Selected antepartal complications.)

After the patient is stabilized, the obstetric team prepares for vaginal or cesarean delivery, depending on the patient's condition and physician management. Ideally, she would deliver vaginally to avoid the complications of surgery. If the cervix is likely to respond to oxytocin—that is, if it is soft, open, and not posterior in position—and the patient and fetus are stable, an induced vaginal delivery is preferred. If assessments reveal fetal distress or an estimated fetal weight of less than 1,500 g, cesarean delivery is preferred.

As a result of the stress of PIH, the patient may have a shorter labor and a precipitous delivery. The neonatal team would need to be present for delivery, especially if the neonate is premature, which is common in patients with severe preeclampsia. If the patient received magnesium sulfate during labor, the nurse prepares for potential neonatal effects. Magnesium sulfate toxicity may occur in the neonate, producing respiratory depression, hypotonia, and hypotension.

Rh isoimmunization

Rh isoimmunization refers to sensitization and immune response of maternal blood antibodies to fetal blood antigens, which can create a serious blood incompatibility between the two during pregnancy. This can lead to erythroblastosis fetalis (hydrops fetalis or hemolytic disease of the newborn).

Erythroblastosis fetalis is a serious hemolytic disease of the fetus and neonate that produces anemia; jaundice; liver, spleen, and heart enlargement; and anasarca (severe generalized edema). It may lead to myocardial failure and also may cause placental hypertrophy, which can contribute to fetal hypoxia and death and accounts for a significant percentage of fetal morbidity and mortality.

Rh isoimmunization results when a patient has Rh-negative blood and her fetus has Rh-positive blood. However, this is becoming more rare because most Rh-negative women now receive $Rh_O(D)$ immune globulin (RhoGAM) during antepartal and postpartal care, which provides passive immunization against the Rh antigen.

Today, hemolytic disease of the newborn occurs more commonly when the patient develops a sensitivity to other foreign blood antigens. This sensitization is known as nonimmune hydrops fetalis. Maternal factors that contribute to development of nonimmune hydrops include multiple gestation; perinatal infections, especially syphilis or cytomegalovirus infection; previous transfusion of blood that contained foreign antigens; diabetes mellitus; thalassemia; or PIH. (For more information about isoimmunization, see Chapter 6, Selected antepartal complications.)

Substance abuse

During pregnancy, substance abuse can lead to serious perinatal risks. Substance abusers tend to have unplanned pregnancies or may be uncertain when the pregnancy began. They may have suboptimal nutrition, smoke heavily, abuse multiple drugs, and seek prenatal care late, if at all. Some may have multiple sex partners, placing them at increased risk for STDs and HIV. Recently it was estimated that more than 50% of the HIV infections among women have been acquired through I.V. drug use.

These actions put the substance abuser and her fetus at risk during the intrapartal period. For example, cocaine use during pregnancy causes maternal and fetal vasoconstriction, tachycardia, and elevated blood pressure. These effects reduce blood flow to the fetus and can induce premature uterine contractions. Hence cocaine use increases the risk of preterm labor, delivery of an LBW or SGA neonate, and abruptio placentae.

Substance abuse also can cause problems that may affect the antepartal period and lead to intrapartal problems. For example, severe nutritional deficiencies and STDs, which are common among women who abuse drugs, can compromise fetal health as well. Substance abuse can produce social isolation, which can affect the patient's ability to cope with labor. Use of nonsterile needles can cause maternal infection or embolization, which can affect maternal and fetal health.

Some states have strict laws regarding substance abuse and child protection. If the patient used or tested positive for drugs during the antepartal or intrapartal periods, many states mandate home environment evaluation and referral of the patient for drug treatment before the neonate can be discharged.

STUDY ACTIVITIES

Short answer

1. On her admission to the labor and delivery area, Marcie Yutaka, a 23-year-old primigravida, is diagnosed in latent phase labor. Her pelvic examination reveals that her cervix is 2 cm, 100% effaced, and 0 station. After several hours, her uterine contractions become more intense and frequent as well as much more painful. Ms. Yutaka requests pain medication. She is reexamined and her condition has not changed. Her membranes are intact and the fetus is stable. What type of uterine dysfunction pattern is Ms. Yutaka experiencing? Briefly describe the expected management for this complication.

_____

_____

2. Dawn Matthews, a 32-year-old gravida 3 para 2002, presents in the labor and delivery area with complaints of constant, severe abdominal pain after a sudden episode of vaginal bleeding at 34 weeks' gestation. Her abdomen is tender, distended, and rigid; fetal assessment reveals severe fetal distress with pronounced tachycardia. Ms. Matthews's vital signs indicate that she is developing shock. What complication should the nurse suspect, and which obstetric intervention should the nurse be prepared for?

_____

3. On her initial antepartal visit, Rebecca Whitfield mentions to the nurse that it is important to her to attempt a vaginal birth after cesarean (VBAC) with this pregnancy. During her last delivery, surgery was performed for a prolapsed umbilical cord. Now, Ms. Whitfield and her husband are hopeful that she will be able to give birth naturally. Briefly list the advantages of a VBAC for this patient.

_____

4. After her admission to the labor and delivery area, Claire Preston develops a blood pressure of 180/110, a pulse of 88 beats/minute, a respiratory rate of 22 breaths/minute, and a temperature of 99.2° F. This 22-year-old primigravida did not receive any prenatal care and arrived on the intrapartal unit complaining of a severe headache, blurry vision, and numbness of her hands. Although she is at 38 weeks' gestation by her last menstrual period, her fetus is estimated to be small, possibly only 5 lb. Ms. Preston is noted to have pronounced, generalized edema and brisk deep tendon reflexes. She also is found to have marked proteinuria on a catheterized urinalysis. Identify the high-risk intrapartal condition that is most likely occurring to Ms. Preston and list the maternal and fetal risks of this condition.

_____

_____

5. Briefly describe the main symptoms of placenta previa and the expected management.

_____

_____

6. Define a umbilical cord prolapse and discuss the implications of this emergency complication.

_____

_____

7. What are the five most common clinical reasons for cesarean deliveries?

_____

8. Why is the substance abuser who admits to cocaine use considered at high risk during the intrapartal period?

_____

True or false

9. Characterized by rapid progression, precipitate labor typically lasts 3 hours or less.
  ☐ True   ☐ False

10. An oxytocin induction or augmentation may cause excessive or tetanic uterine contractions, which compromise uteroplacental perfusion to the fetus.
  ☐ True   ☐ False

11. A classic sign of abruptio placentae is sudden, painless vaginal bleeding after 20 weeks' gestation.
  ☐ True   ☐ False

12. The most common malpresentation is breech.
  ☐ True   ☐ False

13. When a prolapsed umbilical cord is identified, the nurse should immediately try to replace the cord into the uterus.
☐ True   ☐ False

14. Infections are a major cause of maternal, fetal, and neonatal death.
☐ True   ☐ False

ANSWERS   **Short answer**

1. Hypertonic dysfunction, which typically occurs during the latent phase of labor, is characterized by intense painful contractions unaccompanied by normal cervical dilation. Continuous, careful monitoring of labor progress and fetal status is essential because fetal hypoxia may occur. The nurse must be aware of any signs of fetal distress and be prepared to intervene appropriately.

The patient may be given a narcotic analgesic to produce sleep for several hours. Upon awakening, she may be in a normal, progressive labor pattern. Administration of the analgesic may be contraindicated if there was fetal distress or ruptured membranes.

2. Abruptio placentae, a premature separation of some or all of the normally implanted placenta from the uterine wall, is the most likely complication Ms. Matthews is experiencing. The nurse should anticipate obstetric management and prepare for an immediate cesarean section to preserve the life of the fetus and the mother.

3. The advantages of a VBAC over a repeat cesarean delivery would include the potential for a family experience of a normal childbirth, reduced risks of infection and death, less discomfort, less recovery time, and less cost then a surgical delivery.

4. Ms. Preston's history and physical assessment findings are very suggestive of preeclampsia, a form of PIH characterized by hypertension, proteinuria, and edema, leading to oliguria, headache, blurry vision, and increased deep tendon reflexes. If unrecognized and untreated this may progress to eclampsia, causing seizures. Maternal risks include insufficient perfusion of vital organs, including the fetal-placental unit; seizures; hypertonic uterine activity; and abruptio placentae, if the patient develops eclampsia. Preterm labor also may be a risk. Fetal or neonatal risks include prematurity, IUGR, fetal intolerance to labor, and possible magnesium sulfate toxicity, if magnesium sulfate is used to treat PIH during labor.

5. The main symptom of placenta previa is painless vaginal bleeding after week 20 of pregnancy. In some patients, bleeding may not occur until labor begins. Typically the uterus is soft and nontender.

Expected management of any pregnant patient who reports an episode of painless, vaginal bleeding or sudden onset involves hospitalization and ultrasonography to display the location of the placenta. Laboratory studies should include a complete blood count, coagulation studies, and a type and crossmatch if the bleeding is severe. To avoid potentially severe hemorrhage, the patient would not have a manual pelvic examination until the results of the ultrasound are available. Severe hemorrhage warrants immediate emergency delivery.

6. An umbilical cord prolapse occurs when there is displacement of the umbilical cord to a position at or below the fetus's presenting part, most commonly when amniotic membranes rupture before fetal descent. The sudden gush of fluid carries the long, loose cord ahead of the fetus toward and possibly through the cervix, into the vagina. Serious asphyxia may occur when the fetus compresses the cord, interrupting blood flow from the placenta. Umbilical cord prolapse incurs a high infant mortality rate if not detected and treated immediately.

7. The most common clinical reasons for cesarean delivery encompass the following five general categories: dystocia; previous cesarean delivery; breech presentation; fetal distress; and other indications, including active herpes genitalis or condylomata acuminata.

8. The cocaine user is at high risk during the intrapartal period because cocaine causes chronic maternal and fetal vasoconstriction, tachycardia, and elevated blood pressure during pregnancy. These effects reduce blood flow to the fetus and can induce premature uterine contractions. Hence, cocaine use increases the risks of preterm labor and of delivery of a low-birth-weight or small-for-gestational-age neonate, as well as causing abruptio placentae.

True or false

9. True.

10. True.

11. False. Whether an abruption involves a small area of the placenta or total separation, vaginal bleeding after the twentieth week of pregnancy and constant abdominal pain are its classic signs.

12. True.

13. False. Pushing the umbilical cord back into the uterus, once prolapse is determined, is contraindicated. This may traumatize the cord, stop blood flow to the fetus, or start an intrauterine infection.

14. True.

CHAPTER 14

Physiology of the postpartal period

OBJECTIVES
After studying this chapter, the reader should be able to:
1. Describe the return of physiologic function to significant body systems during the postpartal period.
2. Discuss the process of uterine involution.
3. Explain the normal progression of lochia.
4. Outline the hemodynamic events that restore the body to a nonpregnant state.

OVERVIEW OF CONCEPTS
During the postpartal period (puerperium), the changes affecting both the reproductive system and the hormonal processes during pregnancy resolve; eventually, each body system returns to a nonpregnant state. Although officially defined as a 6-week period, the postpartal period spans the time between delivery and the resumption of normal physiologic function. Thus it may vary greatly, especially among breast-feeding women. The patient's physical capabilities and body image must adapt to postpartal changes. The nurse who understands such changes can assess the patient more proficiently and make scientifically grounded decisions, facilitating the patient's return to optimal health.

Reproductive system
The reproductive system recovers from pregnancy and childbirth in a unique and efficient manner. However, some structures retain permanent effects.

Uterus
After delivery of the fetus and placenta, the uterus undergoes a gradual process of involution that leads to its return to a nonpregnant state. These changes involve both the myometrium (uterine muscle) and endometrium (uterine lining).

Involution
Immediately after delivery of the placenta, strong myometrial contractions shrink the uterus to the size of a grapefruit—a reduction of roughly half from the immediate predelivery size. This rapid shrinkage forc-

es the uterine walls into close proximity, causing the center cavity to flatten.

Myometrial contractions (also called "after pains") are irregular in both timing and strength. A multipara usually experiences stronger, more uncomfortable contractions than a primipara, probably because uterine muscles lose elasticity with each pregnancy. Also, a breast-feeding patient has stronger contractions because oxytocin, a hormone that helps regulate milk ejection, stimulates uterine muscles.

Uterine size decreases along with uterine weight. One hour after delivery, the fundus of the uterus is palpable at or just above the umbilicus; each day thereafter, the uterus becomes smaller. By 2 weeks postpartum, the uterus has returned to the pelvic cavity and no longer can be palpated as an abdominal organ. The uterus usually resumes a nonpregnant size and contour by 6 weeks postpartum. (For more information, see *Postpartal changes in fundal height,* page 224.)

Endometrium

In the early stages of involution, myometrial contractions compress blood vessels throughout the decidua and at the placental site, leading to hemostasis (arrest of bleeding). After the first 2 or 3 postpartal days, the decidua basalis differentiates into two distinct layers. Occlusion of decidual blood vessels leads to necrosis of the superficial layer, which is sloughed off as part of the lochial discharge (see *Stages of lochia,* page 225). The deeper decidual layer (basal layer) remains attached to the uterine wall.

By 16 days postpartum, the endometrium is completely restored except at the placental site. Involution of the placental site and restoration of normal tissue here take longer than in the rest of the endometrium. As the placental site heals, regenerating endometrial tissue slowly and progressively replaces the decidua basalis. Healing occurs gradually and without scarring.

Cervix

In a patient who delivered vaginally, cervical muscle tone is poor, and the cervix and lower uterine segment are thin and collapsed. The external os contracts slowly; on the second and third days after delivery, it remains loose and open. By the end of the first week, the os has contracted to 1 cm and cervical tone has improved, making admission of one finger difficult. At this point any cervical edema and hemorrhage have subsided markedly, and the cervical canal (the structure extending from the external os to the interior of the uterus) has begun to reform as the cervix thickens.

Although the cervix resumes its normal functional anatomy by 6 weeks postpartum, it never regains its nulliparous appearance. The external os remains widened and linear, compared to the tiny circular os of the nulliparous patient.

Postpartal changes in fundal height

After delivery, uterine involution—the process that returns the uterus to a normal size—advances so rapidly that the level of the fundus is one fingerbreadth lower than on the previous day.

FUNDAL HEIGHT

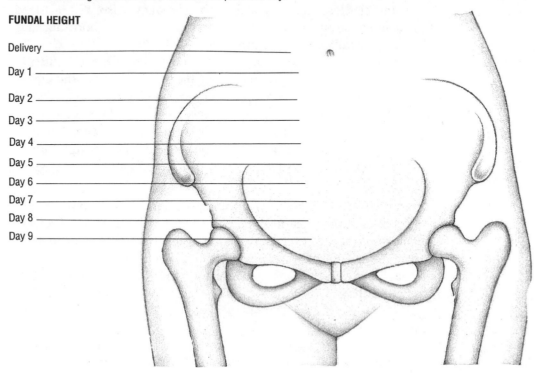

Delivery

Day 1

Day 2

Day 3

Day 4

Day 5

Day 6

Day 7

Day 8

Day 9

UTERINE INVOLUTION

Day 1

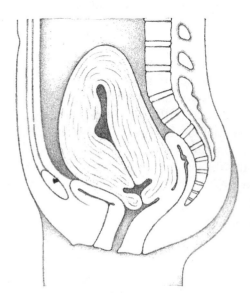

Day 6

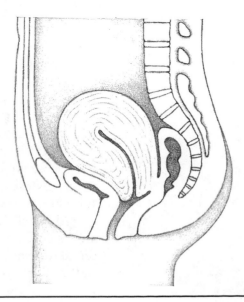

Stages of lochia

Lochia progresses through three stages, each with distinctive characteristics that reflect progressive endometrial healing.

STAGE	USUAL DURATION	DESCRIPTION
Lochia rubra	1 to 4 days postpartum	Bloody, possibly with some mucus, tissue debris, and small clots; may have a slightly fleshy odor
Lochia serosa	5 to 7 days postpartum	Pink-brown, serous, odorless
Lochia alba	1 to 3 weeks postpartum	Creamy white, brown, or almost colorless; may have a slightly stale odor

Lochia

The amount and duration of lochia—postpartal vaginal discharge-correlate with endometrial healing and regeneration. In all patients, lochial flow occurs in three distinct stages. (For more information, see *Stages of lochia*.) Although rates of lochial discharge vary among patients, normal parameters for the amount and duration of lochia during each stage have been established.

Lochia is considered abnormal if it contains large clots (as large as or larger than a fifty-cent piece) or tissue fragments (pieces of tissue, not the tissue debris normal to lochial flow). Also, lochia should not have a foul or offensive odor and should not relapse to a previous stage.

Vagina

After vaginal delivery, the vagina is smooth-walled and somewhat enlarged, with poor muscle tone and significant edema. Gradually, it shrinks and the edema subsides. By the third postpartal week, rugae reappear within the vaginal walls. These rugae remain permanently flattened to varying degrees.

The vaginal epithelium also undergoes notable postpartal changes. Vascular and well-lubricated during pregnancy because of estrogen increase, the epithelium becomes fragile and atrophic by the third or fourth postpartal week. In the patient who is not breast-feeding, atrophy resolves by 6 to 10 weeks postpartum as estrogen normalizes.

Without such complications as hematoma or infection, the perineum heals rapidly. Usually, the introitus and perineum resume a nonpregnant state by 6 weeks postpartum. However, in cases of extreme musculofascial relaxation, extensive laceration, or inadequate perineal repair, the introitus may show residual gaping; typically, this change is permanent.

Breasts

The breast changes initiated during pregnancy—nipple and areola enlargement, maturation of lobes and ducts, and increased vascularity—continue after delivery, particularly in the breast-feeding patient.

In the first 2 postpartal days, breast alveoli (tiny sacs made up of epithelial cells) enlarge. The alveoli—the basic secretory units of the breast—are the site of milk production. Surrounded by a capillary network, alveoli cluster to form lobules. Each lobule is drained by a lactiferous duct. The breast contains 15 to 20 lactiferous ducts, which merge at the nipple and areola to allow emptying of the breast.

Lactation—synthesis and secretion of breast milk—results from an interaction of several hormones. Alveolar growth and development is regulated by estrogen, progesterone, human placental lactogen (hPL), prolactin, cortisol, and insulin. Estrogen stimulates the release of prolactin and sensitizes the mammary gland to prolactin action. The profound drop in serum estrogen and progesterone levels after delivery of the placenta allows prolactin to stimulate lactogenesis (initiation of milk secretion) within the alveoli.

When the neonate sucks on the nipple, nerve endings in the areola transmit sensory messages to the hypothalamus. The anterior pituitary gland then increases the production of prolactin, which stimulates milk production.

When the patient chooses to bottle-feed her neonate, lactation can be suppressed. With suppression, absence of sucking and emptying of the breasts usually leads to breast involution and cessation of lactation within 1 week. No longer stimulated, alveolar cells flatten and stop secreting milk. Mammary blood flow decreases, leading to further involution. Over the next 3 months, connective and adipose tissue replaces some glandular tissue. As involution nears completion, the breasts typically resume their nonpregnancy size. However, a mild alteration in breast shape may be permanent.

Endocrine system

Like the reproductive system, the endocrine system undergoes profound postpartal changes. Many of these changes interrelate with those of the reproductive system.

Placental hormones

With delivery of the placenta, levels of circulating placental hormones drop rapidly. In the patient who is not breast-feeding, estrogen begins to rise to a normal level at approximately 2 weeks postpartum. In the breast-feeding patient, the rise is delayed, leading to such problems as temporary vaginal mucosal atrophy.

Serum progesterone falls below normal luteal-phase levels by the third postpartal day. After the first week, progesterone cannot be detected in the circulation until ovulation returns. Consequently, the first few postpartal menstrual cycles may be irregular and shorter than normal. The two remaining placental hormones—hPL and human chorionic gonadotropin (hCG)—also rapidly diminish.

Hypothalamic–pituitary–ovarian function

Resumption of the menstrual cycle is coordinated by hormones secreted by the hypothalamus (gonadotropin-releasing hormone [GnRH]), pituitary gland (follicle-stimulating hormone and luteininizing hormone), and ovaries (estrogen and progesterone).

Among patients who are not breast-feeding, the average time before the return of ovulation is about 10 weeks; menstruation typically resumes by 6 to 9 weeks. Thus, for most patients who are not breast-feeding, the first postpartal menstrual period may be anovulatory. Breast-feeding delays the return of a normal menstrual cycle; the length of the delay depends on breast-feeding duration and frequency.

Respiratory and cardiovascular systems

After delivery, the respiratory and cardiovascular systems exhibit few subjectively noticeable changes as they resume nonpregnancy status. The postpartal period typically brings complete resolution of pregnancy-related respiratory changes. Thus, associated complaints—such as shortness of breath, chest and rib discomfort, and decreased tolerance for physical exertion—resolve.

Reversal of significant anatomic changes

Full lung expansion returns and the rib cage regains a normal diameter. Cardiac enlargement and displacement reverse as the uterus resumes its normal size and position. Abnormal heart sounds—a result of the anatomic and hemodynamic changes caused by pregnancy—also resolve in the postpartal period.

Reversal of hemodynamic changes

Altered significantly by pregnancy, blood volume and cardiac output quickly resume a nonpregnancy status after delivery. Blood pressure and pulse undergo less dramatic changes.

Blood volume

Increased approximately 45% during pregnancy, blood volume drops sharply just after delivery. Within 4 weeks, it returns to a nonpregnancy level.

Blood pressure and pulse

Immediately after delivery, blood pressure readings should differ only slightly, if at all, from readings taken during the third trimester of pregnancy. A decrease may indicate uterine hemorrhage or excessive blood loss at delivery; an increase may signal a pre-eclamptic tendency, especially if accompanied by headache or visual changes.

For 7 to 10 days after delivery, transient bradycardia (a heart rate of 50 to 70 beats/minute) may occur. This finding is normal and may result from the decrease in cardiac work load that follows delivery. On the other hand, tachycardia (a heart rate above 100 beats/minute) warrants investigation because it may reflect hypovolemia—especially in a patient with a low red blood cell (RBC) count or a decreasing hemoglobin level.

Reversal of varicose conditions

Varicose conditions of the legs, anus (hemorrhoids), or vulva may arise during pregnancy from diminished venous return of the legs, pressure exerted by the fetus, and straining during labor and delivery. In many patients, these conditions improve significantly or regress completely after delivery.

Hematologic system

Levels of blood constituents may vary in the postpartal period. Coagulation, enhanced during pregnancy and delivery, normalizes gradually. However, coagulatory stimulation induced by labor and delivery increases the risk of thromboembolism in the early postpartum period.

Red blood cell parameters

Generally, for a patient who delivered vaginally without complications, hemoglobin level and hematocrit remain near predelivery levels despite normal blood loss at delivery. (This phenomenon results from hemoconcentration—packing of blood cells—which follows postpartal diuresis.) In a healthy patient with adequate nutrition, all RBC parameters typically will return to nonpregnancy levels by 6 weeks postpartum. A significant or progressive decrease in these parameters in the first few postpartal days is abnormal and may indicate excessive or continued blood loss.

A patient lacking the Rh factor (an antigenic substance usually found in RBCs) who delivers an Rh-positive neonate may become sensitized to the Rh antigen in neonatal RBCs; this could cause problems in subsequent pregnancies. An Rh-negative patient must therefore receive $Rh_O(D)$ immune globulin (RhoGAM) at 28 weeks' gestation and again within 72 hours after delivery.

White blood cell count

The WBC count increases in the first 10 to 12 days postpartum, possibly rising as high as $25,000/mm^3$ (the increase is mainly in granulocytes). Although this change reflects a normal stress response, it may complicate diagnosis of a postpartal infection, which also increases the WBC count.

Coagulation factor levels

Postpartal changes in coagulation factors are gradual. Throughout pregnancy, levels of coagulation factors I (fibrinogen), VII, IX, and X rise progressively; during late pregnancy, fibrinolysis (destruction of blood clots) diminishes. These circumstances place the pregnant patient at a progressively increasing risk for thromboembolic disorders.

Delivery stimulates the coagulation system, increasing this risk even further in the early postpartal period. The platelet count returns to a nonpregnancy level by 2 weeks postpartum. However, traumatic delivery, infection, or prolonged immobility may delay the return to normal levels.

Urinary system

Pregnancy affects both the anatomic structure of the urinary tract and the function of the urinary system; delivery may contribute to certain anatomic changes. Unlike most other body systems, the urinary system may show the effects of pregnancy and delivery well into—and even beyond—the postpartal period.

Reversal of anatomic changes

At delivery, fetal passage through the pelvis and vagina causes varying degrees of trauma to the urethra and bladder. A normal amount of trauma leads to edema and microscopic bleeding. Delivery complications (such as precipitous delivery or forceps instrumentation) may cause increased trauma. Especially when accompanied by anesthesia (particularly spinal or epidural anesthesia), delivery trauma may impair bladder tone. If this occurs, the bladder may lose sensitivity, resulting in a diminished voiding urge. This contributes to postpartal urine retention.

Postpartal diuresis may cause bladder overdistention, possibly resulting in muscle damage, atony, and urinary tract infection (from stasis and urine retention). Without such complications, however, the lower urinary tract resumes normal function within 1 or 2 weeks as edema and diuresis resolve, although bladder distention may persist for 3 months.

Urinalysis findings

Mild proteinuria, caused by excretion of protein byproducts of uterine involution, is common after delivery but should disappear by 6 weeks postpartum. Glycosuria, another common postpartal finding, usually resolves by the end of the first week.

Gastrointestinal system

No longer obstructed by the expanding uterus, and with hormone levels declining rapidly, the GI tract quickly resumes normal function after delivery.

Appetite

After vaginal delivery, most patients are extremely hungry from lack of food intake and the exertion of labor and delivery—especially if no anesthesia was used. Appetite tends to subside to a normal level in 1 to 2 days, although a breast-feeding patient may maintain an increased appetite and food intake while breast-feeding.

Bowel motility and evacuation

During pregnancy, GI motility is inhibited by the high serum progesterone level (which relaxes intestinal smooth muscle, decreasing peristalsis) and by increasing uterine size (which compresses the intestines).

With delivery resolving both factors, normal peristalsis and bowel function usually return rapidly.

Typically, bowel evacuation normalizes once bowel motility is restored. Nonetheless, the first bowel movement may be delayed until 2 to 3 days postpartum for reasons unrelated to intestinal function. Also, the patient may avoid bowel evacuation, fearing it will cause pain or damage the episiotomy. Residual dehydration from labor and the subsequent decrease in the fluid content of the stool also may impair bowel evacuation. In many cases, a stool softener, laxative, suppository, or enema must be used to reestablish normal bowel function.

Musculoskeletal system

Although pregnancy-related changes in the musculoskeletal system reverse after delivery, joints and muscles may show some residual effects.

Reversal of postural and joint changes
Delivery removes the mechanical strain on the musculoskeletal system and halts secretion of relaxin. Over the first 6 to 8 postpartal weeks, posture returns to normal and structural changes reverse gradually.

Reversal of muscular changes
During the third trimester, the rectus abdominis muscles may separate, causing diastasis recti abdominis. This condition sometimes can be corrected by postpartal abdominal exercises. However, it may persist indefinitely unless adequate muscle tone is restored. Poor abdominal muscle tone may contribute to back strain and complaints of low backache.

Integumentary system

Pregnancy-related skin changes resolve completely or partially after delivery as hormone levels decrease and the skin no longer is stretched.

Reversal of hormone-related changes
During the postpartal period, pigmentation changes caused by pregnancy—including chloasma (also called melasma, or mask of pregnancy) and linea nigra (a dark midline streak on the abdomen)—reverse gradually. However, they may never disappear completely.

Striae (stretch marks) result from increased corticosteroid levels and mechanical stretching of the skin during pregnancy. These harmless marks commonly appear over the abdomen, back, thighs, and breasts. As body size normalizes, striae shrink and fade from dark red to silvery-white within a year after delivery. Although they become less apparent, they never disappear completely.

Diaphoresis
In the first 2 to 3 days postpartum, many patients experience episodes of profuse diaphoresis (sweating). Associated with the postpartal fluid shift, diaphoresis is a normal mechanism that helps the renal system ex-

crete excess fluid and waste products. It should resolve within the first postpartal week.

STUDY ACTIVITIES

Short answer

1. Following her arrival to the postpartum unit, Josephine Burns, a 22-year-old multipara, requests "something for pain" and tells the nurse that she is having strong cramps that seem almost worse than labor pains. Ms. Burns notes that the pain increases after she breast-feeds her son. How could the nurse explain this?

_____

_____

2. While learning about anticipated postpartum changes during a childbirth education class, Jean DeSanto asks about lochial flow. She explains that a friend had experienced some serious problems from excessive bleeding after her recent delivery; Ms. DeSanto wonders what the signs of abnormal lochia would be. How could the nurse-educator respond?

_____

3. Upon receiving Janice Donohue, a 29-year-old primipara, from the recovery area of Labor and Delivery, the postpartum nurse conducts an initial postpartum assessment. Where should the nurse expect to palpate Ms. Donohue's uterus 2 hours after her normal vaginal delivery? Where would it be found on the first postpartum day?

_____

4. During postpartum discharge instructions, Michelle Ellicot, a 32-year-old para 2002 asks the nurse when her periods will return. She breast-fed her last child and did not get a period until she stopped nursing full time, 1 year postpartum. This time Ms. Ellicot has decided to bottle-feed her new son. How could the nurse answer her question?

_____

5. What are the normal parameters for the amount and duration of lochia for each distinct stage?

_____

_____

6. Describe the factors that might contribute to postpartal urine retention and its significance to nursing care during the early postpartum period.

_____

_____

7. Why do many postpartum patients experience episodes of profuse diaphoresis (sweating) during the early days after delivery?

_____

8. Which of the following postpartum changes are considered abnormal, requiring further medical evaluation?

A. The uterus palpated midway between the symphysis pubis and umbilicus at 2 weeks postpartum

_____

B. The presence of lochia rubra at the end of the first week postpartum

_____

C. A residual gaping of the introitus noted at the 6-week postpartum visit

_____

D. Breast milk leakage 3 months after delivery in a mother who is not breast-feeding

_____

E. Poor abdominal tone and accompanying complaints of low backache at 8 weeks postpartum

_____

True or false

9. Breast changes initiated during pregnancy—nipple and areola enlargement, maturation of lobes and ducts, increased vascularity-continue after delivery, particularly in the breast-feeding patient.
☐ True   ☐ False

10. Although sucking stimulates the hypothalamus, it is the anterior pituitary that increases prolactin, which stimulates milk production.
☐ True   ☐ False

11. The anatomic changes experienced in the cardiac and respiratory systems during pregnancy become permanent after delivery.
☐ True   ☐ False

12. Blood pressure is expected to decrease immediately after delivery and differ significantly from its level in the third trimester of pregnancy.
☐ True   ☐ False

13. Coagulatory stimulation induced by labor and delivery increases the risk of thromboembolism in the early postpartum period.
☐ True   ☐ False

14. As body size normalizes, striae (stretch marks) shrink and fade, eventually disappearing completely.
☐ True ☐ False

ANSWERS **Short answer**

1. Immediately after delivery, strong uterine contractions shrink the uterus to the size of a grapefruit—roughly half of its predelivery size. This rapid reduction in size forces the uterine walls into close proximity, causing the center of the cavity to flatten.

Myometrial contractions are irregular in both timing and strength. Usually a multiparous patient experiences stronger, more uncomfortable contractions because uterine muscles lose elasticity with each pregnancy. Also, a breast-feeding patient has stronger contractions because oxytocin, a hormone that helps regulate milk ejection, stimulates uterine muscles.

2. Although rates of lochial discharge may vary among patients, normal parameters for the amount and duration of each of its three stages have been established. Lochia would be considered abnormal if it contains large clots (as large or larger than a fifty-cent piece) or tissue fragments (pieces of tissue, not the tissue debris normal to lochial flow). Also lochia should not have a foul or offensive odor and should not relapse to a previous stage.

3. The nurse would expect to find the fundus of Ms. Donohue's uterus palpable at or just above the umbilicus. Each day thereafter, the uterus becomes smaller so that the fundus is palpable about one fingerbreadth lower than on the previous day. Thus, the first postpartum day, Ms. Donohue's uterus would be found one fingerbreadth below the umbilicus.

4. Breast-feeding commonly delays the return of a normal menstrual cycle; the length of the delay depends on breast-feeding duration and frequency. For those who are not breast-feeding, the average time before the return of menstruation is 6 to 9 weeks.

5. Lochia progresses through three stages, each with distinctive characteristics that reflect progressive endometrial healing. Lochia rubra usually lasts 1 to 4 days postpartum. It is bloody and may have some mucus, tissue debris, and small clots; it may have a slightly fleshy odor. Lochia serosa follows and lasts 5 to 7 days. It is pink-brown, serous, and odorless. Lochia alba usually lasts 1 to 3 postpartum weeks; it is creamy white, brown, or almost colorless and may have a slightly stale odor.

6. At delivery, fetal passage through the pelvis and vagina causes varying degrees of trauma to the urethra and bladder. A normal amount of trauma leads to edema and microscopic bleeding. Delivery complications (such as precipitous delivery or forceps instrumentation) may cause increased trauma.

Delivery trauma, especially when accompanied by anesthesia, may impair bladder tone. If this occurs, the bladder may lose sensitivity, resulting in a diminished voiding urge that contributes to postpartal urine retention. Also, postpartal diuresis may cause bladder overdistention, possible resulting in muscle damage, atony, and urinary tract infections (from stasis and urine retention).

7. Associated with the postpartal fluid shift, diaphoresis is a normal mechanism that helps the renal system excrete excess fluid and waste products. It should resolve within the first week.

8. A. By 2 weeks postpartum, the uterus should have returned to the pelvic cavity and no longer be palpable as an abdominal organ; B. The normal duration of lochia rubra is 1 to 4 days postpartum; D. With lactation suppression, absence of sucking and emptying of the breasts usually leads to breast involution and cessation of lactation within one week.

True or false

9. True.

10. True.

11. False. After delivery, the respiratory and cardiovascular systems exhibit few subjectively noticeable changes as they resume nonpregnancy status. Full lung expansion returns and the rib cage regains a normal diameter. Cardiac enlargement and displacement reverse as the uterus resumes its normal size and position. Abnormal heart sounds also resolve in the postpartal period.

12. False. Blood pressure readings should differ only slightly, if at all, from readings taken during the third trimester of pregnancy. A decrease may indicate uterine hemorrhage or excessive blood loss at delivery.

13. True.

14. False. Although striae shrink and fade, they never disappear completely. They become silvery-white within a year after delivery.

CHAPTER 15

Health promotion during postpartal adaptation

OBJECTIVES

After studying this chapter, the reader should be able to:

1. Identify the physiologic and psychosocial components of postpartal nursing care.

2. State the indications, actions, and dosages for specific medications commonly used in the postpartal period.

3. Discuss the phases of maternal adaptation to parenthood.

4. Discuss the importance of parent-infant bonding.

5. Describe the optimal conditions for parent-neonate interaction.

6. Identify appropriate parental responses to neonatal communication cues.

7. Describe the teaching needs of the new postpartum family on discharge.

OVERVIEW OF CONCEPTS

Caring for the postpartal patient offers the nurse an opportunity to promote a full and healthy recovery from delivery while helping the patient and her partner make an optimal adaptation to the birth of their child. As early discharge after delivery becomes increasingly common, skillful implementation of the nursing process takes on greater importance as a way for the nurse to meet the patient's physiologic, psychosocial, and teaching needs.

The birth of a child creates major changes in the family. Family members—especially the parents—must adjust to changes in their roles, tasks, and responsibilities. The family as a whole also must adapt to meet the demands of the dependent neonate and the changing needs of individual members.

Care of the postpartal patient

Nursing care during the postpartal period begins with a review of the patient's antenatal, labor, and delivery records. The postpartum nurse receives this information on the patient's transfer from the recovery area of Labor and Delivery. Throughout the patient's stay, the nurse conducts a nursing history, measures vital signs, and evaluates the status of all body systems. In addition, the nurse assesses the patient's and

Postpartal nursing history

A postpartum nursing assessment begins with a chart review. Evaluate the patient's antepartal and intrapartal courses for any risk factors or complications encountered. Document the number of hours or days postpartum. The nursing history should include the following areas:

- *Comfort.* Does the patient have pain or discomfort? Ask her to describe the type of pain, the location, and what makes it feel better.
- *Rest and sleep.* Has the patient been able to rest soundly since delivery? Is she experiencing any difficulties sleeping?
- *Ambulation.* Is the patient able to be fully ambulatory? How frequently is she up? Has she encountered any difficulties, such as dizziness?
- *Appetite.* Has the patient been able to eat since delivery? Is she experiencing any nausea, vomiting, or heartburn? Is she hungry? Is she getting adequate fluids?
- *Voiding.* Has the patient been voiding regularly since delivery? Ask her to describe frequency and amount and any pain (dysuria) or hesitancy encountered.
- *Bowel movements.* Has the patient had a bowel movement since delivery? Was it a normal amount and consistency? Was there any pain or bleeding?
- *Breast-feeding* (if appropriate). Is breast-feeding progressing well, or does she need assistance? Will she have help at home?
- *Additional concerns.* Does the patient have any questions or concerns about herself, her neonate, or others? What is her assessment of her childbirth experience and of her neonate?

family's psychosocial status. (See *Postpartal nursing history*.) After formulating nursing diagnoses, the planning and implementation of the postpartal care plan is instituted.

Assessment

Vital signs

Obtain complete vital signs—temperature, pulse, and respiratory rate—and measure blood pressure on the patient's arrival to the postpartum unit and every hour for the next 2 to 4 hours or until vital signs are stable. Thereafter, obtain vital signs every 4 hours until 24 hours after delivery, then every 8 hours until discharge.

Temperature. Measure the patient's temperature orally. A slight temperature elevation from mild dehydration, caused by labor and delivery, is common during the first 24 hours after delivery. However, suspect infection if the patient has a morbid temperature, defined by the Joint Committee on Maternal Welfare as one that exceeds 100.4° F (38° C) for 2 successive days after delivery, excluding the first 24 hours.

Pulse. During the first postpartal rest or sleep, which usually occurs 2 to 4 hours after delivery, the pulse rate typically decreases.
The hypervolemia of pregnancy protects the postpartal patient to some extent from the detrimental effects of blood loss during delivery. However, an abnormally rapid pulse (tachycardia) may be an early sign of excessive blood loss—especially if the pulse is thready and the patient

Postpartal hemorrhage

A leading cause of maternal mortality, postpartal hemorrhage demands prompt recognition and intervention to avert grave consequences. Postpartal hemorrhage stems from uterine atony, lacerations of the cervix or vagina, or disseminated intravascular coagulation.

The nurse who suspects hemorrhage should notify the physician or nurse-midwife immediately, then continually monitor the patient's vital signs, assess the condition of the uterus, and evaluate the amount and character of lochia. Refer to the chart below to help identify signs of postpartal hemorrhage and prepare for appropriate interventions.

Signs
- Boggy (soft, pliable) uterus
- Excessively large uterus located above the umbilicus at the midline (must be differentiated from a uterus displaced to the right, which results from bladder distention)
- Excessive lochia, possibly containing large blood clots with or without tissue fragments
- Lochia that flows in a steady trickle
- Increased pulse and respiratory rate with decreased blood pressure (may not arise until later, when shock occurs)

Nursing considerations
- Gently massage the uterus to stimulate contractions.
- Assess lochial flow to estimate the type and amount of blood loss and to detect any clots or tissue fragments. If lochia is bright red and flows in a slow trickle and the fundus is firm and located at the midline, suspect cervical or vaginal laceration as the cause of hemorrhage.
- Inspect for accumulated blood posterior to the perineum by turning the patient from side to side and checking for blood on bed sheets and the perineal pad.
- Rapidly infuse oxytocin I.V. or administer carboprost, ergonovine, or methylergonovine by I.M. injection, as prescribed and necessary.
- Place the patient in Trendelenburg's position to facilitate circulation to vital organs.

---

has such signs as pallor, an increased respiratory rate, and diaphoresis. (For more information, see *Postpartal hemorrhage.*)

Respiratory rate. Although the respiratory rate rarely changes significantly after delivery, it may drop slightly (along with the pulse rate) during the first postpartal sleep or if the patient received a narcotic during labor. Assess the patient's respiratory rate, rhythm, and depth. If the respiratory rate increases significantly, however, suspect uterine hemorrhage.

Blood pressure. Postpartal blood pressure should not differ significantly from the patient's average reading. A gradual but persistent drop in blood pressure suggests excessive blood loss. A persistent elevation, especially when accompanied by edema, proteinuria, headache, blurred vision, and hyperactive reflexes, suggests pregnancy-induced hypertension (PIH), a potentially life-threatening disorder. Although most common during the antepartal period, PIH sometimes arises after delivery.

To ensure prompt intervention, immediately report suspicious signs and symptoms to the physician.

Certain drugs used during labor and delivery or the postpartal period may affect blood pressure. For instance, oxytocin, ergonovine, and methylergonovine may increase blood pressure; bromocriptine, used to suppress lactation, may decrease it. (For a review of drugs commonly prescribed during the postpartal period, see *Drugs used during the postpartal period*.)

Reproductive system

Assessment of the reproductive system includes evaluating the patient's breasts, uterus, lochia, perineum, and rectum, which initially are assessed frequently after delivery. Once the patient is stabilized and transferred to the postpartum unit, these areas normally are assessed once during each eight-hour shift, until the patient is discharged.

The nurse must maintain strict principles of hygiene and infection control when performing postpartum assessments. Frequent hand washing while working from the patient's head to her extremities, from the cleanest to the most contaminated areas, will prevent potential infections during a vulnerable period for the new postpartum mother and neonate.

Breasts. With the patient supine and her bra removed, inspect the breasts for symmetry of size and shape. If the patient has chosen to breast-feed her neonate, colostrum initially will be secreted from the breasts.

By the second or third postpartal day, the breast-feeding patient should begin to feel fullness in her breasts and notice some release of mature milk when her breasts are stimulated or when she hears her neonate cry. Mature milk is bluish whereas colostrum is yellow. If the breasts are tense, warm, boardlike, and painful, suspect breast engorgement. Also inspect the nipples for erectility, cracking, and soreness.

Uterus. Assessment of the uterus helps in evaluating the expected progress of involution. Uterine muscle tone should be sufficient for muscles to compress vessels, thereby controlling bleeding.

To ensure accurate assessment of the uterus, ask the patient to void beforehand. Then locate the uterine fundus. Just after delivery, the fundus should be located midline at or slightly above the level of the umbilicus. Each day thereafter, it should descend about one fingerbreadth toward the symphysis pubis until about the tenth postpartal day, when it is no longer palpable as an abdominal organ. Next, assess the consistency of the uterus. It should feel firm; a soft, pliable (boggy) uterus indicates uterine atony (poor muscle tone).

If the patient had a cesarean delivery, take great care when assessing the uterus. With a slow, gentle motion, palpate the abdomen toward the uterus, avoiding sutures or staples. Inspect the incision site every 15 minutes for the first hour, once an hour for the next 4 hours, then at least once every 8 hours. Evaluate the site for color, warmth,

Drugs used during the postpartal period

This chart summarizes the major drugs currently used during the postpartal period.

DRUG	MAJOR INDICATIONS	USUAL ADULT DOSAGES	NURSING IMPLICATIONS
bromocriptine (Parlodel)	Prevention of postpartal lactation	2.5 mg by mouth (P.O.) twice daily with meals for 14 to 21 days	• Monitor blood pressure. Transient hypotension may occur during the first 3 days of therapy. • Check for seizure activity. • Advise the patient to use contraceptive methods other than oral contraceptives during treatment. • Warn the patient to use caution when ambulating. • Do not initiate therapy sooner than 4 hours after delivery and not until signs have stabilized.
carboprost (Prostin/M15)	Postpartal hemorrhage from uterine atony that does not respond to conventional management	250 mcg deep I.M.; may repeat dose at 15- to 90-minute intervals; maximum total dosage should not exceed 2 mg	• Obtain vital signs; assess the amount and character of lochia and the condition of the fundus. • Administer cautiously to the patient with cervical lacerations. • Watch for adverse gastrointestinal (GI) effects. • Do not administer I.V.
codeine	Mild to moderate postpartal pain	15 to 60 mg P.O. every 3 to 4 hours as needed (usually given with 325 to 650 mg of acetaminophen)	• Monitor respiratory and circulatory status and bowel function. • Observe the patient for drowsiness; make sure she is alert when caring for her neonate.
diphenhydramine (Benadryl)	Night-time sedation	25 to 50 mg P.O. at bedtime	• Observe the patient for drowsiness; make sure she is alert when caring for her neonate. • Assess the patient for nausea and dry mouth.
docusate sodium (Colace)	Stool softener	50 to 300 mg P.O. daily or until bowel movements are normal	• Assess the patient for bowel activity, mild abdominal cramping, and diarrhea.
ergonovine maleate (Ergotrate Maleate)	Prevention or treatment of postpartal hemorrhage from uterine atony or subinvolution	0.2 mg I.M. every 2 to 4 hours to a maximum of 5 doses; after initial I.M. dose, may give 0.2 to 0.4 mg P.O. every 5 to 12 hours for 2 to 7 days	• Monitor blood pressure, pulse rate, and uterine response. Report sudden changes in vital signs, frequent periods of uterine relaxation, and any change in the character or amount of lochia. • Contractions begin 5 to 15 minutes after P.O. administration, 2 to 5 minutes after I.M. injection. They may continue 3 hours or more after P.O. or I.M. administration.
ibuprofen (Motrin)	Mild to moderate postpartal pain	400 mg P.O. every 4 to 6 hours	• Assess the patient for signs and symptoms of GI irritation, such as nausea, vomiting, diarrhea, and gastric discomfort. • Warn the patient not to take more than 1.2 g/day without consulting her physician.

(continued)

Drugs used during the postpartal period (continued)

DRUG	MAJOR INDICATIONS	USUAL ADULT DOSAGES	NURSING IMPLICATIONS
meperidine (Demerol)	Moderate to severe postpartal pain (such as after cesarean delivery)	50 to 100 mg P.O., I.M., or subcutaneously (S.C.) every 3 to 4 hours; or by continuous I.V. infusion, 15 to 35 mg/hour as needed or around the clock	• Monitor the patient's pulse rate. • Check for signs of central nervous system (CNS) depression, such as drowsiness or lethargy. Make sure the patient is alert when caring for her neonate. • Assess the patient's pain level. • To avoid toxic metabolites, give the smallest effective dosage.
methylergonovine (Methergine)	Prevention and treatment of postpartal hemorrhage from uterine atony or subinvolution	0.2 mg I.M. every 2 to 4 hours for a maximum of 5 doses; after the initial I.M. dose, may give 0.2 to 0.4 mg P.O. every 6 to 12 hours for 2 to 7 days	• Monitor and record blood pressure, pulse rate, and uterine response. Report any sudden change in vital signs, frequent periods of uterine relaxation, and any change in lochia. • Decrease the dosage if severe cramping occurs. • Contractions begin 5 to 15 minutes after P.O. administration, 2 to 5 minutes after I.M. injection. They continue 3 hours or more.
morphine	Severe pain (such as after cesarean delivery)	4 to 15 mg S.C. or I.M.; may be injected by slow I.V. infusion (over 4 to 5 minutes) diluted in 4 to 5 ml of water for injection	• Monitor for respiratory depression and hypotension. • Check for signs of CNS depression. Make sure the patient is alert when caring for her neonate. • Drug may be injected into the epidural space for prolonged pain relief. Monitor the patient for delayed respiratory depression. • If the patient has pruritus after I.V. or epidural administration, expect to give antihistamines.
oxytocin (Pitocin)	Reduction of postpartal bleeding after expulsion of the placenta	1 to 4 ml (10 to 40 units) in 1,000 ml of dextrose 5% in water or normal saline solution I.V., infused at a rate necessary to control bleeding (usually 20 to 40 mU/minute; or 10 units I.M.	• Administer by I.V. infusion, not I.V. bolus injection. • Record uterine contractions, heart rate, and blood pressure every 15 minutes. • Assess the amount and character of lochia and the condition of the fundus. • Check for increased pulse rate in response to pain from contractions.
simethicone (Mylicon)	Flatulence, functional gastric bloating (such as after cesarean delivery)	40 to 80 mg after each meal and at bedtime	• Make sure the patient chews tablets thoroughly. • Assess the patient for bowel activity and abdominal distention.

edema, discharge, degree of approximation (distance between the edges of the incision), and the condition of sutures, staples, dressing, or supportive abdominal binder.

Lochia. After the patient has delivered, lochia should begin to flow from the vagina. Assess the type and amount of lochia (see *Stages of lochia* in Chapter 14, Physiology of the postpartal period). Lochia should never contain large clots, tissue fragments, or membranes. A foul odor may signal infection (as may absence of lochia). If the patient has a heavy lochial flow, begin a pad count to determine the amount of discharge more precisely. Record the number of pads used and the degree of saturation of each pad.

Perineum. An episiotomy or perineal laceration should appear to be healing with no exudate; the site should be clean and not excessively tender. Assess the approximation of the incision or wound for such abnormalities as redness, warmth, tenderness, edema, ecchymosis, discharge, and hemorrhoids. If the perineum is ecchymotic, extremely painful, and grossly discolored, with a collection of blood under the skin surface, suspect a hematoma and report this to the physician or nurse-midwife.

Rectum. Inspect the rectal area for hemorrhoids, which may cause redness, discomfort, and itching. Hemorrhoids may arise during pregnancy or from the expulsive effort of labor and delivery. Usually, they disappear in the first few postpartal weeks. Document the presence of hemorrhoids and any associated signs and symptoms.

Urinary system

Assessment of urinary elimination patterns is a key component of postpartal nursing assessment. After delivery, the bladder may fill rapidly from postpartal diuresis.

Despite rapid urine production and bladder filling in the early postpartum period, many patients have difficulty voiding. The patient with severe perineal and urethral discomfort may not be able to relax the perineal muscles sufficiently to void; in the postcesarean patient or a patient who received regional anesthesia, the bladder may lack sensitivity to pressure, impairing the urge to void. Failure to void within 6 to 8 hours after delivery may cause excessive uterine bleeding because bladder distention prevents sufficient uterine contraction.

Once the patient is ambulatory and can perform satisfactory self-care, determine her urine output pattern. Ask if she is experiencing urinary frequency, burning, or urgency.

Circulatory system

The postpartal patient may be predisposed to thromboembolic disease as a result of the hypercoagulability caused by decreased plasma volume after delivery. To check for this condition, which most often affects the lower extremities as thrombophlebitis, have the patient lie supine with both legs extended. Inspect the legs for symmetry of shape and size, and palpate the thighs and calves to detect areas of warmth, edema, tenderness, redness, or hardness. Attempt to elicit Homans' sign (pain in the calf when the foot is dorsiflexed).

Neurologic system

If the patient complains of headache, try to determine the onset, intensity, duration, and location of the headache and find out if any specific factors seem to trigger or relieve it. Check for other signs and symptoms associated with PIH—edema, proteinuria, blurred vision, decreased blood pressure, and hyperactive reflexes.

In a patient who received some types of regional anesthesia, such as a spinal block, headache may result from loss of cerebrospinal fluid through the dural puncture site—a condition called postspinal headache. During the first 4 hours after delivery, the patient who received regional anesthesia should regain full sensory and motor function.

Gastrointestinal system

Assess the patient's progress toward establishing normal bowel function and document this progress daily. Bowel sounds generally resume gradually the first postpartum day. Postcesarean patients may have diminished bowel sounds accompanied by abdominal distention and lack of peristalsis.

Assess abdominal shape, consistency, and tone. During the postpartal period, the abdomen typically is nontender, slightly distended, and soft, with poor muscle tone. The abdomen has become so stretched during pregnancy that the rectus abdominis muscles, which lie vertically, side by side, separate at the midline. This condition, called diastasis recti abdomina, rarely warrants treatment.

Hematologic system

Usually, a complete blood count is performed 24 to 48 hours after delivery. Typically, the white blood cell (WBC) count is elevated, sometimes reaching 25,000/mm^3—especially if the patient had a prolonged labor. Consequently, an elevated WBC count is not a reliable marker of postpartal infection. However, when accompanied by other potential infection signs, an infection should be ruled out.

Compare the postpartal hemoglobin level and hematocrit to the corresponding predelivery levels. If the postpartal hemoglobin level is more than 3 g/dl below the predelivery level, the patient is at risk for anemia; if it is 5 g/dl or more below the predelivery level, suspect heavy blood loss.

Immune system

Detection of postpartal infection is a primary nursing concern. In most cases, such infection involves the reproductive system. Besides regularly assessing the patient's temperature, observe closely for subtle signs and symptoms of infection, such as chills, malaise, and pallor. Also review the patient's chart for risk factors for puerperal infection, such as prolonged labor, prolonged time since rupture of the membranes, vaginal or cervical lacerations, and retention of placental fragments.

NURSING DIAGNOSES

Postpartal patient

The following are potential nursing diagnoses for problems and etiologies that the nurse may encounter when caring for a patient during the postpartal period. Specific nursing interventions for many of these diagnoses are provided in *Postpartum planning and implementation,* pages 244 and 245.
• Altered urinary elimination related to perineal and urethral edema and ecchymosis
• Anxiety related to new role development
• Constipation related to poor intestinal tone, diminished food intake, and immobility
• High risk for injury related to blood loss, fatigue, limited food intake, or medication effects
• Impaired skin integrity related to the perineal wound
• Ineffective breathing pattern related to immobility following cesarean delivery
• Knowledge deficit related to self-care or parenting skills
• Pain related to the perineal wound, uterine contractions, or breast engorgement

---

The patient who received regional anesthesia has an increased risk of infection because of the invasive administration route used. Carefully and regularly inspected the spinal or epidural site for redness, warmth, edema, pain, and tenderness; promptly report any of these signs to the physician.

Review the patient's chart to assess her Rh status (to determine the potential for isoimmunization) and rubella status (to determine her immunity for future pregnancy protection).

Nursing diagnoses
After gathering assessment data, review it carefully to identify pertinent nursing diagnoses for the patient. (For a partial list of applicable diagnoses, see Nursing Diagnoses: *Postpartal patient.*)

Planning and implementation
After assessing the patient and formulating nursing diagnoses, develop and implement a plan of care. (See *Postpartum planning and implementation,* pages 244 and 245.)

During discharge teaching it is imperative that the patient be advised to report any postpartal warning signs to her health care provider. These could herald the onset of serious complications during the postpartal period; they warrant further medical assessment and treatment as soon as possible, prior to her follow-up visit 6 weeks after delivery. (For details, see *Postpartal warning signs,* page 246.)

Evaluation
The following examples illustrate appropriate evaluation statements for the postpartal patient:
• The patient's uterus remained firm and was involuting normally on discharge.
• The patient had a normal lochial flow with no large clots, tissue fragments, or membranes.

Postpartum planning and implementation

Below are appropriate nursing goals with nursing interventions.

GOAL	NURSING INTERVENTIONS
Ensure safety	• Assist the patient out of bed and provide instructions on use of bed rails. • Advise the patient to avoid sleeping with the neonate in bed to avoid a fall. • If the patient has impaired motor or sensory function from anesthesia or analgesia, assess functional ability prior to allowing her to leave the bed for the first time.
Provide for adequate rest and sleep	• Promote adequate rest to facilitate recovery and healing. Limit phone calls and visitors, if necessary.
Provide for sufficient nutrition and fluids	• Provide nourishment as soon as the patient is stable and hungry after delivery, regardless of the time of day. A light meal is recommended, and increased oral fluids are especially important to reduce the potential for dehydration or infection. • Teach the patient about dietary sources of iron, and administer iron supplementation. • Monitor for signs of intolerance to low hemoglobin levels (tachycardia, shortness of breath, headache).
Promote self breast care for breast-feeding mothers	• Facilitate successful breast-feeding by encouraging feedings every 2 to 4 hours, helping the patient develop proper nursing techniques, and providing information or resources for the patient's enhanced understanding and support. • Encourage good hand washing, nipple and breast care, and the wearing of a good support bra.
Ensure lactation suppression, as indicated	• Encourage the patient to wear a snug support bra or breast binder and to avoid any stimulation of the breasts and nipples. • Administer bromocriptine, as ordered.
Promote uterine involution and prevent hemorrhage	• Encourage the patient to void within the first 4 to 8 hours. Failure to void within 8 hours or bladder distension necessitate catheterization. • Provide and teach the patient gentle uterine massage to help restore firm tone. • If necessary, administer oxytocin to ensure uterine tone.
Relieve uterine discomfort	• Administer a mild analgesic or a nonsteroidal anti-inflammatory drug, as ordered. • Encourage frequent voiding to avoid bladder distension and cramping.
Reduce perineal discomfort	• Initially apply an ice pack to the perineum, followed by warm sitz baths, and a topical spray or perineal cream with an anesthetic or witch hazel pads. • If necessary, administer a mild analgesic to reduce perineal discomfort. • Stress the importance of perineal hygiene, especially after voiding or bowel movements.
Alleviate hemorrhoidal discomfort	• Apply witch hazel pads or an anesthetic or steroid cream. • Administer antihemorrhoidal suppositories to help relieve discomfort. • If ordered, instruct the patient to lie on her side and to take sitz baths. Administer a mild analgesic.
Promote bladder and bowel function	• Encourage early ambulation to the bathroom with assistance. If the patient is confined to bed, offer a bedpan. • Provide increased fluids. • Irrigate the perineum while guarding against bladder distention with delayed voiding. • Promote a high-fiber diet, encourage relaxation during bowel movements, and provide a stool softener or a rectal suppository to promote bowel evacuation.

Postpartum planning and implementation *(continued)*

GOAL	NURSING INTERVENTIONS
Ensure sound immunologic status	• Monitor closely for signs of infection and prevent dehydration. • Institute measures to improve nutritional status and healing. • If the neonate is Rh-positive and the patient is Rh-negative, administer Rh immune globulin (RhoGAM) within 72 hours of delivery. • Administer a rubella vaccine prior to discharge, as ordered.
Implement patient discharge teaching	• Focus on the patient's self-care as well as neonatal care. The former should include such topics as postpartal danger signs, rest, nutrition, postpartum exercises, resumption of sexual activity, family planning methods, community resources, and referrals for postpartum follow-up visits at 4 to 6 weeks. (See *Postpartal warning signs*, page 246.)
Special post-operative measures	
Enhance respiratory capacity	• Monitor the patient's respiratory rate and effort. • Encourage her to cough and deep-breathe hourly and to turn from side to side every 1 to 2 hours to promote oxygenation. • Teach the patient incentive spirometry, if ordered, to facilitate full lung expansion and mobilize secretions.
Alleviate abdominal distention and flatus accumulation	• Encourage slow resumption of oral intake—beginning with ice chips and progressing to a liquid, then regular diet—and early ambulation to promote resumption of normal bowel activity and subsequent flatus expulsion. • Administer oral simethicone, if ordered, to reduce flatus formation and abdominal distention. Also administer rectal suppositories to promote bowel activity. • If necessary, assist with rectal tube insertion to help expel flatus.

• The patient demonstrated adequate healing of the episiotomy, with no exudate.
• The patient can state when to return to her nurse-midwife or physician for the postpartal examination.

Documentation

Thorough documentation not only allows the nurse to evaluate the effectiveness of the care plan, but it also makes this information available to other members of the health care team, helping to ensure consistency of care. Documentation for the postpartal patient should include:

• vital sign trends
• physical findings from the examination of the breasts, abdomen, and extremities
• location and condition of the fundus
• amount, color, and consistency of lochia
• appearance of the perineum, episiotomy, or surgical incision
• bowel and bladder elimination status
• patient's comfort level and any necessary interventions to improve it

Postpartal warning signs

During the discharge teaching, the nurse reinforces the importance of the patient informing the physician or nurse-midwife promptly if the following conditions occur:
• Heavy vaginal bleeding or passage of clots or tissue fragments
• A fever of 100.2° F or higher
• A red, warm, painful area in either breast or nipple
• Excessive breast tenderness not relieved by a support bra, analgesia, or warm compresses
• Nausea and vomiting, severe headache
• Pain on urination or voiding only small amounts of urine
• A warm, red, tender area on either leg, especially the calf

---

• patient's activity level and rest and sleep patterns
• nature of the patient's interaction with the neonate
• patient teaching provided and the patient's understanding of this teaching

Transition to parenthood

Parenting is a complex process encompassing various tasks, attitudes, and responsibilities through which an adult takes on the care of a dependent child. The parent-child dyad is the most basic and complex relationship within the family, profoundly affecting the child's development.

Psychosocial status

The postpartal nurse has a unique opportunity to assess the patient's and her partner's response to childbirth and to evaluate their interaction with the neonate.

Initial psychosocial assessment focuses on the patient. Eventually, the nurse broadens the assessment to include the father and other family members.

Evaluating maternal emotional status

The patient's emotional status can affect her interaction with the neonate and her adaptation to her role. The patient's mood, attitude, energy level, feelings about the childbirth experience, level of confidence in caregiving, and sense of satisfaction with her neonate influence her emotional status.

A patient who feels overwhelmed by becoming a mother may seem withdrawn. With such a patient, check for other signs that indicate a potential for maladaptive parenting, such as depression, low self-esteem, lack of support, and a seeming preoccupation with physical discomfort.

Evaluate for signs and symptoms of postpartal "blues," such as crying spells, irritability, insomnia, and poor appetite. The nurse who detects postpartal emotional problems should expect the patient to be referred to a counselor, psychiatric nurse clinician, or psychiatrist for early treatment.

Parental adaptation

As parents begin their relationship with the neonate, adjustments must be made to family relationships, interactions, and lifestyle. The adjustments each parent makes influence the welfare of the family as a whole.

Maternal adaptation

Many factors affect the mother's adaptation to the birth of a child. Energy level, attitude, degree of confidence in care-giving skills, and psychological status can help or hinder adaptation. Rubin, one of the first nurses to study parental behavior, identified three distinct phases of behavior that occur as a woman adapts to the parental role. These phases move from "taking in" to "taking hold" to "letting go" and establish a progressive framework for understanding early maternal adaptation behaviors.

Paternal adaptation

The father's role and tasks within the family have evolved to include more active participation in child care and nurturing. Fathers use the same progressive touching pattern typical of mothers. Also, they tend to talk rapidly in response to such neonatal behaviors as vocalization, whereas mothers are more likely to touch the neonate. When both parents are with the neonate, the father touches, vocalizes, and holds the neonate more than the mother does but smiles at the neonate less.

Acquaintance, attachment, and bonding

The development of a healthy parent-child relationship in the early postpartal days and weeks increases the chance for optimal child growth and development. Poor attachment and bonding can lead to such disorders as vulnerable child syndrome, child abuse, failure to thrive, and a disturbed parent-child relationship.

During the immediate postpartal period, parents and neonate typically become acquainted—they interact to gain information about each other. Acquaintance behaviors include eye contact, touching, verbalizing, and exploring. Acquaintance is a prerequisite of attachment and bonding—terms now used interchangeably to describe the process in which parent and child form an enduring relationship.

Parent-neonate interaction

Positive interaction between the parents and neonate promotes healthy bonding. Such interaction depends on the ability of both parties to send, receive, and interpret messages correctly.

Neonatal attentiveness and temperament

A neonate who is attentive and responsive rewards the parent's interactive efforts; this in turn encourages the parent to continue such interaction. Thus, the more attentive and responsive the neonate, the more frequently the parent will interact. Temperament also plays a part. A neonate who smiles frequently, eats well, is easy to console, and remains alert for long periods is more pleasant to interact with than one who is irritable and hard to console.

Communication cues and reciprocity

Parental sensitivity to neonatal cues is essential to the developing parent-child relationship. Parents typically vary in their ability to interpret neonatal cues and respond appropriately. Communication cues can be verbal or nonverbal. Verbal cues used by neonates include crying and cooing; nonverbal cues include reaching movements, facial expressions, staring, and gaze aversion.

The process by which the neonate gives cues and the parent interprets and responds to these cues is known as reciprocity. Through reciprocity, the interaction is maintained and the parent-neonate relationship develops. Reciprocity may take several weeks to develop.

Verbal communication and entrainment

At first, parent-neonate communication takes on unique qualities. To soothe a neonate, parents frequently speak softly and slowly; to gain the neonate's attention, they use fast, high-pitched speech.

Healthy neonates move in rhythm with adult speech. This phenomenon, known as entrainment, is essential to parent-infant bonding, rewarding the parent and encouraging further communication. Entrainment continues as the child learns speech.

Promoting parental psychosocial adaptation

During the early postpartum period, the nurse has an opportunity to assist the new mother and her partner in adjusting to their new roles. Encourage the new parents to express their feelings—both positive and negative—about the childbirth experience, their neonate, and their expectations of parenthood and of each other. This helps prepare them for new parenthood and for future pregnancies. Provide positive feedback whenever possible and enhance the parent's sense of confidence and competence in neonatal caregiving.

Encourage the new parents to attend infant care classes, or provide instructions on bathing, feeding, and diapering. Support groups for new parents also help smooth the transitions at home. Special arrangements can be made to include any siblings in classes to help them prepare for their new role adjustments.

Nursing diagnoses

The following are potential nursing diagnoses for problems and etiologies that the nurse may encounter when caring for the family of a patient during the postpartal period. Specific nursing interventions for many of these diagnoses are provided in *Postpartum planning and implementation*, pages 244 and 245.

• Family coping: potential for growth, related to the birth of a new family member

- Ineffective individual coping related to parenting tasks and responsibilities
- Knowledge deficit related to parenting tasks, infant care, and community resources
- Parental role conflict related to the birth of a new family member.

Evaluation

The following examples illustrate appropriate evaluation statements for the postpartal patient:

- The patient showed positive interaction with the neonate.
- The patient has responded appropriately to neonatal communication cues.
- The patient showed increasing proficiency and confidence in caregiving skills.

Documentation

Thorough documentation not only allows the nurse to evaluate the effectiveness of the care plan, but it also makes this information available to other members of the health care team, helping to ensure consistency of care. Documentation of nursing care for the postpartal family should include:

- the quality of parent-neonate interaction
- the patient's ability to interpret and respond appropriately to neonatal communication cues
- the patient's emotional status, including any signs of postpartal depression
- the patient's caregiving skills.

STUDY ACTIVITIES

Short answer

1. Erin O'Neill, a 22-year-old primipara, delivered her daughter Sarina 14 hours ago by normal vaginal delivery. The nurse noted on her chart that Ms. O'Neill had a normal labor and delivery with a midline episiotomy and a 350 cc blood loss. No risk factors had been identified during her pregnancy or delivery, and her early postpartum course was uneventful. She is breast-feeding her neonate. Ms. O'Neill reports she had a good night's sleep and she has been up to the bathroom without assistance, voiding without difficulties. What other parameters should the nurse assess in order to complete this nursing history on the first postpartum day?

2. Keisha Taylor, a 16-year-old primigravida, appears very self-absorbed and withdrawn to the nurse conducting her initial postpartum assessment. She is 3 hours postpartum after an 18-hour labor and seems interested only in talking about the delivery. Ms. Taylor's mother, her support person in labor, admits to being unsure of her daughter's feelings about being a new mother. Ms. Taylor has never taken care of babies before. What factors commonly affect a new mother's adaptation to the birth of a child?

_____

3. Briefly discuss comfort measures that would be used to achieve the postpartum nursing goal of "reduced perineal discomfort."

_____

4. What topics should the postpartum nurse include during patient discharge teaching?

_____

5. List the postpartum warning signs that must be reinforced when the nurse completes the discharge teaching with a new mother.

_____

_____

Multiple choice

6. What is the most likely reason for a temperature of 99.8° F during the first 24 hours postpartum?
  A. Puerperal infection
  B. Mastitis
  C. Dehydration
  D. Chorioamnionitis

7. Certain drugs used during the postpartal period may affect blood pressure. Which drug would decrease a postpartum patient's blood pressure?
  A. Oxytocin
  B. Bromocriptine
  C. Ergonovine
  D. Methylergonovine

8. In the early postpartum period prior to the patient's discharge, the nurse should expect to palpate the fundus:
  A. Above the symphysis pubis
  B. Halfway between the symphysis and the umbilicus
  C. At the umbilicus
  D. Three fingerbreadths above the umbilicus

9. Normal lochial findings in the first 24 hours include:
  A. Bright red blood
  B. Large clots or tissue fragments
  C. A foul odor
  D. The complete absence of lochia

True or false

10. If the perineum is ecchymotic, extremely painful, and grossly discolored, with a collection of blood under the surface, a hematoma should be suspected.

□ True   □ False

11. Failure to void within 6 to 8 hours after delivery may cause excessive uterine bleeding because bladder distention prevents sufficient uterine contraction.

□ True   □ False

12. Methergine, used in the prevention and treatment of postpartal hemorrhage from uterine atony or subinvolution, can be administered I.M., I.V., or by mouth.

□ True   □ False

13. The process by which the neonate gives cues and the parent interprets and responds to these cues is known as attachment.

□ True   □ False

ANSWERS   **Short answer**

1. The nursing history also should include assessment of the patient's comfort, appetite, difficulties with breast-feeding, bowel movements, and any concerns that Ms. O'Neill might have about herself, her daughter, or others.

2. A new mother's energy level, attitude, degree of confidence in caregiving skills, and psychological status can help or hinder her adaptation to the birth of a child.

3. To reduce the perineal discomfort for a perineal laceration or an episiotomy, the nurse initially applies an ice pack to the perineum, followed by warm sitz baths, a topical spray or anesthetic cream for the perineum, or witch hazel pads. A mild analgesia also may reduce perineal discomfort. In addition, perineal hygiene is stressed, especially after voiding or having a bowel movement.

4. When implementing patient discharge teaching with a postpartum patient, the nurse should focus on the patient's self-care as well as neonatal care. The former should include such topics as postpartal danger signs, rest, nutrition, postpartum exercises, resumption of sexual activity, family planning methods, community resources, and referrals for postpartum follow-up visits at 4 to 6 weeks.

5. During the discharge teaching, the nurse reinforces the importance of the patient informing the physician or nurse-midwife promptly if the following conditions occur: heavy vaginal bleeding or passage of clots or tissue fragments; a fever of 100.2° F or higher; a red, warm, painful area in either breast or nipple; excessive breast tenderness not relieved by a support bra, analgesia, or warm compresses; nausea and vomiting, or a severe headache; pain on urination or voiding only small amounts of urine; and a warm, red, tender area on either leg, especially the calf.

Multiple choice

6. C. A slight temperature elevation from dehydration is common during the first 24 hours after delivery.

7. B. Bromocriptine used to suppress lactation can cause a decrease in blood pressure.

8. C. The uterus should be palpated at the level of the umbilicus.

9. A. Lochia should never contain large clots, tissue fragments, or membranes. A foul odor may signal infection, as may absence of lochia.

True or false

10. True.

11. True.

12. False. Methergine can be safely administered only I.M. or by mouth and is never given I.V.

13. False. Attachment and bonding are used interchangeably to describe the process in which parent and child form an enduring relationship. Reciprocity is the process by which the neonate gives cues and the parents interpret them.

CHAPTER 16

Selected postpartal complications

OBJECTIVES

After studying this chapter, the reader should be able to:

1. Recognize signs and symptoms of selected postpartum complications and initiate appropriate nursing measures in order to reduce risks of further complications.

2. Identify the major causes of puerperal infection.

3. Discuss the nursing assessment that is essential to distinguish between uterine atony and birth canal injuries.

4. Explain the potential for developing urinary tract infections during the early postpartum period and their significance to a patient's recovery.

5. Identify the assessment data that suggest thrombophlebitis and its potentially life-threatening complication, a pulmonary embolism.

6. Describe the patient teaching to prevent mastitis in a breast-feeding mother.

7. Discuss nursing considerations for a diabetic patient during the postpartum period.

8. List the nursing measures to be instituted for a postpartum patient suspected of developing pregnancy-induced hypertension.

9. Describe the postpartal care needs of a substance-abusing patient.

OVERVIEW OF CONCEPTS

The first 6 weeks of the postpartal period is a time of significant physiologic and psychological stress. Fatigue caused by labor, blood loss during delivery, and other conditions brought on by childbirth can cause complications—some of them critical—in the postpartal patient. Prevention of such complications is a major focus of nursing care. Once a complication occurs, of course, the nurse must work to promote the patient's recovery and ensure that the problem does not jeopardize the developing mother-neonate relationship.

Puerperal infection

Puerperal infection—an infection of the reproductive tract occurring during the postpartal period—is a leading cause of childbearing-associated death throughout the world. Childbirth reduces resistance to infec-

Types of puerperal infection

A puerperal infection develops from a local lesion or its extension. With a local lesion, the infection remains within the original infection site. The vagina, the cervix, a hematoma, an episiotomy, and any laceration of the vulva, vagina, or perineum are potential entry points for pathogenic organisms. An operative incision (as in a cesarean delivery) also may be the source of infection; the morbidity rate from puerperal infection is two to four times higher after cesarean than after vaginal delivery.

Extension occurs when a localized infection spreads to other areas via the blood or lymphatic vessels, leading to such infections as endometritis salpingitis, parametritis, peritonitis, or thrombophlebitis. Postpartal extension infections such as parametritis, peritonitis, or thrombophlebitis may lead to systemic infection of the bloodstream, resulting in bacteremic shock. In this condition, vascular resistance decreases, causing a severe blood pressure decline and the threat of imminent death. Bacteremic shock most frequently stems from gram-negative organisms.

Assessment

Review the patient's history for risk factors (see *Risk factors for puerperal infection*). Because puerperal infection is associated with temperature elevation, monitor vital signs regularly. Suspect an infection if the patient has a morbid temperature, defined by the Joint Committee on Maternal Welfare as one that exceeds 100.4° F (38° C) for 2 successive days after delivery, excluding the first 24 hours.

Complaints of chills, malaise, anorexia, or vomiting with generalized pain or discomfort are signs and symptoms that commonly accompany infection. Assess the postpartum patient for lower abdominal pain or uterine tenderness as well as severe afterpains. Assess uterine tone and fundal height and evaluate lochial discharge, noting the amount, color, consistency, and odor. Also obtain information about the patient's sleep and rest patterns, hydration, and nutritional status.

Laboratory analysis typically reveals an elevated white blood cell count and an increased erythrocyte sedimentation rate if infection is present. Blood and vaginal cultures may be ordered to isolate the causative organism.

For a localized wound infection, inspect for localized areas of edema, erythema, and tenderness; purulent drainage; gaping of wound edges; and dysuria. Stay alert for complaints of pain in a specific area. Lochial evaluation is very important.

Nursing diagnoses

After gathering all of the assessment data, review it carefully to identify pertinent nursing diagnoses for the patient. (For a partial list of applicable diagnoses, see Nursing Diagnoses: *Postpartal complications,* page 256.)

Planning and implementation

Prevention is the best intervention for puerperal infections. Careful aseptic technique, especially thorough hand washing, is crucial. To prevent cross-

Risk factors for puerperal infection

The nurse should stay alert for signs and symptoms of infection in a postpartal patient with any of the risk factors presented below.

Prenatal risk factors
- History of venous thrombosis
- Anemia
- Poor nutrition
- Lack of prenatal care

Intrapartal risk factors
- Numerous vaginal examinations during labor, especially after rupture of the membranes
- Intrauterine fetal monitoring
- Prolonged labor
- Prolonged rupture of membranes
- Chorioamnionitis (inflammation of the amniotic membranes)
- Episiotomy
- Lacerations of the vaginal wall or perineum
- Operative procedures (forceps or cesarean delivery)
- Manual removal of placenta

Postpartal risk factors
- Inadequate infection control
- Postpartal hemorrhage
- Retained placental fragments

Nursing diagnoses

After gathering all of the assessment data, review it carefully to identify pertinent nursing diagnoses for the patient. (For a partial list of applicable diagnoses, see Nursing Diagnoses: *Postpartal complications,* page 256.)

Planning and implementation

Prevention is the best intervention for puerperal infections. Careful aseptic technique, especially thorough hand washing, is crucial. To prevent cross-contamination among patients, make sure each patient has her own sanitary supplies and that nondisposable items are cleaned after each use.

Teach the patient techniques that help prevent infection. (Teaching is important even if an infection is diagnosed.) To prevent contamination of the vagina with rectal bacteria, instruct her to use a front-to-back motion when applying perineal pads and cleansing the vulvar and perineal area.

Expect to administer antimicrobial and antipyretic therapy if an infection is diagnosed. Many patients require a combination of oral and I.V. antibiotics. The physician also may order analgesics to help relieve general malaise, headache, and backache. For a localized wound infec-

NURSING DIAGNOSES

Postpartal complications

The following are potential nursing diagnoses for problems and etiologies that the nurse may encounter when caring for a patient with a postpartal complication. Specific nursing interventions for many of these diagnoses are provided in the "Planning and implementation" section of this chapter.

- Altered peripheral tissue perfusion related to hypovolemia
- Anxiety related to perceived health status
- Body image disturbance related to birth canal injury
- High risk for injury related to seizure secondary to eclampsia
- Interrupted breast feeding related to postpartal complication
- Knowledge deficit related to aseptic technique and perineal hygiene
- Knowledge deficit related to dietary and insulin requirements
- Knowledge deficit related to etiology and treatment of the postpartal complication
- Pain related to birth canal injury
- Sexual dysfunction related to altered body structure secondary to a birth canal injury
- Sleep pattern disturbance related to the need for frequent monitoring

---

tion, the physician may incise the infected area or remove sutures to promote drainage.

Independent nursing actions for the patient with a puerperal infection focus on alleviating signs and symptoms and helping to meet the patient's psychosocial needs. Offer comfort measures, ensure adequate rest, and provide a relaxed, quiet environment to counter malaise.

Allow the patient and neonate to spend as much time together as possible. Teach the patient and her family about her condition and treatment, and provide emotional support and encouragement. To help them work through anxiety and discouragement, encourage them to express their feelings.

Evaluation

The following examples illustrate appropriate evaluation statements for the patient with a postpartal infection:

- The patient expressed an understanding of infection control measures.
- The patient demonstrated how to perform perineal hygiene.

Documentation

To help ensure consistency of care, the nurse should include the following in documentation for the patient with a postpartal complication:

- the patient's vital signs
- the patient's comfort level
- changes in status
- color, amount, consistency, and odor of lochia
- appearance of the affected area
- the patient's understanding of the treatment course
- laboratory results

• the patient's feelings about her condition
• the patient's ability to care for and interact with the neonate.

Birth canal injuries
Many patients suffer lacerations of the cervix and vagina during childbirth.

Cervical lacerations
Cervical lacerations up to 2 cm long can be sustained during childbirth. Normally, if they are not bleeding, they heal uneventfully within 6 to 12 weeks and cause no further problems.

Deep cervical lacerations, an occasional result of precipitous labor, may lead to serious hemorrhage because of increased vascularity of the cervix and fragility of surrounding tissues. The tear may involve one or both sides of the cervix, possibly reaching up to or beyond the vaginal junction. Primiparous patients typically suffer more cervical lacerations than multiparous patients.

Vaginal and perineal lacerations and hematomas
Shallow lacerations of the anterior vagina near the urethra are relatively common intrapartal events. Typically, these injuries are accompanied by perineal lacerations; a deep perineal laceration may involve the anal sphincter, extending through the vaginal walls. Lacerations of the middle and upper portion of the vagina are less common than anterior lacerations and usually result from forceps delivery; these wounds may lead to copious blood loss.

Occasionally, trauma resulting from labor and delivery can create a concealed vascular lesion. The injury leads to a collection of extravasated blood as blood escapes into the connective tissue beneath the vaginal mucosa (vaginal hematoma) or beneath the skin of the vaginal mucosa.

Assessment
Injury to the birth canal may cause a wide range of signs and symptoms. Prompt detection is necessary to prevent further complications. Key factors to assess for include vital sign measurements and their trends, fundal height and tone (to evaluate for uterine atony), the amount and color of vaginal bleeding, the presence of increasing anxiety or apprehension, and increasing pain or discomfort. Also stay alert for signs of shock.

Signs and symptoms of a deep cervical laceration include bright red (arterial) vaginal bleeding with a firmly contracted uterus. The cervix appears lacerated, edematous, bruised, and ulcerated. An extensive sublabial laceration usually is apparent; this wound may bleed spontaneously and interfere with normal voiding. A vaginal laceration may bleed and is only visible on pelvic examination.

If the patient has severe perineal pain with sensitive ecchymosis, suspect vulvar hematoma. A vaginal hematoma, on the other hand, may manifest as severe rectal pain or pressure and inability to void. A vaginal hematoma is more difficult to visualize than a vulvar hematoma.

The Redness, Edema, Ecchymosis, Discharge, Approximation (REEDA) scale may be used to assess the condition of the perineum. This scale, which provides a means for objective assessment, evaluates the five components of healing (as its name suggests). Daily documentation allows tracking of the healing.

Nursing diagnoses

For a partial list of applicable diagnoses, see Nursing Diagnoses: *Postpartal complications,* page 256.

Planning and implementation

Depending on their size and location, some perineal and vaginal lacerations heal on their own. The nurse provides pain relief measures and teaches the patient how to manage pain through the use of ice packs to the perineum, sitz baths, topical or oral medications, and conscious relaxation techniques. If the patient has difficulty voiding, an indwelling catheter is inserted, as prescribed, until healing begins.

An extensive perineal or vaginal laceration that bleeds profusely requires suturing, as does a deep cervical laceration. Because of their location, labial lacerations are difficult to repair and cause much discomfort during healing. To prevent serious blood loss or infection from a hematoma, the physician may incise and evacuate (drain) the hematoma. Because these procedures also may cause an infection, encourage aseptic technique during subsequent perineal care and teach the patient to perform consistent perineal hygiene.

Evaluation

For the patient with birth canal injuries, appropriate evaluation statements may include general ones for any postpartal complication (see "Puerperal infection" earlier in this chapter) as well as the following:
• The patient demonstrated an understanding of the operative procedures accomplished.
• The patient's behavior reflected increasing comfort levels.

Documentation

Documentation for the patient with a birth canal injury should include the general documentation for any postpartal complication (see "Puerperal infection" earlier in this chapter) as well as:
• the appearance of the perineum
• the presence of edema or ecchymosis
• bowel status, including bowel movements
• the patient's comfort level
• the patient's concerns about healing.

Urinary tract disorders   Because of normal postpartal diuresis, urine production increases markedly in the first 48 hours after delivery; urine output typically measures

500 to 1,000 ml/voiding. This increase in urine production heightens the risk of urinary tract infection (UTI). Other conditions that are common during the postpartal period, such as increased bladder filling and reduced sensitivity to the voiding urge, also may lead to urinary tract problems.

Bladder distention

This condition may follow urine retention, which results from increased bladder capacity and decreased sensitivity to the voiding urge (such as from bladder edema or anesthetics used during delivery). Also, the patient with a distended bladder may void incompletely, leading to urine stasis—a condition that fosters bacterial growth and subsequent UTI. Bladder distention, in turn, may prevent uterine contractions and subsequent vessel compression, causing hemorrhage.

Cystitis

This inflammatory condition of the bladder and ureters may result from retention of stagnant urine in the bladder, catheterization, or bladder trauma during delivery. Usually, the infecting organisms ascend from the urethra to the bladder, then spread to the kidneys.

Pyelonephritis

This diffuse pyogenic inflammation of the kidney occurs when a bladder infection spreads to the ureters and kidneys.

Assessment

Bladder distention causes a boggy (soft) uterus that is displaced upward and to the right. Bladder distention with overflow is characterized by frequent voiding of small amounts (less than 75 ml). With cystitis, expect urinary urgency and frequency, dysuria, discomfort over the bladder area, hematuria, and a low-grade fever. With pyelonephritis, expect urinary urgency, dysuria, nocturia, cloudy urine, chills, and flank pain accompanied by a temperature of 102° F or higher.

Nursing diagnoses

For a partial list of applicable diagnoses, see Nursing Diagnoses: *Postpartal complications,* page 256.

Planning and implementation

Expect to administer antimicrobial therapy, provide comfort measures (such as sitz baths), and apply topical antiseptics. Catheterization may be necessary to prevent stagnant urine from accumulating in the bladder. Ensure a fluid intake of more than 3,000 ml/day, and record fluid intake and output. As prescribed, collect urine specimens for culturing.

Evaluation

For the patient with a urinary tract disorder, appropriate evaluation statements may include general ones for any postpartal complication (see "Puerperal infection" earlier in this chapter) as well as the following:

• The patient expressed an understanding of perineal care.
• The patient's voiding patterns have returned to preinfection status.

Documentation

Documentation for the patient with a urinary tract disorder should include the general documentation for any postpartal complication (see "Puerperal infection" earlier in this chapter) as well as voiding patterns, including urinary frequency and amount.

Venous thrombosis

Venous thrombosis (thrombus formation in a vein) affects less than 1% of postpartal patients. Conditions that predispose the postpartal patient to this disorder include hydramnios, preeclampsia, cesarean delivery, and immobility. Since early ambulation has become the norm, the frequency of venous thrombosis has decreased dramatically.

Typically, thrombophlebitis lasts 4 to 6 weeks, with symptoms subsiding gradually. In severe cases, potentially fatal abscesses develop. Thrombophlebitis is most common in a superficial vein (superficial thrombophlebitis) but may develop in a deep leg vein (deep-vein thrombophlebitis, or DVT). Typically, superficial thrombophlebitis manifests on the third or fourth postpartal day.

Assessment

With superficial thrombophlebitis, the affected vessel feels hard and thready or cordlike and is extremely sensitive to pressure. The surrounding area may be erythematous and feel warm; the entire limb may be pale, cold, and swollen. The patient may have a low-grade fever.

In a patient with suspected DVT or one who is at risk for DVT, perform a general assessment, including temperature measurement. Stay alert for complaints of cramping or aching pain in a specific region, especially if that region appears stiff, swollen, and red. Attempt to elicit Homans' sign; however, be aware that a negative Homans' sign does not rule out DVT. Other manifestations of DVT include malaise; edema of the ankle and leg with taut, shiny skin over the edematous area; fever; and chills. Measure leg, calf, and thigh circumferences to document any edema.

Nursing diagnoses

For a partial list of applicable diagnoses, see Nursing Diagnoses: *Postpartal complications,* page 256.

Planning and implementation

Preventing and detecting pulmonary embolism are the highest priorities when caring for the postpartal patient with venous thrombosis. Monitor the patient for dyspnea, a low-grade fever, tachycardia, chest pain, a productive cough, pleural friction rub, and signs of circulatory collapse.

As prescribed, administer an anticoagulant, and monitor for therapeutic efficacy and adverse effects of the drug. Observe closely for signs of bleeding, and teach the patient about the drug's purpose, adverse effects, and interactions with any other medications she is receiving. For thrombophlebitis, also expect to administer antibiotics.

Do not massage or rub the affected extremity and caution the patient never to do this, especially if she has phlebothrombosis. Because the thrombus is loosely attached to the vessel wall, rubbing can dislodge it, increasing the risk of embolism.

Management of the patient with superficial thrombophlebitis typically involves local heat application, elevation of the affected limb, bed rest, analgesics, and use of elastic stockings to help prevent blood from pooling in the legs. If these interventions are ineffective, the physician may prescribe an anticoagulant. For DVT, treatment typically includes I.V. heparin therapy, bed rest, analgesics, elevation of the affected limb, and elastic stockings.

Evaluation

For the patient with venous thrombosis, appropriate evaluation statements may include general ones for any postpartal complication (see "Puerperal infection" earlier in this chapter) as well as the following:
- The patient's condition remained stable, with no signs of pulmonary embolism.
- The patient's leg circumference decreased.
- The patient expressed an understanding of the purpose, dosage, and adverse effects of anticoagulant medication and the necessity for continued medical supervision.

Documentation

Documentation for the patient with venous thrombosis should include the general documentation for any postpartal complication (see "Puerperal infection" earlier in this chapter) as well as clotting times and other laboratory values, such as prothrombin time and partial thromboplastin time.

Mastitis This inflammation of the breast occurs in 2% to 3% of breast-feeding patients. The most common cause is infection by *Staphylococcus aureus* bacteria; other causative organisms include beta-hemolytic streptococci, *Haemophilus influenzae, H. parainfluenzae, Escherichia coli,* and *Klebsiella pneumoniae.* The pathogenic organism usually enters through a crack or abrasion in the nipple; however, mastitis can occur even in patients with intact nipples.

Assessment

Signs and symptoms of mastitis typically do not arise until 2 to 3 weeks after delivery. A portion of the breast is firm, tender, reddened, and warm; axillary lymph nodes may become enlarged. The patient reports chills, malaise, headache, nausea, and aching joints. Typically, the body temperature measures 102° to 104° F (38.8° to 40° C). A culture of either breast milk or the neonate's throat will identify the causative organism; elevated leukocyte and bacterial counts indicate infectious mastitis.

Nursing diagnoses

For a partial list of applicable diagnoses, see Nursing Diagnoses: *Postpartal complications*, page 256.

Planning and implementation

Because this infection usually manifests itself after discharge, teach the patient how to prevent and detect mastitis when preparing her for discharge. The first line of defense against mastitis is prevention of cracked nipples. Advise the patient not to use soap or alcohol to clean the nipples because these substances have a drying effect. Instead, she should use plain water, allow the nipples to air dry, then apply a breast cream that does not contain lanolin. Instruct her to remove the neonate from her breast carefully at the end of a feeding session to avoid undue tension on the tissues. Because mastitis also may result from milk duct blockage and resulting milk stasis, advise the patient to breast-feed frequently and to call the physician or nurse-midwife if her breasts become severely engorged.

Treatment for mastitis includes a full course of organism-specific antibiotic (usually lasting 10 days), bed rest for at least 48 hours, close monitoring, and patient teaching.

Evaluation

For the patient with mastitis, appropriate evaluation statements may include general ones for any postpartal complication (see "Puerperal infection" earlier in this chapter) as well as the following:
- The patient demonstrated an understanding of breast care.
- The patient expressed an understanding of warning signs of mastitis.

Documentation

Documentation for the patient with mastitis should include the general documentation for any postpartal complication (see "Puerperal infection" earlier in this chapter) as well as appearance of the affected area and the patient's understanding of the treatment course.

Diabetes mellitus

As previously discussed, diabetes mellitus refers to a group of endocrine disorders characterized by impaired carbohydrate metabolism secondary to insufficient insulin secretion or resistance to insulin.(See Chapter 6, Selected antepartal complications.)

In the early postpartal period, the diabetic patient may need little or no exogenous insulin because the rapid decline in placental hormones and cortisol reduces the opposition to insulin that is already available. However, as hormone levels begin to stabilize, the need for exogenous insulin increases. Throughout the postpartal period, the insulin dosage must be readjusted to achieve diabetic control in patients with insulin-dependent and noninsulin-dependent diabetes. Patients diagnosed with gestational diabetes usually resume a normal glucose status postpartally.

Assessment

If the patient is diabetic, she is at increased risk for developing postpartal complications, including infection, hemorrhage, hypoglycemia, and hyperglycemia. Also, the risk of preeclampsia is four times greater in diabetic patients than in the general population.

Infection in the diabetic patient typically involves the urinary tract. If the patient had a cesarean delivery, monitor her closely for infection at the incision site and the indwelling catheter site. If she delivered vaginally, assess episiotomy healing and evaluate lochia for signs of infection (such as foul odor or a yellow or greenish color).

Hyperglycemia or hypoglycemia may develop as plunging levels of placental hormones alter postpartal glucose metabolism. Strong postpartal emotions and the work of labor contribute to glucose alterations. To detect hyperglycemia, monitor signs of excessive thirst, hunger, dramatic weight loss, and polyuria. Left untreated, hyperglycemia may lead to diabetic ketoacidosis. Also check for indications of hypoglycemia, tremulousness, cold sweats, piloerection, hypothermia, and headache. Confusion, hallucinations, bizarre behavior, and, ultimately, seizures and coma may occur in late hypoglycemia.

Nursing diagnoses

For a partial list of applicable diagnoses, see Nursing Diagnoses: *Postpartal complications,* page 256.

Planning and implementation

Nursing care centers on monitoring serial blood glucose measurements and observing for signs of hypoglycemia and hyperglycemia, preventing or controlling complications of diabetes, and teaching the patient about her insulin needs. Also, ensure proper nutrition and promote mother-infant bonding.

If the patient had gestational diabetes, advise her to inquire about a follow-up oral glucose tolerance test 6 to 8 weeks postpartum. Inform her that she may develop gestational diabetes in future pregnancies. Thus, early prenatal care would be advisable.

Evaluation

For the patient with diabetes mellitus, appropriate evaluation statements may include general ones for any postpartal complication (see "Puerperal infection" earlier in this chapter) as well as the following:
• The patient's blood glucose level remained within normal limits.
• The patient showed no signs or symptoms of hypoglycemia or hyperglycemia.
• The patient remained free of infection.

• The patient expressed an understanding of the effects of nutrition, rest, and breast-feeding on her insulin requirements.

Documentation

Documentation for the patient with diabetes mellitus should include the general documentation for any postpartal complication (see "Puerperal infection" earlier in this chapter) as well as:
• serial blood glucose levels
• insulin administered
• signs or symptoms of hypoglycemia or hyperglycemia
• signs or symptoms of preeclampsia, infection, or hemorrhage
• patient teaching about diet, exercise, insulin dosage and schedule, blood glucose monitoring schedule, signs and symptoms to report to the physician, and the need for regular follow-up medical care.

Pregnancy-induced hypertension

As previously discussed, pregnancy-induced hypertension (PIH) refers to hypertensive disorders that develop between the twentieth week of pregnancy and the end of the first postpartal week. Preeclampsia refers to hypertension with albuminuria or edema. Eclampsia occurs in a preeclamptic patient and involves seizures, possibly with coma; untreated, eclampsia usually is fatal.

Although the cause of PIH is unknown, inadequate prenatal care may be a contributing factor. Other possible predisposing factors include primigravidity, multiple gestation, preexisting diabetes mellitus or hypertension, and hydramnios. (For details, see Chapter 6, Selected antepartal complications.)

Assessment

Evaluate the patient for continued or current evidence of PIH. Usually, signs and symptoms of PIH subside rapidly after delivery. However, in the at-risk patient, blood pressure is monitored closely during the first 24 hours postpartum. Suspect PIH if systolic pressure rises at least 30 mm Hg and diastolic pressure increases at least 15 mm Hg above the baseline values determined in pregnancy. Such an increase in blood pressure may signify an impending seizure.

With mild preeclampsia, generalized edema and proteinuria are experienced in addition to hypertension. With severe preeclampsia, blood pressure increases more sharply and the patient typically complains of a severe, persistent headache and visual disturbances, such as blurring. She also may have epigastric pain, hyperreflexia, vomiting, apprehensiveness, photophobia, and sensitivity to noise.

Inspect the patient's hands and feet for edema, which may make visualization of the joints impossible. Be sure to assess fluid intake and urine output, sometimes by employing an I.V. and Foley catheter. Urine output may drop below 30 ml/hour even if the patient is receiving I.V. fluids. Weigh the patient daily to assess postpartal diuresis.

Promptly report to the physician urine output below 30 ml/hour, proteinuria, and other suggestive findings.

In the preeclamptic patient, blood volume may increase without an accompanying increase in hemoglobin; thus, an accurate hemoglobin measurement is important. The physician usually orders clotting studies to rule out disseminated intravascular coagulation (DIC), a grave bleeding disorder resulting from damage to vessel walls. Such damage is a characteristic feature of preeclampsia and may predispose the patient to DIC. (See Chapter 6, Selected antepartal complications.)

Nursing diagnoses

For a partial list of applicable diagnoses, see Nursing Diagnoses: *Postpartal complications,* page 256.

Planning and implementation

Postpartum nursing management for preeclampsia and eclampsia focuses on preventing seizures and monitoring signs and symptoms of these disorders to prevent further complications. The ultimate goal is to stabilize the patient by intervening appropriately, providing optimal environmental conditions, and promoting psychosocial adjustment.

If the patient was diagnosed as preeclamptic during pregnancy, the physician may order I.V. magnesium sulfate postpartally to decrease the seizure threshold, provide sedation, and dilate blood vessels. A narcotic also may be prescribed. Immediately report to the physician any change in the patient's condition. To help ensure patient safety in case of a seizure, make sure bed rails are padded, an airway is at the bedside, and emergency equipment (including oxygen and suction apparatus) is readily available.

Maintaining an optimal environment is crucial for the patient with PIH. Minimize external stimulation. Once the patient shows signs of improvement, visitors, telephone, and television can be reintroduced gradually. When providing care, be thorough and efficient so as to disturb the patient as little as possible.

The patient who is not critically ill probably will express concern about her own and the neonate's physical safety. Offer reassurance and coordinate nursery contact with the patient.

Evaluation

For the patient with PIH, appropriate evaluation statements may include general ones for any postpartal complication (see "Puerperal infection" earlier in this chapter) as well as the following:
• The patient's blood pressure maintained normal limits.
• The patient remained free of seizures.
• The patient maintained normal reflexes (2 +).
• The patient's edema decreased.
• The patient maintained a urine output greater than 30 ml/hour.

Documentation

Documentation for the patient with PIH should include the general documentation for any postpartal complication (see "Puerperal infection" earlier in this chapter) as well as:
- daily weight
- consciousness level
- fluid intake and urine output
- presence of urinary protein
- signs of edema
- status of deep tendon reflexes.

Substance abuse

In some patients, substance abuse is not detected until the postpartal period, when the neonate shows neurobehavioral problems.

Assessment

Because postpartal hospital stays are short, the nurse must remain alert for and report possible signs of substance abuse. Physical signs include chronic nasal congestion, dilated pupils, anorexia, tachycardia, irregular pulse, and needle marks on the skin. (Physical signs in the neonate also may be present.) Psychosocial signs include memory loss, mood swings, hostile or violent behavior, and low self-esteem. The substance-dependent patient may develop cardiovascular and central nervous system complications. Cocaine and other vasoconstrictive drugs may cause a transient increase in blood pressure and pulse.

To help detect recently ingested drugs, the physician may order toxicologic urine and blood screening. During assessment, try to establish a rapport and convey a caring, nonjudgmental attitude.

Nursing diagnoses

For a partial list of applicable diagnoses, see Nursing Diagnoses: *Postpartal complications,* page 256.

Planning and implementation

The substance-abusing postpartal patient may be difficult to care for—irritable, manipulative, angry, defensive, and fearful—and typically requires a multidisciplinary treatment approach. Besides the nurse and physician, a social worker, child protection worker, and community health worker may be involved in her care. Treatment depends on her willingness to admit her problem and comply with a treatment program, such as Alcoholics Anonymous or Narcotics Anonymous.

The increasing problem of maternal substance abuse has sparked debate on such issues as the rights of substance-abusing patients and their neonates and the responsibilities of all parties involved in their care. Most states allow a substance-abusing patient to be discharged from the health care facility with her neonate unless she has previously abused a child or unless health care professionals have sufficient reason to believe the neonate is at high risk for neglect or abuse. Early consultation with a social worker can initiate child welfare visits if the neonate is determined to be at risk; a history of substance abuse usually is sufficient documentation to initiate such visits.

Evaluation
For the substance-abusing patient, appropriate evaluation statements may include general ones for any postpartal complication (see "Puerperal infection" earlier in this chapter) as well as the following:
• The patient acknowledges substance abuse.
• The patient expressed readiness to enter a treatment program.

Documentation
Documentation for the substance-abusing patient should include the general documentation for any postpartal complication (see "Puerperal infection" earlier in this chapter) as well as:
• signs and symptoms of drug withdrawal or continued drug use
• response to prescribed analgesics
• extent of the patient's interaction with the neonate, her partner, and the health care team
• absence or presence of signs of mother-infant bonding
• expressions of willingness to be treated for substance abuse.

STUDY ACTIVITIES

Short answer
1. On her first postpartum day, Delores Asta, a 35-year-old multipara, developed a temperature of 101.4° F that prevented her discharge. No other signs of infection were apparent. On the following morning during the postpartum nursing assessment, Ms. Asta complains of malaise, a severe headache, feeling "achy," and intermittent chills. What other information should the nurse collect and what should be suspected?

_____

_____

2. A chart review reveals that Ms. Asta had no prenatal care and was noted to be anemic during her assessment on admission. She reported leaking amniotic fluid for at least 24 hours prior to the onset of her labor, which then brought her to the hospital. Due to her history and an unsure gestational age, an intrauterine fetal monitor was used. After a long labor, she was delivered by forceps due to exhaustion and fetal distress. List the factors that placed Ms. Asta at risk.

_____

3. Ms. Asta is eager to get home to her other children and asks the nurse why she can't leave, even if she does have a "little fever" and "touch of the flu." Why is this a significant postpartum problem? What could be the potential results of this problem if left untreated?

_____

_____

4. On discharge from the birthing suite, Jewel Davis reminds the nurse that she had developed mastitis with her last baby after nursing her for a month. She wants to prevent the problem this time and is very sure she wants to breast-feed her new son. What patient teaching should the nurse provide Ms. Davis?

_____

_____

5. Ginny Weir, a known cocaine addict, has delivered her third child prematurely. She is difficult to care for because she is irritable, angry, and manipulative. How should the postpartum nurse plan for Ms. Weir's care? How best could the nurse approach this patient?

_____

6. What preventive nursing measures can be employed to keep patients from developing puerperal infections?

_____

_____

7. If a patient is 2 hours postpartum after a difficult forceps delivery and is noted to have heavy, bright red vaginal bleeding with a firmly contracted uterus, what complication should the nurse suspect?

_____

8. When an early postpartum patient exhibits a systolic blood pressure rise of 30 mm Hg and a diastolic rise of at least 15 mm Hg above her baseline prenatal values, what condition should the nurse evaluate this patient for? What other signs and symptoms might be present to guide this assessment?

_____

_____

9. Why is bladder distention considered a problem in a patient who had epidural anesthesia and a vacuum extraction delivery?

_____

True or false

10. In the early postpartum period, the diabetic patient may need little or no exogenous insulin because the rapid decline in placental hormones and cortisol reduces opposition to the insulin that is already available.

☐ True   ☐ False

11. The REEDA scale is used to assess the patient's breasts when signs of mastitis are suspected.
☐ True   ☐ False

12. Once the patient has delivered, there is no further risk of developing pregnancy-induced hypertension.
☐ True   ☐ False

13. Signs and symptoms of mastitis typically do not arise until 2 to 3 weeks after delivery.
☐ True   ☐ False

14. Prevention is the best intervention for puerperal infections.
☐ True   ☐ False

ANSWERS   **Short answer**

1. In addition to monitoring her vital signs, the nurse should assess Ms. Asta for lower abdominal pain or uterine tenderness, the presence of severe after pains, and uterine tone and fundal height. She should also evaluate lochial discharge, noting the amount, color, consistency, and odor, and evaluate the patient's sleep and rest patterns, hydration, and nutritional status. Laboratory analysis may be ordered, including white blood cell count and sedimentation rate. Blood and vaginal cultures also may be ordered to isolate the causative organism.

2. Ms. Asta's risk factors include her lack of prenatal care, anemia, prolonged rupture of membranes, long labor, intrauterine fetal monitoring, and forceps delivery. The nurse should stay alert for signs and symptoms of infection in a postpartal patient with these risk factors.

3. Puerperal infection is a leading cause of childbearing-associated death throughout the world. A puerperal infection develops from a local lesion or its extension. With a local lesion, the infection remains within the original infection site. If untreated, a localized infection may extend to other areas via the blood or lymphatic vessels, causing such infections as endometritis, peritonitis, or thrombophlebitis. These extension infections, then, may lead to systemic infection of the bloodstream, resulting in bacteremic shock and the threat of imminent death.

4. The nurse should teach Ms. Davis that the first line of defense against mastitis is prevention of cracked nipples. Ms. Davis should be advised against using soap or alcohol to clean her nipples because these substances have a drying effect. Instead, she should use plain water, allow the nipples to air dry, and apply a breast cream that does not contain lanolin. To avoid undue tension on the tissues, Ms. Davis should be instructed to remove her son from her breast carefully at the end of a feeding session. She also should be told to breast-feed frequently and to call her physician or nurse-midwife if her breasts become severely engorged.

5. When dealing with a patient such as Ms. Weir who is a known substance abuser, the nurse should attempt to establish rapport and convey a caring, nonjudgmental attitude. This type of patient typically requires a multidisciplinary treatment approach. Besides the nurse and physician, a social worker, child protection worker, and community health worker may be involved in Ms. Weir's care.

6. Careful aseptic technique, especially thorough hand washing, is crucial to preventing puerperal infections. To prevent cross-contamination among patients, the nurse makes sure each patient has her own sanitary supplies and that nondisposable items are cleaned after each use. Also, the patient is taught techniques that help prevent infection. To prevent contamination of the vagina with rectal bacteria, she is instructed to use a front-to-back motion when applying perineal pads and cleansing the vulvar and perineal areas.

7. The nurse should suspect a deep cervical laceration, signs and symptoms of which include bright red (arterial) vaginal bleeding with a firmly contracted uterus. An extensive or deep cervical laceration that bleeds profusely requires suturing.

8. The nurse should suspect PIH if the systolic pressure rises at least 30 mm Hg and diastolic pressure increases at least 15 mm Hg about baseline prenatal values. Such an increase in blood pressure may signify an impending seizure. With mild preeclampsia, generalized edema and proteinuria are experienced in addition to hypertension. With severe preeclampsia, blood pressure increases more sharply and the patient typically complains of a severe, persistent headache and visual disturbances. She also may have epigastric pain, hyperreflexia, vomiting, apprehensiveness, photophobia, and sensitivity to noise.

9. Bladder distention may follow urine retention, which results from increased bladder capacity and decreased sensitivity to the voiding urge (such as from anesthetics used during delivery). The patient with a distended bladder may void incompletely, leading to urine stasis—a condition that fosters bacterial growth and subsequent UTI. Bladder distention may prevent uterine contractions and subsequent vessel compression, causing hemorrhage.

True or false
10. True.
11. False. The REEDA scale is used to assess the perineum for five components of healing (redness, edema, ecchymosis, discharge, and approximation).
12. False. Pregnancy-induced hypertension refers to hypertensive disorders that develop between the twentieth week of pregnancy and the end of the first postpartal week.
13. True.
14. True.

CHAPTER 17

Physiology of neonatal adaptation

OBJECTIVES   After studying this chapter, the reader should be able to:
1. Identify the unique anatomic structures of fetal circulation.
2. Distinguish between fetal and neonatal circulation.
3. Discuss the status of the integumentary, neurologic, and reproductive systems at birth.
4. Identify the neonate's four defenses against heat loss.
5. Describe the biological adaptations necessary in the hematopoietic, renal, gastrointestinal, hepatic, and endocrine systems to ensure successful transition to extrauterine life.
6. Discuss the capacity of the neonate's immune system to prevent infection.
7. Identify the sensory capacities of the healthy neonate.

OVERVIEW OF CONCEPTS   For the neonate, birth begins a critical 24-hour phase, called the transitional period, that encompasses adaptation from intrauterine to extrauterine life. The transitional period imposes changes in all body systems and exposes the neonate to a wide range of external stimuli. Conditions that prevent successful adaptation to extrauterine life pose a serious threat.

Two-thirds of all neonatal deaths occur in the first 4 weeks after birth, reflecting the potential difficulties that the neonate must overcome during this period. By becoming familiar with the normal events of transition, the nurse recognizes signs of poor adaptation and intervenes promptly when they occur.

Biological characteristics of adaptation   Crucial physiologic adjustments take place in all body systems after birth. The cardiovascular and pulmonary systems undergo immediate, drastic changes as soon as the umbilical cord is clamped and respiration begins. Although cardiovascular and pulmonary changes occur simultaneously, they are discussed separately to facilitate understanding.

Cardiovascular system

Fetal circulation involves certain unique anatomic features—the ductus venosus, the foramen ovale, and the ductus arteriosus—that shunt most blood away from the liver and lungs and separate the systemic and pulmonary circulations. To ensure the neonate's survival, fetal circulation must convert to neonatal circulation during the transitional period (see *Fetal circulation* in Chapter 1, Conception and fetal development).

Conversion from fetal to neonatal circulation

Beginning at birth, fetal shunts undergo changes that establish neonatal circulation. (For an illustration of blood flow in the neonate, see *Neonatal circulation*.) As the umbilical cord is clamped and the neonate draws the first breath, systemic vascular resistance increases and blood flow through the ductus arteriosus is reduced. This results in functional closure of the foramen ovale. (Functional closure refers to cessation of blood flow, resulting from pressure changes, that renders a structure nonfunctional.) Within several months, the foramen ovale undergoes anatomic closure (structural obliteration from constriction or tissue growth).

Onset of respiratory effort and the effects of increased partial pressure of arterial oxygen (PaO_2) constrict the ductus arteriosus, which functionally closes 15 to 24 hours after birth. By age 3 to 4 weeks, this shunt undergoes anatomic closure.

Clamping of the umbilical cord halts blood flow through the ductus venosus, functionally closing this structure. The ductus venosus closes anatomically by the first or second week. Because anatomic closure lags behind functional closure, fetal shunts may open intermittently before closing completely. Clinically insignificant functional murmurs or transient cyanosis may result. Both cyanosis and murmurs in the neonate should be carefully monitored and evaluated so that any underlying abnormalities can be detected.

Respiratory system

Throughout gestation, biochemical and anatomic respiratory features develop progressively, preparing the fetus for the abrupt respiratory changes brought on by birth. The reduction of surface tension created by the secretion of a phospholipid, surfactant, in the neonate's lungs facilitates gas exchange, decreases inflation pressures needed to open the airways, improves lung compliance, and decreases labor of breathing.

Onset of neonatal respiration

The fetal lungs contain fluid secreted by the lungs, amniotic cavity, and trachea. For the neonate to assume the tasks of ventilation and oxygenation, air must rapidly replace lung fluid. In the healthy neonate, replacement occurs with the first few breaths.

The time needed to clear the lungs varies from 6 to 24 hours after vaginal delivery of a healthy, full-term neonate. Inadequate lung fluid

Neonatal circulation

With birth comes functional closure of the fetal shunts (ductus venosus, foramen ovale, and ductus arteriosus) that direct blood flow away from the lungs and liver and separate the systemic and pulmonary circulations. As the shunts close, blood flows from the pulmonary arteries to the lungs and through the portal system to the liver. Neonatal circulation then follows the same path as normal adult circulation. The boxed illustrations show the shunts as they previously existed.

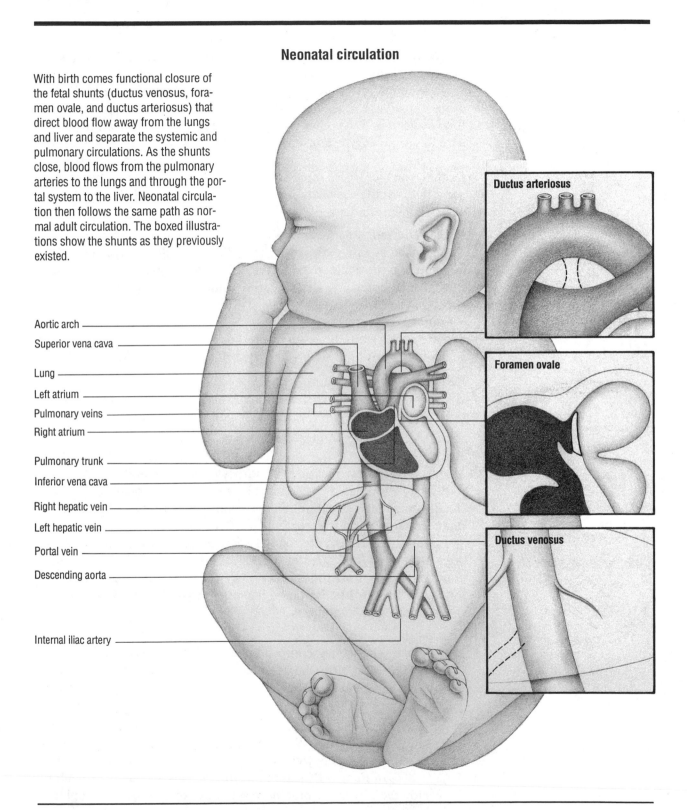

Aortic arch

Superior vena cava

Lung

Left atrium

Pulmonary veins

Right atrium

Pulmonary trunk

Inferior vena cava

Right hepatic vein

Left hepatic vein

Portal vein

Descending aorta

Internal iliac artery

Ductus arteriosus

Foramen ovale

Ductus venosus

removal may cause transient tachypnea, a common problem in neonates.

Normally, the neonate breathes within 20 seconds of delivery, stimulated by the medullary respiratory center of the brain.

Asphyxia—the combination of hypoxemia, hypercapnia, and acidosis—provides the strongest stimulus for the first breath. Because the final stage of delivery interrupts gas exchange, even the healthy neonate has some degree of asphyxia at birth.

Other stimuli that help trigger breathing include cord occlusion, thermal changes (from rapid heat loss caused by increased energy expenditure), tactile stimulation, and other environmental changes (such as bright lights and noise).

Neonatal respiratory function

The respiratory rate varies over the first day, stabilizing by about 24 hours after birth. Maintained by the effects of biochemical and environmental stimulation, the neonate's respiratory functioning requires:
• a patent airway
• a functioning respiratory center
• intact nerves from the brain to chest muscles
• adequate calories to supply energy for the labor of breathing.

Hematopoietic system

Like other body systems, the hematopoietic system is not fully developed at birth. This system defends the body against infection and disposes of cell breakdown products.

Red blood cells

Erythropoiesis—production of erythrocytes, or red blood cells (RBCs)—is stimulated by the renal hormone erythropoietin. At birth, the increased oxygen saturation that follows the onset of respiration inhibits erythropoietin release, reducing RBC production.

Fetal RBCs have a life span of about 90 days, compared to 120 days for normal RBCs. As fetal RBCs deteriorate, the neonate's RBC count decreases, sometimes resulting in physiologic anemia before stabilization. By age 2 to 3 months, however, the RBC count rises to within acceptable neonatal limits.

Hemoglobin

Blood's oxygen-carrying component, hemoglobin is produced by developing RBCs. After birth, the hemoglobin value decreases simultaneously with the RBC count.

White blood cells

White blood cells (WBCs), or leukocytes, serve as the neonate's major defense against infection. WBCs exist in five types: neutrophils, eosinophils, basophils, lymphocytes, and monocytes. Neutrophils account for 40% to 80% of total WBCs at birth; lymphocytes account for roughly 30%. However, by age 1 month, lymphocytes outnumber neutrophils.

Neutrophils and monocytes are phagocytes—cells that engulf and ingest foreign substances.

Thrombocytes

Thrombocytes (platelets) are crucial to blood coagulation. The neonate usually has an adequate platelet count and function.

Hepatic system

The neonate's hepatic system—responsible for bilirubin clearance, blood coagulation, carbohydrate metabolism, and iron storage—is immature, yet functions adequately.

Bilirubin clearance

As RBCs age, they become fragile and eventually are cleared from the circulation. The resultant by-product, a yellow bile pigment called bilirubin, then binds to plasma albumin. In this water-insoluble state, it is called indirect (unconjugated) bilirubin.

Indirect bilirubin must be conjugated—converted to direct bilirubin—for excretion. Conjugation occurs in the liver with the assistance of the enzyme glucuronyl transferase; a water-soluble bilirubin form results. The bilirubin compounds resulting from breakdown are excreted in the urine and stool.

Jaundice. If unconjugated bilirubin accumulates faster than the liver can clear it, the neonate may develop the yellow pallor known as jaundice. Slow or ineffective bilirubin clearance results in some degree of jaundice in approximately half of full-term neonates and 90% of preterm neonates. Fortunately, most full-term neonates avoid toxic bilirubin accumulation because they have adequate serum albumin binding sites and sufficient liver production of glucuronyl transferase. Factors that may increase the risk of hyperbilirubinemia (an elevated unconjugated bilirubin level) include asphyxia, cold stress (ineffective heat maintenance), hypoglycemia, and maternal salicylate ingestion.

Four types of jaundice occur in the neonate: physiologic jaundice, pathologic jaundice, breast milk jaundice (BMJ), and breast-feeding-associated jaundice (BFAJ). (See *Jaundice in the neonate,* page 276.)

Bilirubin encephalopathy (kernicterus). Unconjugated serum bilirubin levels of approximately 20 mg/dl or higher may lead to bilirubin encephalopathy, a life-threatening condition. To assess the risk for bilirubin encephalopathy, consider the neonate's condition and gestational and chronological ages in conjunction with the bilirubin level. The condition may be treated with phototherapy or exchange transfusions.

Blood coagulation

Neonates are especially at risk for hemorrhagic disease of the newborn because, for the first few days after birth, the gastrointestinal tract lacks the bacterial action to synthesize adequate vitamin K. Vitamin K catalyzes synthesis of prothrombin by the liver, activating key coagulation factors in the blood that prevent spontaneous hemorrhage. All neo-

Jaundice in the neonate

Four distinct types of jaundice occur in the neonate. The nurse must be aware of the distinctions between each in order to provide prompt intervention, prevent complications and be able to explain the appropriate facts to the parents.

TYPE	ONSET	PEAK LEVEL	DURATION	CAUSES	TREATMENT
Physiologic jaundice	48 to 72 hrs	4 to 12 mg/dl by 3 to 5 days	Increases by ≤5 mg/dl/day	Ends by day 7	• Decreased hepatic circulation • Increased bilirubin load • Reduced hepatic bilirubin • Uptake from the plasma • Decreased bilirubin conjugation • Decreased bilirubin excretion
Pathologic jaundice	First 24 hours	≥13 mg/dl	Must be treated to resolve	• Blood group or blood type incompatibilities • Hepatic, biliary or metabolic abnormalities • Infection	• Phototherapy • Exchange transfusions
Breast milk jaundice (BMJ)	Becomes apparent about 5 to 6 days, peaks between days 10 and 15	15 to 25 mg/dl	May persist for several weeks; in rare cases, several months	Breast milk enzyme "beta-glucuronidase" causes increased intestinal bilirubin absorption, thus blocking bilirubin excretion	• Controversial — conservative treatment temporarily stopping breast-feeding until bilirubinemia declines, usually in 24 to 48 hours • Breast pumping advised; others say *no* treatment necessary
Breast-feed-ing-associat-ed jaundice (BFAJ)	Becomes apparent at 48 to 72 hours	15 to 19 mg/dl by 72 hours	Increases by <5 mg/dl/day If level approaches 18 to 20 mg/dl	Variable	• Poor caloric intake that leads to decreased hepatic transport and removal of bilirubin from body

nates now receive a prophylactic injection of vitamin K soon after delivery to help prevent hemorrhage.

Carbohydrate metabolism

The major energy source during the first 4 to 6 hours after birth for the neonate is glucose stored in the liver as glycogen. The increased metabolic demands of labor, delivery, and the first few hours after birth cause rapid glycogen depletion (approximately 90% of liver glycogen is used within the first 3 hours). If the neonate does not receive exogenous glucose, glycogenolysis (breakdown of glycogen into a usable glucose form) occurs. Until the neonate takes in sufficient nutrition, glycogenolysis causes release of glucose into the bloodstream to maintain a serum glucose level of approximately 60 mg/dl. However, such stresses as hypothermia, hypoxia, and delayed feeding may rapidly exhaust glycogen stores, leading to hypoglycemia.

Renal system

A relatively immature renal system makes the neonate susceptible to dehydration, acidosis, and electrolyte imbalance if vomiting and diarrhea occur.

The neonate usually voids within 24 hours of birth. The first urine may appear rust-colored and cloudy from urate and mucus, although this has no clinical significance. The neonate's urine usually is odorless; specific gravity ranges from 1.005 to 1.015.

As the neonate's fluid intake increases, urine output increases, and urine becomes clear or light straw in color. The breast-fed neonate may require 10 to 12 diaper changes daily. The bottle-fed neonate typically requires about 6 diaper changes daily.

Loss of fluid through urine, feces, insensible (imperceptible) losses, intake restrictions related to small gastric capacity, and increased metabolic rate contributes to a reduction of 5% to 15% of the birth weight over the first 5 days of extrauterine life. However, in the period before the mother's milk supply is established, increased extracellular fluid volume protects the breast-fed neonate from dehydration. The neonate should regain the birth weight within 10 days.

Gastrointestinal system

Despite a relatively immature GI system, the healthy neonate can ingest, absorb, and digest nutrients. In most cases, feedings should begin as soon as the neonate is physiologically stable and exhibits adequate coordination of the sucking and swallowing reflexes. Gastric capacity is between 40 and 60 ml on the first day after birth; it increases with subsequent feedings. Because of this limited capacity, nutrient needs must be met through frequent small-volume feedings. Gastric emptying time—typically 2 to 4 hours—varies with the volume of the feeding and the neonate's age. Peristalsis is rapid.

Many neonates regurgitate a small amount of ingested matter (1 to 2 ml) after feedings because of an immature cardiac sphincter (a muscular ring constricting the esophagus). Persistent, forceful, or large-volume regurgitation is abnormal and warrants investigation.

GI enzymes and weight gain

The neonate's ability to digest nutrients depends on enzyme action and gastric acidity. Milk digestion begins in the stomach and continues in the small intestine. Secretions from the pancreas, liver, and duodenum aid digestion. Enzyme deficiencies initially limit the neonate's absorption of complex carbohydrates and fats. Typically, the infant doubles the birth weight by age 5 to 6 months and triples it by the first birthday.

Vitamin K synthesis

Synthesis of vitamin K through bacterial action is another important GI function. Although initially sterile, the GI tract establishes normal colonic bacteria within the first week after birth, allowing adequate vitamin K synthesis.

Neonatal stools

Initially, the neonate's intestines contain meconium, a thick, dark-green, odorless fecal substance consisting of amniotic fluid, bile, epithelial cells, and lanugo—the fine, soft hair covering the fetus's shoulders and back. Typically, the neonate passes the first meconium stool within 24 hours of birth.

After enteric feedings begin, fecal color, odor, and consistency change. Transitional stools usually appear on the second or third day after feedings begin. These greenish-brown stools have a higher water content than meconium. The type of feeding determines the characteristics of subsequent stools. The formula-fed neonate passes pasty, pale-yellow stools with a strong odor. Stools from the breast-fed neonate are golden-yellow, sweet smelling, and more liquid.

Food ingestion causes relaxation and contraction of intestinal colonic muscles, commonly leading to a bowel movement during or after a feeding. Typically, the breast-fed neonate has more frequent bowel movements than the formula-fed neonate because breast milk digests more rapidly than formula.

Immune system

With the neonate's birth comes exposure to pathogens (for example, bacteria) not normally present in utero. Such exposure activates components of the immune response. The first year is the period of greatest vulnerability to serious infections.

Immune response

The various elements of the immune system recognize, remember, respond to, and eliminate foreign substances called antigens. Primarily proteins, antigens may invade the body's protective barriers (such as the skin and mucous membranes) or arise from malignant cell transformation. The immune system is deficient at birth.

When local barriers and inflammation fail to fight off antigenic invasion, the immune system initiates a humoral or cell-mediated response. The response is carried out by the mononuclear phagocytic system, which includes cells in the thymus, lymphoid tissue, liver, spleen, and bone marrow. Cells involved in the immune response include lymphocytes (specifically, T cells and B cells), granulocytes, monocytes, RBCs, and platelets.

Neurologic system

Although not fully developed, the neonate's neurologic system can perform the complex functions required to regulate neonatal adaptation—stimulate initial respirations, maintain acid-base balance, and regulate body temperature. The neonate's neurologic function is controlled primarily by the brain stem and spinal cord. The autonomic nervous system and brain stem coordinate respiratory and cardiac functions. All cranial nerves are present at birth; however, the nerves are not yet fully sheathed with myelin, a substance essential for smooth nerve impulse transmission.

At birth, the brain measures about one-fourth the size of the adult brain. The brain grows and matures in a cephalocaudal (head-to-toe) direction.

The brain needs a constant supply of glucose for energy and a relatively high oxygen level to maintain adequate cellular metabolism. For this reason, the neonate must be assessed and monitored carefully to detect impaired gas exchange or signs of hypoglycemia.

Nerve tract development

Sensory, cerebellar, and extrapyramidal nerve pathways are the first to develop. This accounts for the neonate's strong sense of hearing, taste, and smell. The cerebellum governs gross voluntary movement and helps maintain equilibrium. The extrapyramidal tract controls reflexive gross motor movement and postural adjustment by regulating reciprocal flexion and extension of muscle groups, thus maintaining smooth, coordinated movement.

Neonatal reflexes

The neonate's reflexes—categorized as feeding, protective, postural, and social—include such primitive reflexes as sucking and rooting (which causes the neonate to turn toward and search for the nipple). Crucial to survival, these reflexes serve as the basis for neonatal neurologic examination. Persistence of the neonatal reflexes beyond the age at which they normally disappear may indicate a neurologic abnormality.

Endocrine and metabolic systems

At birth, the endocrine system is anatomically mature but functionally immature. Complex interactions between the neurologic and endocrine systems help coordinate adaptation to extrauterine life.

Hormonal roles

Many neonatal adaptations are regulated by hormones secreted by the endocrine glands, including growth hormone, thyroid-stimulating hormone, adrenocorticotropic hormone, cortisol, and catecholamines.

Metabolic changes at birth

Withdrawal of maternally supplied glucose and calcium necessitates significant and immediate metabolic changes to ensure successful neonatal adaptation. During the first few hours after birth, serum glucose and calcium levels change rapidly.

Glucose. At birth, the neonate's serum glucose level usually measures 60% to 70% of the maternal serum glucose level. Over the next 2 hours, this level falls, stabilizing between 35 and 40 mg/dl. Unless the neonate experiences cold stress, delayed feeding, metabolic abnormalities, or sepsis, serum glucose rises to about 60 mg/dl by 6 hours after birth.

Calcium. The serum calcium level decreases at birth but usually stabilizes between 24 and 48 hours after birth. A level below 7 mg/dl reflects hypocalcemia.

Thermoregulation

Body temperature maintenance—essential for successful extrauterine adaptation—is regulated by complex interactions between environmental temperature and body heat loss and production. The neonate has limited thermoregulatory capacity, achieved by body heating and cooling mechanisms. When the neonate no longer can maintain body temperature, cooling or overheating results; exhaustion of thermoregulatory mechanisms brings death. Neonatal morbidity and mortality can be favorably influenced by the nurse who takes steps to prevent cold stress.

Heat loss can occur through four mechanisms: evaporation, conduction, radiation, and convection. In *evaporation,* fluids from the neonate's body (insensible water, visible perspiration, and pulmonary fluids) turn to vapor in dry air. The drier the environment, the greater the heat loss. In *conduction,* the warm neonate comes into direct contact with a cooler surface and heat is transferred away from the body, creating heat loss. In *radiation,* a cooler, solid surface not in direct contact with the neonate draws heat away from the body. This occurs regardless of the ambient temperature surrounding the neonate. In *convection,* the neonate's body surface loses heat to cooler environmental air. (For more information see *Preventing heat loss* in Chapter 19, Care of the healthy neonate.)

Neutral thermal environment (NTE). A neonate's NTE requires the least amount of energy to maintain a stable core temperature. For an unclothed, full-term neonate on the first day after birth, NTE ranges from 89.6° to 93.2° F (32° to 34° C). Within this narrow environmental temperature range, oxygen consumption and carbon dioxide production are lowest and core temperature is normal.

Defenses against hypothermia. In a cold environment or in other stressful circumstances, the neonate defends against heat loss through vasomotor control, thermal insulation, muscle activity, and nonshivering thermogenesis. Defined as the production of heat through lipolysis of brown fat, nonshivering thermogenesis is the neonate's most efficient heat production mechanism because it increases the metabolic rate minimally. Named for its rich vascular supply, dense cellular content, and numerous nerve endings, brown fat is deposited around the neck, head, heart, great vessels, kidneys, and adrenal glands; between the scapula; behind the sternum; and in the axillae.

The brain, liver, and skeletal muscles take part in nonshivering thermogenesis. In response to heat loss, sympathetic nerves stimulate the release of norepinephrine, the major mediator of nonshivering thermogenesis. Norepinephrine stimulates oxidation of brown fat, causing increased heat production. Heat produced by brown fat oxidation is distributed throughout the body by the blood, which absorbs heat as it flows through fatty tissue.

Integumentary system

The healthy neonate is moist and warm to the touch. Lanugo—fine, downy hair—may appear over the shoulders and back.

As with adults, the neonate's skin serves as the first line of defense against infection. The outermost skin layer, the stratum corneum, is initially fused with the vernix caseosa. A greasy white substance produced by sebaceous glands in utero, the vernix caseosa coats the fetal skin and protects it from the amniotic fluid. (Due to its protective properties, the remaining vernix caseosa should not be scrubbed off the neonate.) With maturation, the stratum corneum becomes an effective protective barrier.

In many neonates, vasomotor instability, capillary stasis, and high hemoglobin levels lead to acrocyanosis, characterized by bluish discoloration of the hands and feet. Acrocyanosis, a common condition, should not be confused with central cyanosis, which reflects impaired gas exchange. In central cyanosis, the neonate's skin and mucous membranes turn blue.

Musculoskeletal system

Ossification (bone development) is incomplete at birth but proceeds rapidly afterward. The neonate's skeleton consists mainly of bone. Six thin, unfused bones comprise the neonate's skull; these bones accommodate subsequent brain and head development. Fibrous joints called sutures mark the intersection of these bones. Fontanels, soft-tissue areas covered with tough membranes, separate the sutures. Typically, vaginal delivery causes the sutures to override ("molding"), a spontaneously resolving condition. (See Chapter 7, Physiology of labor and childbirth, for more details.)

The muscles are anatomically complete at term birth. Muscle mass, strength, and size increase with age. Increasing muscle strength is crucial to the development of postural control and mobility.

Reproductive system

The reproductive system is anatomically and functionally immature at birth. However, the female's ovaries contain all potential ova, which decrease in number from birth to maturity by roughly 90%. In approximately 90% of males, the testes have descended into the scrotum by birth, although no sperm appear until puberty.

High maternal estrogen levels may cause transient adverse effects in the neonate. For example, breast hypertrophy with or without witch's milk (a thin, watery secretion similar to colostrum) may appear in both the male and female neonate. The female may have pseudomenstruation, a mucoid or blood-tinged vaginal discharge caused by the sudden drop in hormone levels after birth. Clinically insignificant, breast hypertrophy and pseudomenstruation resolve spontaneously.

Normally, the male neonate has adhesions of the prepuce (penile foreskin) that prevent separation of the prepuce and glans. During fetal development, prepuce tissue is continuous with the epidermal glans covering.

Behavioral characteristics of adaptation

The neonate has remarkable sensory, cognitive, and social abilities at birth which allow spontaneous interaction, even in the first few days of life.

Neonate-environment interactions

Able to see, hear, and differentiate among tastes and smells, the neonate responds to touch and movement, defends against overstimulation, and gives verbal signals (such as crying) that, when interpreted by a responsive caregiver, can satisfy the neonate's needs.

Neonatal sensory capacities

Using the sensory capacities—vision, hearing, touch, taste, and smell—the neonate perceives, interacts with, modifies, and learns from the environment. Combined with the neonate's attractive physical features, these sensory capacities play a major role in parent-infant bonding.

Vision. Although the neonate can see, visual acuity is limited to a distance of approximately 9″ to 12″. The neonate has a preference for geometric shapes, such as squares, rectangles, or circles roughly 3″ in diameter. Black and white images hold the neonate's gaze longer than color images.

The neonate can conjugate the eyes (move them in unison) at or just after birth. However, immature neuromuscular control limits visual accommodation (the ability to adjust for distance) for the first 4 weeks after birth. Incomplete muscle control of ocular movements sometimes causes transient strabismus (deviation of the eyes, or "crossed" eyes).

The neonate apparently finds the human face intriguing and typically fixes the eyes and gazes intently at a face in proximity, as during feeding or cuddling. Such behavior strongly reinforces parent-infant bonding. Visual acuity improves quickly; by age 6 months, adult-level visual acuity is achieved.

Hearing. The neonate can hear at birth. Hearing is well established after aeration of the eustachian tube and drainage of blood, vernix caseosa, amniotic fluid, and mucus from the outer ear. Shortly after birth, the neonate turns toward sounds and startles in response to loud noises.

Touch. The neonate has well-developed tactile perception, which serves as a stimulus for the first breath. The most sensitive body areas include the face (especially around the mouth), hands, and soles.

Until recently, experts believed that incomplete nerve myelination prevented the neonate from experiencing pain, except perhaps to a limited degree. However, research has demonstrated that physiologic changes associated with pain in the neonate include increased blood pressure and pulse during and after a painful procedure. Also, painful stimuli have elicited simple motor responses (flexion and adduction of extremities), distinct facial expressions (pain, sadness, surprise), and characteristic crying.

Handling of the neonate provides sensory stimulation from motion as well as from touch. Such stimulation elicits alertness and orienting responses. These responses, in turn, influence neonatal development and parent-neonate interaction. However, the neonate may tire if handled too much.

Taste. The neonate differentiates among tastes by the first or second day after birth. A sweet solution, for example, elicits satisfied sucking; a sour solution induces a grimace and cessation of sucking; and a bitter solution provokes an angry facial expression, cessation of sucking, and, in many cases, turning away of the head.

Smell. Although little research has been conducted on neonatal olfaction, the neonate is known to react to strong or noxious odors by averting the head from the odor. Sensitivity to olfactory stimuli increases over the first 4 days after birth.

Characteristic patterns of sleep and activity

During the transitional period, the neonate experiences a series of changes encompassing state of consciousness, behavioral response to stimuli, and physiologic parameters. Various neonatal sleep and awake states also have been identified.

Periods of neonatal reactivity

The neonate's initial hours are characterized by a predictable, identifiable series of behavioral and physiologic characteristics. This series collectively has been described as the periods of neonatal reactivity.

All neonates experience the same sequence of periods. However, when each period begins and how long it lasts varies from one neonate to another. Maternal medication, anesthesia, labor duration, and any stress affecting the neonate may influence the duration of a given period. (See "Periods of reactivity" and *Assessment findings during periods of reactivity* in Chapter 18, Neonatal assessment.)

Sleep and awake states of the neonate

The neonate's state of consciousness has been classified into six states: two sleep states—deep sleep and light sleep—and four awake states—drowsy state, alert state, active state, and crying state. The sleep and awake states encompass the behavioral states used in the Brazelton Neonatal Behavioral Assessment Scale (BNBAS). Developed to measure a neonate's capabilities, the BNBAS assesses neonatal behavioral responses and elicited responses as well as behavioral states. (For details on the BNBAS, see Chapter 18, Neonatal assessment.)

The neonate's ability to regulate the state of consciousness reflects central nervous system integrity. The state of consciousness may be affected by medication, hunger, diurnal cycles, stress (such as from noise, pain, and bright lights), and any other physical discomfort. Normally, the neonate in a sleep state responds to stimuli with increased activity, whereas a neonate in the crying state responds with decreased activity.

STUDY ACTIVITIES   **Short answer**

1. JoNelle Davidson, a 38-year-old primipara, delivered her son, Robert, at 35 weeks' gestation after spontaneous rupture of membranes and a sudden onset of labor. At birth, Robert showed some evidence of asphyxia, though he responded well to minimal resuscitation. He weighed 2,495 g (5 lb, 8 oz). When he was received in the nursery, it was noted that he was slightly hypothermic and hypoglycemic. Measures were taken immediately to correct these problems and stabilize this neonate. Robert was determined to be preterm and appropriate for gestation age. Two days later, Ms. Davidson has become alarmed when she notices that Robert is very yellow. He is diagnosed with physiologic jaundice. What factors in Robert's history contributed to his condition?

_____

2. A neonatologist comes in to speak with Ms. Davidson about Robert's condition. Phototherapy is recommended to treat his jaundice. His unconjugated bilirubin has already reached a level of 18 mg/dl at 52 hours of life. In trying to weight the benefits versus the risks of phototherapy, Ms. Davidson asks what could happen if Robert was left untreated. What is the potential consequence of untreated hyperbilirubinemia?

_____

3. On the fourth postpartum day after a cesarean section for a persistent breech presentation, Joan Gabriel, a 22-year-old primipara, is worried about her daughter's weight. During discharge instructions, she asks the nurse why her infant has lost an entire half pound from her initial birth weight and whether the cause could be insufficient breast milk. How could the nurse explain expected neonatal weight loss (assessed as within normal limits) to this new mother? What guidelines should be given about her daughter's subsequent weight gain?

_____

4. As the nurse is preparing to give vitamin K to the neonate in the delivery room, Andrea Woodsdale, a 25-year-old multigravida, questions whether it's really necessary for her son to receive an injection so soon after birth. How could the nurse explain the necessity of vitamin K at this time?

_____

5. Identify the unique anatomic structures of fetal circulation and the basic difference between fetal and neonatal circulation.

_____

6. What five stimuli help trigger the neonate to breathe within 20 seconds of delivery?

_____

7. Identify the functions of the neonate's neurologic system that help regulate adaptation during the transition period.

_____

8. List the four functions of the neonate's hepatic system.

_____

9. The neonate's respiratory function stabilizes by about 24 hours after birth and is maintained by the effects of biochemical and environmental stimulation. What four physiologic conditions must be present in order for the neonate's respiratory functioning to proceed?

_____

Matching related elements

Heat loss, which begins at birth, can occur through four specific mechanisms. Match the mechanism on the left with its proper description on the right.

10. ___ Evaporation

A. The neonate's body surface loses heat to cooler environmental air.

11. ___ Conduction

B. Fluids from the neonate's body (insensible water, visible perspiration, and pulmonary fluids) turn to vapor in dry air. The drier the air, the greater the heat loss.

12. ___ Convection

C. A cooler, solid surface not in direct contact with the neonate draws heat away from the body, regardless of the ambient temperature surrounding the neonate.

13. ___ Radiation

D. The warm neonate comes into direct contact with a cooler surface and heat is transferred away from the body, creating heat loss.

True or false

14. Although physiologic anemia may initially result in the neonate as any remaining fetal red blood cells (RBCs) deteriorate, by age 2 to 3 months the neonate's RBC count rises to acceptable limits.
☐ True   ☐ False

15. The renal system is mature at birth, which makes the neonate invulnerable to dehydration, acidosis, and electrolyte imbalance if vomiting and diarrhea occur.
☐ True   ☐ False

16. Unless the neonate experiences cold stress, delayed feeding, metabolic abnormalities, or sepsis, serum glucose rises to about 60 mg/dl 6 hours after birth.
☐ True   ☐ False

ANSWERS **Short answer**

1. Factors that may increase the risk of hyperbilirubinemia (an elevated, unconjugated bilirubin level) include Robert's prematurity (90% of all preterm neonates develop jaundice), asphyxia, cold stress (hypothermia), and hypoglycemia.

2. Unconjugated serum bilirubin levels of 20 mg/dl or higher may lead to bilirubin encephalopathy (kernicterus), a life-threatening condition. The neonate's condition and gestational and chronological ages must be considered in conjunction with the bilirubin level.

3. The nurse could explain to Ms. Gabriel that the loss of fluid through urine, feces, insensible losses, intake restrictions related to small gastric capacity, and increased metabolic rate all contribute to a normal reduction of 5% to 15% of her daughter's birth weight over the first 5 days of life. However, as Ms. Gabriel's milk supply is established, increased extracellular fluid volume protects the neonate from dehydration. She can expect to see her daughter regain her birth weight within 10 days. Her daughter's weight should double by age 5 to 6 months and triple by the end of the first year.

4. For the first few days after birth, the neonate's GI tract lacks the bacterial action to synthesize adequate vitamin K. Vitamin K catalyzes synthesis of prothrombin by the liver, which activates key coagulation factors in the blood that prevent spontaneous hemorrhage. Thus, all neonates now receive a prophylactic injection of vitamin K soon after delivery to help prevent serious hemorrhagic disease of the newborn.

5. Fetal circulation involves unique anatomic features that shunt most blood away from the liver and lungs; hence, the systemic and pulmonary circulations are separate. The ductus venosus, the foramen ovale, and the ductus arteriosus are fetal shunts that all close, converting to an integrated neonatal circulation during the transition period.

6. Asphyxia—the combination of hypoxemia, hypercapnia, and acidosis—provides the strongest stimulus for the first breath. Other stimuli include cord occlusion, thermal changes (from rapid heat loss cause by increased energy expenditure), tactile stimulation, and other environmental changes (such as bright lights and noise).

7. The neurologic system regulates the neonate's adaptation by stimulating initial respirations, maintaining acid-base balance, coordinating cardiac and respiratory functions, and controlling body temperature.

8. The neonate's hepatic system is responsible for bilirubin clearance, blood coagulation, carbohydrate metabolism, and iron storage.

9. Respiratory functioning requires a patent airway, a functioning respiratory center, intact nerves from the brain to chest muscles, and adequate calories to supply energy for the labor of breathing.

Matching related elements
10. C.
11. A.
12. D.
13. B.

True or false
14. True.
15. False. The renal system is relatively immature at birth, which makes the neonate susceptible to dehydration, acidosis, and electrolyte imbalance.
16. True.

CHAPTER 18

Neonatal assessment

OBJECTIVES

After studying this chapter, the reader should be able to:

1. Describe general guidelines to follow when assessing the neonate.

2. Discuss the characteristics of each period of neonatal reactivity and understand how these characteristics may affect assessment findings.

3. Identify the proper sequence to use for the comprehensive assessment.

4. Discuss the essential elements of neonatal gestational-age, physical, and behavioral assessments.

OVERVIEW OF CONCEPTS

The neonate undergoes many physiologic changes during the neonatal period—the first 28 days after birth. The nurse plays a critical role in the neonate's transition by conducting a thorough, systematic assessment that provides baseline information about the neonate's physiologic status and the adequacy of neonatal adaptation. Besides knowing how to conduct such an assessment, the nurse also must understand the significance of assessment findings. Early detection of a potential or actual problem reduces the risk of complications; in some cases, it may mean the difference between life and death.

General assessment guidelines

The nurse must adapt the assessment to the neonate's tolerance, delaying any maneuvers that could compromise the neonate and combining overlapping portions of the various assessments to help conserve the neonate's energy.

Assessment sequence

Neonatal assessment proceeds from an immediate determination of the Apgar score to a complete physical assessment. The immediate assessment—determination of the Apgar score—takes place in the delivery area. Once stabilized in the delivery area, the neonate customarily is transferred to the nursery for observation. Some facilities have rooming-in privileges for the mother and neonate after a brief observation.

Within the next few hours, the nurse conducts a complete physical assessment to determine how well the neonate is adapting to the extrauterine environment and to check for obvious problems and major anomalies. This assessment includes evaluation of general appearance, vital sign measurement, and anthropometric measurements. The nurse then estimates the neonate's gestational age and, if indicated, conducts a formal gestational-age assessment, using a special assessment tool, to determine gestational age precisely. Based on education and experience, the nurse may assist with a behavioral assessment.

Health history

Obtain a complete history of the antepartal and intrapartal periods from the maternal and delivery room records, then review it for any problems that the patient might have experienced. Determination of preterm or post-term status usually is established by the time of delivery. However, the maternal history may be reviewed for factors that increase the risk of a gestational-age variation so that the health care team can anticipate potential perinatal problems more accurately. (For further information see Chapter 21, Care of high-risk neonates.)

The prenatal history also may suggest a birth-weight variation. Such variations include small for gestational age (SGA), defined as a birth weight that falls below the 10th percentile for gestational age on the Colorado Intrauterine Growth Chart, and large for gestational age (LGA), defined as a birth weight that exceeds the 90th percentile for gestational age on the growth chart. Like a gestational-age variation, a birth-weight variation increases the risk of perinatal problems.

Periods of neonatal reactivity

During the first hours after birth, the neonate experiences gradual, predictable changes in physiologic characteristics and behavioral responses, reflecting the periods of neonatal reactivity. The two reactivity periods are separated by a sleep stage (considered a discrete period of reactivity by some authorities).

With each period of reactivity, vital signs, state of alertness, and responsiveness to external stimuli change. The nurse must be able to recognize the characteristics of each period and use them when interpreting assessment findings (for key features associated with each reactivity period, see *Assessment findings during periods of reactivity,* page 290.) Although a specific assessment for these periods of reactivity is not necessary, stay alert for deviations from normal findings because such deviations may signify a disorder.

Initial physical assessment
During the initial physical assessment of the neonate, the nurse evaluates the neonate's general appearance, assesses vital signs, and takes anthropometric measurements. To prevent the neonate from becoming tired or stressed, conduct this assessment as swiftly and systematically as possible.

Assessment findings during periods of reactivity

The nurse should consider the period of reactivity when assessing the neonate — especially when using the Brazelton Neonatal Behavioral Assessment Scale to evaluate behavior. This chart shows the normal assessment findings associated with each reactivity period.

PARAMETER	FIRST PERIOD	SECOND PERIOD
Skin color	Fluctuates from pale pink to cyanotic (blue)	Fluctuates from pale pink to cyanotic, with periods of mottling
Alertness level	Awake and alert, progressing to sleep	Hyperactive, with exaggerated responses
Cry	Rigorous, diminishing as sleep begins	Periodic
Respiratory rate	Up to 80 breaths/minute when crying	40 to 60 breaths/minute, with periods of more rapid respirations
Respiratory effort	Irregular and labored, with nasal flaring, expiratory grunts, and retractions	Usually unlabored
Heart rate	Up to 180 beats/minute when crying	120 to 160 beats/minute, with periods of more rapid beating
Heart rhythm	Fluctuating, progressing to regular	Fluctuating as the neonate falls asleep, progressing to regular
Bowel sounds	Absent	Present
Stool	May not be passed	Meconium stool passed
Voiding	Rare	Usually begins
Mucus production	Minimal, diminishing gradually	Present, may be excessive
Sucking reflex	Strong, diminishing as sleep begins	Strong

General appearance

By assessing general appearance, the nurse quickly gauges the neonate's maturity level (a reflection of gestational age) and may detect obvious problems. Features to assess in the general survey include posture, head size, skin color and tone, activity, maturity, body symmetry, cry, and state of alertness (for details on evaluating general appearance, see "Complete physical assessment" later in this chapter).

Vital signs and blood pressure

After assessing general appearance, measure vital signs (temperature, respiratory rate, and pulse rate) and blood pressure—not a routine vital sign but usually included. Measure the neonate's core (internal, formerly called rectal) temperature first. Axillary temperature also accurately reflects core temperature; research has found that rectal and axillary temperatures differed by only 0.2° F.

Axillary temperature should measure 96.8° to 98.6° F (36° to 37° C), although the more acceptable range is 97.5° to 99° F (36.4° to

37.2° C). Axillary temperature above 99° F (37.2° C) reflects hyperthermia or fever; below 96° F (35.5° C), poor peripheral perfusion or prematurity.

The respiratory rate varies with the state of alertness and period of reactivity; thus, it may fluctuate widely in the first hours after birth. After the first period of reactivity, the respiratory rate typically measures 40 to 60 breaths/minute. If it exceeds 60 breaths/minute, or if the neonate has apneic episodes lasting longer than 15 seconds accompanied by duskiness or cyanosis, suspect respiratory distress, sepsis, or transient tachypnea.

In the first few hours after birth, the pulse rate fluctuates from 120 to 160 beats/minute but may increase to 180 beats/minute when the neonate is crying. The neonate's cardiopulmonary rates and rhythms may be irregular and high during the periods of reactivity, especially during the first few minutes after birth. Even nasal flaring and grunting may be noted immediately following birth. The neonate may or may not be crying. Report these irregularities if they continue, even though they represent only the normal transition to postnatal life for some neonates. For other neonates, however, they may be the earliest signs of respiratory difficulties or cardiac problems.

Neonatal blood pressure rises during periods of heightened activity; usually, it is relatively high for the first two weeks. The most accurate way to measure blood pressure is with a Doppler probe, an electronic instrument that eliminates the need for a stethoscope.

Anthropometric measurements

The nurse takes anthropometric measurements (weight, head-to-heel length, head and chest circumference, and crown-to-rump length). Birth weight averages 2,500 to 4,000 g (5 lb, 8 oz to 8 lb, 13 oz). In the term neonate, head-to-heel length ranges from 45 to 55 cm (18″ to 22″); head circumference averages 33 to 35.5 cm (13″ to 14″), with a range of 32 to 36.8 cm (12½″ to 14½″). Chest circumference usually measures about 2 cm less than head circumference, averaging 30 to 33 cm (12″ to 13″). Crown-to-rump length approximates head circumference.

Gestational-age assessment

Gestational-age assessment determines the neonate's physical and neuromuscular maturity, helping health care providers anticipate perinatal problems associated with preterm or post-term status. Correlation of gestational age with birth weight may suggest perinatal problems related to SGA or LGA status (see *Classifying the neonate by gestational age and birth weight,* page 292.)

Gestational age should be assessed for any neonate, but especially one who weighs less than 2,500 g (5 lb, 8 oz) or who has a suspected alteration in the intrauterine growth pattern. Gestational-age assessment tools rely on external physical features and neurologic maturity—not birth weight—as indices of growth and maturation.

Classifying the neonate by gestational age and birth weight

Organ system maturity depends largely on gestational age. Thus, the greater a neonate's gestational age, the more fully developed the organ systems. The premature neonate is one born before 37 weeks from the first day of the mother's last menstrual period. Low birth weight (LBW) is 2,500 g or less; neonates may be subdivided into term and preterm LBW neonates.

An additional classification—very low birth weight (VLBW)—has been added to describe the neonate weighing 500 g to 1,499 g. Most VLBW neonates have a gestational age of 23 to 30 weeks. VLBW neonates have had a tremendous impact on medical research and have sparked important advanc-

es in neonatal care—even though they account for only a tiny percentage of neonates.

Currently, neonates are evaluated according to the Colorado Intrauterine Growth Chart, developed by Battaglia and Lubchenco, which correlates gestational age with birth weight. After weighing the neonate and determining gestational age, the examiner plots these two parameters on the graph. The neonate whose weight falls between the 10th and 90th percentiles for gestational age on this chart is classified as appropriate for gestational age. One whose birth weight falls outside this range is considered to be small or large for gestational age, with an increased risk for certain perinatal problems.

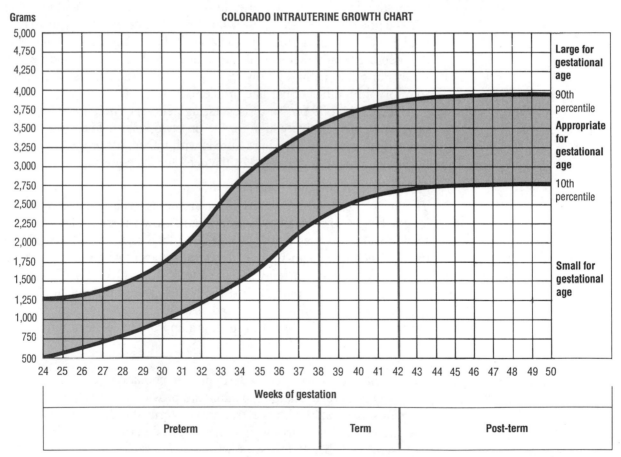

Battaglia, F.C., and Lubchenco, L.O. (1967). A practical classification of newborn infants by weight and gestational age. Journal of Pediatrics, 71, 159-163. Graph used with permission from Mosby, Inc.

The most common gestational-age assessment tools are the Dubowitz tool and the Ballard tool. The Dubowitz tool includes 11 external and 10 neurologic signs. With early patient discharge now routine, the Dubowitz tool has become somewhat impractical because the neurologic part of the examination must be delayed.

The Ballard tool, an abbreviated version of the Dubowitz tool, consists of 7 physical maturity and 6 neuromuscular maturity criteria. This tool is refined periodically in response to research. The 1988 revision incorporates criteria for gestational-age assessment of neonates at 24 to 44 weeks' gestation. (For more information, see *Ballard gestational-age assessment tool,* page 294.)

The examiner also plots gestational age against length and head circumference on an appropriate growth chart to determine whether these measurements fall within the normal range—the 10th to 90th percentile for the corresponding gestational age.

Complete physical assessment

When conducting the complete physical assessment, the nurse may use a systematic, head-to-toe approach tailored to the neonate's size and age or may assess heart and lung sounds first because these assessments require a quiet neonate. Ensure thermoregulation by placing the neonate under a radiant heat warmer and examining only one area at a time.

Check vital signs before the examination begins; if they are unstable or if the neonate has a temperature below 96° F (35.5° C), do not proceed with the examination. Instead, swaddle the neonate securely. Because the period of reactivity affects assessment findings, record the neonate's behavioral state and age (in hours or days after birth) at the time of the examination.

Physical examination

Examine the neonate's skin for temperature, color, turgor, and variations. The skin should feel warm to the touch, with a temperature ranging from 96° to 98° F (35.5° to 36.5° C), or 0.9° F (0.5° C) below core temperature. Evaluate any generalized edema, which may indicate a cardiac or renal problem. Skin variations are common in neonates; most are minor and do not require treatment. Common variations include the following:
- milia—minute, white, epidermal cysts caused by sebaceous gland obstruction; commonly seen on the face
- erythema toxicum neonatorum—pink, papular rash covering the thorax, back, abdomen, and groin; commonly occurs within 24 to 48 hours after birth
- nevus flammeus (port wine stain)—flat, capillary hemangioma; color of this permanent birthmark ranges from pale red to deep red-purple

Ballard gestational-age assessment tool

To use this tool, the examiner evaluates and scores the neuromuscular and physical maturity criteria, totals the scores, then plots the sum in the maturity rating box to determine gestational age. Unlike portions of the Dubowitz neurologic examination, the Ballard neuromuscular examination can be done even if the neonate is not alert.

	−1	0	1	2	3	4	5
NEUROMUSCULAR MATURITY							
Posture	–						–
Square window (wrist)	>90°	90°	60°	45°	30°	0°	–
Arm recoil	–	180°	140° to 180°	110° to 140°	90° to 110°	<90°	–
Popliteal angle	180°	160°	140°	120°	100°	90°	<90°
Scarf sign							–
Heel to ear							–
PHYSICAL MATURITY							
Skin	Sticky, friable, transparent	Gelatinous, red, translucent	Smooth, pink; visible vessels	Superficial peeling or rash; few visible vessels	Cracking; pale areas; rare visible vessels	Parchmentlike; deep cracking; no visible vessels	Leathery, cracked, wrinkled
Lanugo	None	Sparse	Abundant	Thinning	Bald areas	Mostly bald	–
Plantar surface	Heel-toe 40 to 50 mm:−1; <40 mm:−2	>50 mm; no crease	Faint red marks	Anterior transverse crease only	Creases over anterior two-thirds	Creases over entire sole	–
Breast	Imperceptible	Barely perceptible	Flat areola, no bud	Stippled areola; 1- to 2-mm bud	Raised areola; 3- to 4-mm bud	Full areola; 5- to 10-mm bud	–
Eye and ear	Lids fused, loosely:−1; tightly:−2	Lids open; pinna flat, stays folded	Slightly curved pinna; soft, slow recoil	Well-curved pinna; soft but ready recoil	Formed and firm; instant recoil	Thick cartilage; ear stiff	–
Genitalia, male	Scrotum flat, smooth	Scrotum empty; faint rugae	Testes in upper canal; rare rugae	Testes descending; few rugae	Testes down; good rugae	Testes pendulous; deep rugae	–
Genitalia, female	Clitoris prominent; labia flat	Prominent clitoris; small labia minora	Prominent clitoris; enlarging minora	Majora and minora equally prominent	Majora large; minora small	Majora cover clitoris and minora	–

MATURITY RATING

Score	−10	−5	0	5	10	15	20	25	30	35	40	45	50
Weeks	20	22	24	26	28	30	32	34	36	38	40	42	44

Adapted from Ballard, J.L., Khoury, J.C., Wedig, K., et al. (1991). New Ballard Score, expanded to include extremely premature infants. *Journal of Pediatrics,* 119(3), 417-423. Used with permission from Mosby, Inc.

- telangiectatic nevi (stork bite)—flat, deep pink, localized areas of capillary dilation; typically appear on the upper eyelids, across the nasal bridge and occipital bone, or along the neck.

Assess the neonate's head and neck for size, shape, and symmetry. Palpate the suture lines and the anterior and posterior fontanels. Examine the hair for distribution, texture, and color. To help assess cardiovascular status, palpate the carotid pulses, which should be equal and strong bilaterally.

Examine the neonate's face for symmetry of features. Observe the appearance of the mouth, chin, cheeks, and oral cavity. Inspect the oral mucous membranes, which should be moist, and inspect for the intactness of the hard and soft palates. Evaluate the neonate's eyes for symmetry, spacing, and movement. Note the color of the sclerae and conjunctivae and the pupillary response to light. Inspect the ears for symmetry, shape, and size. Also check the neonate's gross hearing ability; a loud noise should elicit the startle reflex or crying. Assess the nose for location, size, and patency of nares (nostrils); the neonate is an obligate nose breather who depends on patent nares.

Assess the size and symmetry of the thoracic cavity and chest excursion. In the SGA or preterm neonate, expect decreased chest circumference.

Inspect the abdomen for shape and symmetry. Check the umbilical cord remnant, which should appear bluish-white, contain two arteries and one vein, and be free of drainage. Auscultate for bowel sounds, which normally begin a few hours after birth. Then palpate and percuss the abdomen for abnormalities. Assess the neonate's back for spinal alignment, enlargement, or masses. Examine the sacrum for dimpling or a tuft of hair and observe for bulges. Palpate the vertebral column for enlargement and signs of pain.

Examine the anus and genitalia for abnormalities, keeping in mind that genital appearance depends on gestational age. The urinary meatus should be midline, the perineum smooth, and the anus midline and patent. In the male neonate, palpate the scrotal sac to determine if the testes are descended.

Inspect the extremities for length, symmetry, and size—relative to each other and to the body as a whole. Test the neonate's range of motion. Inspect the hands and feet for number of digits, palmar and plantar creases, and such abnormalities as syndactyly (webbing).

Some neurologic characteristics will have been evaluated during the gestational age assessment, preceding the complete physical assessment. To conserve the neonate's energy, do not reevaluate these characteristics during the complete physical assessment.

The neonate's posture typically reflects fetal positioning, gestational age, or delivery method. The healthy term neonate has a flexed posture and shows muscle resistance when the examiner extends the extremities. However, with breech delivery or in utero positioning, the legs may remain extended for a few days after birth. With some neonates born in a breech position, the legs are flexed back as far as the ears. Also check for tremors of the extremities. Tremors may stem from hypoglycemia, cold stress, or neurologic immaturity.

Next, assess reflexes—both localized and mass (full body) reflexes (see *Assessing neonatal reflexes*). Localized reflexes include the sucking, rooting, gag, blink, pupillary, grasp, and Babinski reflexes. Mass reflexes include the startle, Moro, fencing, Galant, and stepping reflexes.

Finally, assess the neonate's cry. The cry should be loud and strong, even in a preterm neonate (unless respiratory problems are present). A high-pitched cry or catlike cry suggests increased intracranial pressure; a grunting or low-pitched cry, respiratory distress syndrome; a weak, soft cry, brain damage. Duration of the cry varies with temperament.

Behavioral assessment

The behavioral assessment allows the nurse to evaluate the neonate's behavioral capacities and interaction with the environment. The Brazelton Neonatal Behavioral Assessment Scale (BNBAS), developed by pediatrician T. Berry Brazelton in 1973, is the most commonly used behavioral evaluation tool. To score the BNBAS reliably, the examiner must take an intensive 2-day course.

The nurse without such preparation may want to use the BNBAS as a guideline for assessing neonatal behavior in a more general way, without scoring the neonate. Areas evaluated by the BNBAS include the neonate's behavioral state (level of wakefulness) and behavioral responses, including elicited responses.

Behavioral state

The BNBAS assessment begins by observing the neonate's behavioral state (degree of alertness). The neonate experiences six behavioral states.

Deep sleep is a quiet period during which the neonate makes few or no spontaneous movements; any movements that occur are brief and jerky. No rapid eye movements (REMs) are detected. Respirations are even and regular. The neonate can be aroused from this state only for a few moments.

In *light sleep,* the neonate can be aroused and brought to wakefulness easily; REMs can be detected. The arms or legs may move occasionally, and movements are smoother than during deep sleep. The breathing pattern varies as the neonate drifts from light sleep to drowsiness.

The *drowsy state* is characterized by an attempt to become fully alert. Movements become more frequent and regular, and the eyes open periodically. Although the neonate responds to auditory and tactile stimuli, the response may be sluggish until the next state approaches.

Assessing neonatal reflexes

To evaluate neurologic status during the complete physical assessment, the nurse should test neonatal reflexes. The chart below describes some testing methods and normal responses. A weak, absent, or asymmetrical response is considered abnormal. The grasp, Babinski, Moro, fencing, and Galant reflexes normally disappear a few weeks or months after birth.

REFLEX	TESTING METHOD	NORMAL RESPONSE
Babinski	Stroke one side of the neonate's foot upward from the heel and across the ball of the foot.	Neonate hyperextends the toes, dorsiflexes the great toe, and fans the toes outward.
Fencing (tonic neck)	With a swift motion, turn the neonate's head to either side.	Neonate extends the extremities on the side to which the head is turned and flexes the extremities on the opposite side.
Galant	Using a fingernail, gently stroke one side of the neonate's spinal column from the head to the buttocks.	Neonate's trunk curves toward the stimulated side.
Grasp	Palmar: Place a finger in the neonate's palm.	Neonate grasps the finger.
	Plantar: Place a finger against the base of the neonate's toe.	Neonate's toes curl downward and grasp the finger.
Moro	Suddenly but gently drop the neonate's head backward (relative to the trunk).	Neonate extends and abducts all extremities bilaterally and symmetrically; forms a "C" shape with the thumb and forefinger; and adducts, then flexes, the extremities.
Rooting	Touch a finger to the neonate's cheek or the corner of mouth. (The mother's nipple also should trigger this reflex.)	Neonate turns the head toward the stimulus, opens the mouth, and searches for the stimulus.
Stepping (automatic walking)	Hold the neonate in an upright position and touch one foot lightly to a flat surface (such as the bed).	Neonate makes walking motions with both feet.

In the *alert state,* the neonate seems to be transfixed by external stimuli and has limited motor activity.

The *active state* is characterized by regular eye and body movements in response to external stimuli.

In the *crying state,* the neonate responds to both internal and external stimuli, cries vigorously and without interruption, and makes thrusting movements.

The neonate should move successively through these states, although the time spent in each may vary widely from one neonate to the next. The sleep-awake pattern also varies, depending on gestational age and other factors. The typical neonate sleeps 10 to 20 hours daily, with deep sleep accounting for only about 4 hours of total sleep. A neonate affected by maternal drug use may have an extremely labile sleep-awake pattern.

Behavioral responses

Neonatal behavioral responses fall into six categories: habituation, orientation, motor maturity, variations, self-quieting ability, and social behaviors.

Habituation

A protective mechanism, habituation refers to the process of becoming accustomed (habituating) to environmental stimuli, such as noise and light. A neonate's ability to become habituated to a stimulus varies with the behavioral state. A slowed or diminished response commonly reflects neurologic immaturity or impaired neurologic function.

Orientation

This term refers to the neonate's responsiveness to visual and auditory stimuli. Normally, the neonate orients to (follows) a visual or auditory stimulus by moving both the head and eyes. No response or lack of head movement is abnormal. Also observe for nystagmus (rapid, darting eye movements) and for gaze aversion after direct eye contact—both normal responses.

Motor maturity

Best assessed with the neonate in the alert state, motor maturity refers to posture, muscle tone, muscle coordination and movements, and reflexes. In the term neonate, asymmetrical or absent movement of an extremity calls for further investigation, as do muscle flaccidity or hypotonia, extreme tremors, and excessive jerking movements.

Variations

This term refers to the frequency of changes in activity level, state, and skin color. Document these changes throughout the behavioral assessment.

Self-quieting ability

To test this, observe how soon and how effectively the neonate self-quiets when crying. Attempts to self-quiet include such behaviors as moving the hands toward the mouth, sucking on the fist, changing position, and attending to auditory or visual stimuli. Consolability is documented in terms of whether and to what degree the neonate self-quiets after introduction of a visual or an auditory stimulus.

Social behaviors

Neonatal social behaviors include reflexive smiling, cuddling, and other distinct behavioral cues. Such cues—signals that indicate the neonate's needs—include crying to be fed and stopping sucking when hunger has been sated. These behaviors should be tested with the neonate in the alert or active state.

STUDY ACTIVITIES   **Short answer**

1. During an orientation to the newborn nursery, the neonatal nurse-educator describes some general guidelines for the new graduate nurses to follow as they are taught to perform an accurate neonatal assessment. This includes the period from the immediate determination of the Apgar score in the delivery area through a complete physical assessment in the nursery. Briefly identify the basic components of a thorough neonatal nursing assessment.

_____

_____

2. Justin Jones was delivered vaginally at 37 weeks' gestation after a rapid 3-hour labor. His mother's prenatal course was uneventful, and an ultrasound had been conducted early in the pregnancy for accurate dating. His Apgar scores are 8 and 9. He is vigorous and weighs in at 2,250 g. He measures 42 cm in length, with a 32 cm head measurement and a 30 cm chest.

Using the Ballard gestational-age assessment tool, the nurse evaluates Justin's neuromuscular and physical maturity at 6 hours of life. The physical findings include: _skin_—cracking, pale areas, rare veins visible; _lanugo_—mostly bald; _plantar surface_—creases over anterior two thirds; _breast_—raised areola, 3 to 4 mm bud; _eye and ear_—formed and firm, instant recoil; _genitalia_—testes down, good rugae. The neuromuscular findings include: _posture_—slight flexion of arms, full flexion of legs; _square window_—30° angle formed between hypothenar eminence and forearm; _arm recoil_—brisk recoil to complete flexion; _popliteal angle_—120° angle behind knee; _scarf sign_—elbow at midline; _heel to ear_—90° distance of foot from ear, knees flexed.

What is Justin's gestational age, according to these findings? Where would he fall on the Colorado Intrauterine Growth Chart in relation to his weight? Why is this assessment important to Justin's care?

_____

_____

3. Describe the features to be assessed in the neonate's general appearance survey and why these are important.

_____

4. Why must the nurse be alert to the neonate's specific period of reactivity when conducting the initial physical assessment?

_____

5. What are the parameters for a normal respiratory rate in a neonate who is several hours old? Briefly describe some common abnormal respiratory findings that should prompt the nurse to suspect other problems that warrant further assessment.

_____

6. When should the nurse delay an initial physical assessment on the neonate?

_____

Matching related elements

When evaluating neurologic status, the nurse should test neonatal reflexes. Match the following normal neonatal responses with their appropriate reflex:

7. ___ Babinski

A. Neonate grasps a finger placed in its palm; toes curl downward and grasp the examiner's finger

8. ___ Fencing

B. Neonate turns the head toward the stimulus, opens the mouth, and searches for the stimulus

9. ___ Grasp

C. Neonate extends the extremities on the side to which the head is turned and flexes the extremities on the opposite side

10. ___ Moro

D. Neonate makes walking motions with both feet

11. ___ Rooting

E. Neonate extends and abducts all extremities bilaterally and symmetrically; forms a "C" shape with the thumb and forefinger; and abducts, then flexes, the extremities

12. ___ Galant

F. Neonate hyperextends the toes, dorsiflexes the great toe, and fans the toes outward

13. ___ Stepping

G. Neonate's trunk curves toward the stimulated side.

True or false

14. Normally the chest circumference of the neonate is 2 centimeters greater then the head circumference.
☐ True   ☐ False

15. Crown-rump length approximates the neonate's head circumference.
☐ True ☐ False

16. The neonate's umbilical cord stump contains two arteries and one vein.
☐ True ☐ False

17. In the first few hours, the neonate's pulse rate fluctuates from 120 to 160 beats/minute but may increase to 210 beats/minute when crying.
☐ True ☐ False

18. The neonate's posture typically reflects fetal positioning, gestational age, or the delivery method.
☐ True ☐ False

19. A high-pitched or catlike cry suggests prematurity.
☐ True ☐ False

20. Habituation is a protective mechanism that refers to the neonatal behavioral response of becoming accustomed to environmental stimuli.
☐ True ☐ False

ANSWERS **Short answer**

1. After the immediate assessment of the Apgar score in the delivery area, the neonate is customarily transferred to the nursery for observation. Within the next few hours, the nurse conducts a complete physical assessment to determine how well the neonate is adapting to the extrauterine environment and to check for obvious problems and major anomalies. This assessment includes evaluation of general appearance, vital sign measurements, and anthropometric measurements. The nurse then conducts a gestational-age assessment and may assist with a behavioral assessment.

2. Justin's physical scores include: *skin*, 3; *lanugo*, 4; *plantar surface*, 3; *breast*, 3; *eye and ear*, 3; and *genitalia*, 3, for a total physical maturity score of 19. Neuromuscular findings include: *posture*, 3; *square window*, 3; *arm recoil*, 4; *popliteal angle*, 2; *scarf sign*, 3; and *heel to ear*, 3, for a total neuromuscular score of 18. His total score is thus 37, and his maturity rating is 39 weeks.

According to the Ballard tool, Justin is 2 weeks ahead of his estimated gestation. However, when this is plotted, his weight falls below the 10th percentile for his gestational age on the Colorado Intrauterine Growth Chart. Thus he is classified as small for gestational age (SGA).

A neonate who falls outside the normal range is considered at an increased risk for certain perinatal problems associated with such a variation and would require more close observation.

3. Features to be assessed in the general survey include posture, head size, skin color and tone, activity, maturity, body symmetry, cry and state of alertness. By assessing general appearance, the nurse can gauge the neonate's maturity level (a reflection of gestational age) and may detect obvious problems.

4. With each period of reactivity, vital signs, state of alertness, and responsiveness to external stimuli change. The nurse must be able to recognize the characteristics of each period and use them when interpreting assessment findings. The nurse should stay alert for deviations from normal findings because such deviations may signify a disorder.

5. After the first period of reactivity, the normal respiratory rate typically measures 40 to 60 breaths/minute. If it exceeds 60 breaths/minute, or if the neonate has apneic episodes lasting longer than 15 seconds accompanied by duskiness or cyanosis, the nurse should suspect prematurity, respiratory distress, sepsis, or transient tachypnea.

6. Prior to a physical examination, the nurse checks vital signs. If these are unstable or the neonate has a temperature below 96° F (35.5° C), the examination should be delayed and the neonate swaddled securely.

Matching related elements
7. F
8. C
9. A
10. E
11. B
12. G
13. D

True or false
14. False. The neonate's chest circumference usually measures 2 cm less then the neonate's head circumference.
15. True.
16. True.
17. False. The pulse should increase only to 180 beats/minute to be considered normal.
18. True.
19. False. A high-pitched or catlike cry suggests increased intracranial pressure. Premature neonates, unless respiratory problems are present, should have a strong and loud cry.
20. True.

CHAPTER 19

Care of the healthy neonate

OBJECTIVES After studying this chapter, the reader should be able to:

1. Identify the essential components of nursing care of the healthy neonate.

2. Identify factors affecting neonatal thermoregulation.

3. Describe the information to include in a teaching plan for new parents to promote confidence in their caregiving abilities.

4. Discuss nursing strategies that promote a positive parent-infant interaction.

OVERVIEW OF CONCEPTS The neonate undergoes various physiologic changes during the neonatal period—the first 28 days after birth. To make a successful transition, the neonate must adapt to these changes effectively, especially during the first 24 hours (known as the transitional period). The nurse plays a crucial role during the neonatal period by promoting a stable physiologic status. Nursing goals include maintaining oxygenation, hydration, nutrition, elimination, hygiene, and thermoregulation; preventing and detecting complications; and ensuring environmental safety.

Neonatal nursing care also calls for a family-centered approach that helps ease the neonate's transition to the home and promotes a positive parent-infant interaction. The nurse must assess parent-teaching needs regarding neonatal care and identify risk factors for poor parent-infant bonding. Parent teaching can be enhanced if the nurse serves as a caregiver role model and provides positive reinforcement during the parents' supervised attempts at caring for their child.

While providing care, the nurse must remain aware of cultural differences that may affect the parents' neonatal care decisions—for example, cultural attitudes toward circumcision. Considering these differences when planning, promoting, and implementing holistic neonatal and family care is essential.

Assessment During the first few days after the neonate's birth, the nurse should conduct a comprehensive physical assessment. Throughout the neonate's hospitalization, however, the nurse should conduct ongoing evaluations to ensure optimal neonatal adaptation and to detect changes in the neonate's status. The nurse evaluates the neonate continually for obvious or subtle changes from baseline clinical findings (including heart and respiratory rate and rhythm, skin color, cry, response to stimuli, alertness level, and irritability level) or laboratory values. The nurse also assesses for indications of neonatal distress, which could lead to serious complications. These include:

• abdominal distention
• apprehensive facial expression
• bile-stained emesis
• cyanosis (other than acrocyanosis or periorbital cyanosis)
• excessive mucus production or meconium in the nasal passages
• frequent apneic episodes
• hypotonia during active and alert periods
• jaundice
• labored respirations accompanied by skin or mucous membrane color changes
• lethargy during periods of expected activity
• meconium-stained skin
• persistent, pronounced increase or decrease in heart and respiratory rates from baseline vital signs
• temperature instability.

Nursing diagnoses

After gathering assessment data, review it carefully to identify pertinent nursing diagnoses for the neonate. (For a partial list of applicable diagnoses, see Nursing Diagnoses: *Healthy neonate.*)

Planning and implementation

After assessing the neonate and formulating nursing diagnoses, develop and implement a plan of care. For the healthy neonate, the plan centers on promoting optimal neonatal adaptation and parent-neonate interaction and includes such routine therapeutic interventions as umbilical cord care and vitamin K administration.

The American Academy of Pediatrics recommends that the neonate be kept in a transitional care nursery or under close observation in a birthing suite during the transitional period. Then the neonate may be returned to the mother's room to avoid further separating mother and neonate. This area should have oxygen and suction outlets, resuscitation equipment, and multiple electrical outlets with safety grounds.

Ensuring oxygenation

At birth, the neonate must begin breathing through the nose and drawing air into the lungs. Closure of the fetal shunts (ductus arteriosus, ductus venosus, and foramen ovale) after birth changes the circulatory direction and facilitates peripheral circulation and alveolar gas exchange. Maintaining adequate oxygenation is crucial to ensure successful respiratory adaptation.

A few hours after birth, the gastrointestinal (GI) tract begins secreting gastric juices; this leads to increased saliva and mucus production.

NURSING DIAGNOSES:

Healthy neonate

For the healthy neonate, the nurse may find the following examples of nursing diagnoses appropriate.
- Altered nutrition: less than body requirements, related to decreased oral intake and increased caloric expenditure
- Altered parenting related to the addition of a new family member
- Altered urinary elimination related to renal immaturity
- Altered peripheral tissue perfusion related to transition to the extrauterine environment
- Anxiety (parental) related to lack of confidence in parenting ability
- High risk for altered body temperature related to radiant, conductive, convective, or evaporative heat loss or gain
- High risk for altered parenting related to lack of knowledge about neonatal care
- High risk for fluid volume deficit related to insensible fluid losses
- High risk for infection related to circumcision site
- High risk for infection related to immunologic immaturity
- High risk for infection related to umbilical cord healing
- Hypothermia related to cold stress
- Ineffective airway clearance related to the presence of mucus
- Ineffective breathing pattern related to respiratory dysfunction

Mucus production peaks in the first 2 to 3 days after birth. Suctioning with a bulb syringe or sterile catheter may be necessary to prevent aspiration of mucus. A bulb syringe may be kept at the bedside; clean it with warm, soapy water after each use to reduce the risk of bacterial growth.

An irregular respiratory pattern, including periodic breathing and slight chest retractions, is common in the first few hours after birth while the neonate adapts to the new environment. Changes in the respiratory pattern that persist for several hours or become increasingly severe may indicate respiratory distress. If skin or mucous membrane color changes from pink to dusky or cyanotic, check for grunting, nasal flaring, crackles, rhonchi, and other abnormal signs. Immediately report any significant deviations from normal cardiopulmonary parameters, and assess vital signs continually to help prevent complications.

Maintaining thermoregulation

The term neonate has protective mechanisms to promote heat conservation—layers of adipose tissue and areas of brown fat, most prominent over the scapula and flank. Brown fat supplies fatty acids for heat production (thermogenesis), a process that begins when the neonate starts to lose heat. To maintain a stable core temperature, the body breaks down fats, burns calories, consumes oxygen, and increases the metabolic rate.

The preterm neonate, in contrast, has insufficient adipose tissue and brown fat insulation and may suffer cold stress from heat loss. The posture of the preterm neonate also contributes to heat loss. Unlike the term neonate—who assumes a fetal position to reduce the exposed surface area and thus minimize convective heat loss—the preterm neonate lies flaccid with arms and legs extended, exposing a greater surface area.

Cold stress may occur in any neonate who is exposed to a cold environment without adequate protection or whose caloric expenditure exceeds caloric consumption. When oxygen and nutritional reserves are depleted, the neonate loses protein and muscle tissue as well as weight. Anabolic metabolism ensues, leading to metabolic acidosis. (See *Preventing heat loss.*)

Even if the neonate is placed under a radiant warmer and dried to reduce heat loss, wide temperature fluctuations are common in the first few hours after birth. If the neonate has been in an open warmer for 2 to 3 hours and the axillary temperature measures over 97.6° F (36.5° C), wrap the neonate in a blanket and place in an open, clear bassinet. Monitor skin temperature, which should measure 97.5° to 99° F (36.4° to 37.2° C), or 0.2 to 0.9° F below the core temperature.

Observing and intervening for cold stress. Signs of cold stress include an accelerated respiratory rate, labored respirations, and an increased metabolic rate accompanied by hypoglycemia (indicating greater use of glucose stores). Evaluate signs of hypoglycemia, such as a serum glucose level below 30 mg/dl before the third day after birth or below 40 mg/dl on or after the third day. Other signs of hypoglycemia include tremors, seizures, irritability and lethargy (from breakdown of fats and proteins to maintain body heat), and apnea or bradycardia (from changes in arterial oxygen saturation and a shift to anaerobic metabolism). Neurologic immaturity may prevent homeostasis in the hypoglycemic neonate, leading to unstable vital signs.

Maintaining optimal hydration and nutrition. Hydration and nutrition are vital to immune system development and maintenance. The American Academy of Pediatrics recommends that the initial feeding never be delayed more than 6 hours after birth. If the mother plans to breast-feed, the neonate can be put to the breast in the delivery room.

Assessing the adequacy of fluid intake. To maintain adequate output and hydration, frequently compare fluid intake to urine output. The term neonate requires a fluid intake of 140 to 160 ml/kg/day to maintain hydration. This requirement increases with illness, preterm birth, and excessive evaporative or radiant fluid loss. Urine output should measure 1 to 2 ml/kg/hour. In the first 24 hours after birth, the neonate may void only once or twice, although output from these first voidings exceeds output from later voidings.

The formula-fed neonate who requires a diaper change every 2 to 4 hours is receiving adequate fluids. (Diapers should be moderately saturated six to ten times per 24 hours.) The breast-fed neonate usually voids slightly less frequently but at least six to eight times a day. With any neonate, scanty or infrequent voiding (less than five times a day)

Preventing heat loss

Preventing heat loss is an important part of neonatal nursing care. Heat loss can occur through four mechanisms—conduction, convection, evaporation, and radiation. The chart below describes some nursing measures that help prevent heat loss by each mechanism.

Conductive heat loss
- Preheat the radiant warmer bed and linen.
- Warm the stethoscope before use.
- Wrap the neonate in a warm blanket or allow the mother to hold the neonate to provide the warming effect of skin contact.
- Pad the scale with paper or a preweighed, warmed sheet to weigh the neonate.
- Check the temperature of any surface before placing the neonate on it.

Convective heat loss
- Place the neonate's bed out of direct line with an open window, a fan, or an air-conditioning vent.
- Cover the neonate with a blanket when moving the neonate to another area.
- Raise the sides of the radiant warmer bed to prevent exposing the neonate to air currents.
- Avoid using fans in the delivery room or nursery.

Evaporative heat loss
- Dry the neonate immediately after delivery.
- When the neonate is not in a warming bed, keep the neonate dry and swaddled in warmed blankets.
- Remove wet blankets.
- Delay the bath until the neonate's temperature is stable.
- When bathing the neonate, expose only one body part at a time; wash each part thoroughly, then dry it immediately.
- When assessing the neonate, uncover only the specific area to be assessed.
- Place a cap on the neonate's head in the delivery room.

Radiant heat loss
- Use a radiant heat warmer for initial postdelivery stabilization.
- Place the neonate in a double-walled incubator.
- Keep the neonate away from areas with cold surfaces (such as a cold formula bottle or a window in winter).

suggests impaired fluid intake or a urinary problem. Document this finding and notify the physician.

Giving the first feeding. For the first feeding, the bottle-fed neonate usually is given sterile water because it is less irritating than formula or glucose water if it is aspirated. If the neonate takes the sterile-water feeding without problems, glucose water or formula then may be given. In some facilities, the neonate is given a few milliliters of sterile water followed by 15 to 30 ml of glucose water to prevent hypoglycemia.

During the first feeding, assess the neonate's sucking ability and observe how well the neonate coordinates the sucking, swallowing, and gag reflexes. Immediately after the feeding, check for salivation, mucus production, aspiration, and regurgitation. The neonate produces more saliva and mucus in the first few hours after birth than at later times. Consequently, regurgitation—especially of a combination of mucus and feeding matter—is common. To promote digestion, place the neonate in a right side–lying position, which allows food to move more easily through the stomach and into the GI tract for absorption.

To prevent aspiration and facilitate digestion, place the neonate in semi-Fowler's position after feeding. The neonate who becomes cyanotic or extremely fatigued during a feeding may have a cardiac or respiratory problem. A respiratory rate above 60 to 80 breaths/minute increases the risk of aspiration.

If aspiration or regurgitation occurs, stop the feeding immediately and allow the neonate to rest before attempting further feeding. Document the incident thoroughly, and report it for further assessment.

Supporting the parents' choice of feeding method. Optimal nutrition may be achieved by breast-feeding, bottle-feeding, or both. Support the parents' choice of feeding method. Their choice may be based on such factors as economic and financial considerations, the mother's occupational status, and sociocultural influences as well as neonatal health implications.

Promoting adequate urinary and bowel elimination

Urinary and bowel elimination must be adequate to maintain hydration and nutrition. Elimination patterns are established in the first few days after birth. Although the kidneys begin functioning in utero (fetal urine is the major component of amniotic fluid), the neonate's kidneys do not concentrate urine as effectively as an adult's.

Monitoring for voiding onset. Despite the limitations described above, voiding should begin by 48 hours after birth. (Some neonates even void on the delivery table.) Over 90% of term neonates void within 24 hours of birth; all but 1%, within 48 hours. Failure to void within 48 hours may indicate a renal disorder, inadequate fluid intake, increased water loss, or fluid retention (edema).

Assessing urine characteristics. Initially, urine should be cloudy and amber (from urinary protein, blood, and mucus); specific gravity should measure 1.005 to 1.015. In the female neonate, blood in the urine represents pseudomenstruation; in the circumcised male neonate, blood originates from the surgical site.

A deviation from the usual urinary pattern may warrant further investigation. If the neonate is losing excessive fluids, check skin turgor and assess the fontanels and eye area. With dehydration, skin turgor is decreased and the anterior fontanel and eye orbits appear sunken. Edema, indicated by shiny, taut skin, may suggest fluid retention caused by a cardiac or renal disorder. All of these signs warrant further evaluation to help prevent complications.

Assessing bowel elimination patterns. The first stool (usually passed in the delivery room or within 48 hours after birth) consists of meconium, a thick, dark green, sticky, odorless material made up of amniotic fluid and shed GI mucosal cells. Failure to pass meconium within 48 hours may indicate anal or bowel malformation or Hirschsprung's disease, a congenital disorder characterized by incomplete bowel innervation.

Once feeding patterns have been established, stools change in color and consistency, the GI tract starts to secrete digestive enzymes, and intestinal bacteria (especially *Escherichia coli*) start to colonize. Transitional stools— thinner, lighter green, and seedier than meconium—

then appear. After 2 or 3 days, stools change again, taking on distinctive characteristics that vary with the feeding method.

Feeding method affects stool consistency and output. The stool of a breast-fed neonate is looser and paler yellow than that of a formula-fed neonate. Also, the breast-fed neonate typically passes 2 to 10 stools daily; the formula-fed neonate usually passes 1 stool daily or every other day.

Assess for deviations in stool pattern or consistency. If the neonate has diarrhea, a condition that increases fluid loss, assess for signs of dehydration (described above). If the neonate fails to pass stool or passes a hard, ribbonlike stool, suspect an intestinal obstruction. Also assess for abdominal distention, and palpate the abdomen for fecal masses. Observe the neonate during and just after feeding; an abdominal obstruction may cause vomiting and irritability at these times. Report any problem with stools, feedings, and related changes in the neonate's status so that prompt diagnosis and treatment can begin.

Providing hygienic care

Maintaining hygiene is an important aspect of neonatal care. The epidermal layer of the skin protects against traumatic injury, helps minimize heat loss, and serves as a barrier against bacterial infection by maintaining the pH of the skin at 4.9.

Bathing the neonate. To guard against heat loss during bathing, bathe the neonate only after temperature and vital signs have stabilized—especially if the core temperature is below normal. In the first hour or so after birth, use a soft sterile cotton cloth soaked with warm water to remove dried blood, meconium, and debris arising from delivery; then dry the skin thoroughly. Removing these contaminants reduces the risk of infection by the hepatitis B, herpes simplex, and human immunodeficiency viruses. It is not necessary to remove the vernix caseosa, the grayish-white substance that covers the skin of the term neonate.

Proceed from head to toe, washing the cleanest areas first to reduce the risk of infection from any contaminated areas. The neonate is not usually immersed in a tub; this could cause chilling or infection of the umbilical cord or an unhealed circumcision. During bathing, inspect the neonate's body for such variations as skin tags, unusual hair distribution, palmar creases, and other minor abnormalities. These variations may indicate more serious abnormalities.

Preventing and detecting complications

Document and report subtle changes in the neonate's condition immediately to prevent and detect complications. Also monitor laboratory values.

Respiratory dysfunction. The most common neonatal complication, respiratory dysfunction may be mild (such as transient tachypnea) or severe (such as respiratory distress syndrome). Assess for changes in the respiratory rate and effort or accompanying skin color changes, such as duskiness or cyanosis. If cyanosis is present, supplemental oxygen may be necessary. Be sure to allow the neonate to rest between nursing procedures to minimize oxygen consumption.

Hypocalcemia. The neonate who experienced birth asphyxia, is premature, or was born of an insulin-dependent diabetic mother is at risk for hypocalcemia (a serum calcium level below 7 mg/dl). Signs of hypocalcemia include twitching of extremities, cyanosis, apneic episodes, seizures, and listlessness.

Physiologic jaundice. Physiologic jaundice (yellow skin discoloration accompanied by an increased serum bilirubin level) is a common neonatal complication resulting from hepatic immaturity. It develops in the full-term neonate 48 to 72 hours after birth. Suspect physiologic jaundice if the neonate's skin appears abnormally yellow. To verify the disorder, apply pressure to the tip of the neonate's nose. With jaundice, a yellow tinge appears instead of the normal blanching as circulation is impeded. (This test is accurate in dark-skinned as well as light-skinned neonates.)

If the neonate has jaundice, pathologic jaundice must be ruled out. Unlike physiologic jaundice, pathologic jaundice develops within 24 hours.

Infection. Infection, another common complication, stems from immunologic immaturity. Thorough hand washing significantly reduces the risk of neonatal infection. Before and after performing any nursing procedure, wash the hands. Also emphasize to parents the importance of frequent hand washing and proper hand-washing technique.

Because the neonate does not have localized immune reactions, infection may cause only subtle, nonspecific signs. Such signs may include a high, low, or unstable body temperature; a weak or high-pitched cry; pallor; cyanosis; feeding problems or fatigue after feedings; diminished peripheral perfusion causing reduced skin temperature; sudden onset of apneic or bradycardic episodes; and early onset jaundice.

Ensuring environmental safety

Consider safety when providing all care measures, such as feeding, bathing, and weighing. Never look away or leave the neonate unattended while bathing or weighing. Before leaving the neonate's bedside, make sure the crib side rails are secured and in the locked position.

When the neonate is ready for discharge, confirm that an infant car seat (not a carrier seat, which cannot be locked into place) is available for the trip home. Most states require such seats or seat belts for all children.

Providing care for the family

Nursing care must involve the entire family—not just the neonate. By facilitating bonding and offering parent teaching, the nurse can help prepare the family for the neonate's discharge.

Providing parent teaching. Ongoing parent teaching is an essential part of discharge planning. Such teaching includes bathing, providing cord and diaper rash care, changing diapers, observing stool and voiding patterns, ensuring environmental safety, and integrating the neonate into the family.

The nurse also should serve as a caregiver role model for the parents and reinforce their caregiving behaviors. Active parental involvement in neonatal care before discharge has been found to lead to a strong parent-infant bond. Encourage the parents to ask questions about their child or the required care. Also urge them to interact with their child to enhance bonding. Explain how to detect early signs of potential problems, such as cold stress, infection, and dehydration, to help prevent life-threatening complications. The parents may be eager for their child to establish regular sleep-awake and eating patterns. However, inform them that a neonate typically sleeps 10 to 20 hours a day at first. Also emphasize that sleep patterns vary and that a deviation from the typical pattern does not necessarily indicate an abnormality.

The mother may have an increased need for support after discharge and might benefit by having relatives or friends available to help her. This is especially important for the single mother who may have to serve as the sole caregiver.

Performing routine therapeutic interventions

Routine nursing care of the healthy neonate includes umbilical cord care, vitamin K administration, circumcision care, and collection of urine specimens.

Providing umbilical cord care. Immediately after birth, the umbilical cord is moist, making it an excellent breeding ground for bacteria. To promote drying of the cord and prevent infection, keep the cord clean by wiping the surface gently with an alcohol swab or a cotton ball saturated with isopropyl alcohol. The base of the cord is most likely to become infected. To ensure the base is coated with alcohol, lift the cord away from the abdomen when wiping.

Note any drainage, such as blood, urine, or pus, appearing at the cord, so that cultures can be taken and antibiotic therapy initiated, if necessary.

Typically, the umbilical cord dries and falls off within 2 weeks after birth. To keep the area as dry and bacteria-free as possible, avoid giving the neonate tub baths.

Administering vitamin K. The neonate naturally has a vitamin K deficiency, which results partly from lack of intestinal bacterial flora necessary to synthesize vitamin K, until enteral feedings are established and milk or formula is digested. Without sufficient vitamin K, the liver cannot synthesize coagulation factors, which predisposes the neonate to hemorrhage. The American Academy of Pediatrics recommends a prophylactic I.M. injection of 1 mg of vitamin K_1 (phytonadione) during the first hour after birth.

Caring for a circumcision site. Circumcision, the surgical removal of the prepuce (foreskin) that covers the glans penis, has become controversial. The traditional rationale for the procedure was that it promotes hygiene and helps prevent penile and cervical cancers, urinary tract infections, and sexually transmitted diseases. However, some medical authorities believe that no known medical reason exists for performing circumcision during the neonatal period. The American Academy of Pediatrics states that there is no medical indication for circumcision.

The main advantage of circumcision is hygienic. The circumcised penis is easier to keep clean. Because the neonate's tight skin makes foreskin retraction difficult, bacterial growth is less common with a circumcised penis. The major disadvantage of circumcision is the pain and discomfort it causes.

Apply petrolatum gauze over the penis to prevent bleeding and protect it. Change the gauze with each diaper. The gauze is necessary for only 2 to 3 days after the procedure.

Collecting urine specimens. Urine specimens sometimes must be collected from healthy neonates for urine cultures, for routine urinalysis, or to determine urine specific gravity, pH (by dipstick testing), protein, ketones, glucose, bilirubin, or blood. To obtain urine for a specific gravity measurement or dipstick test, withdraw the specimen from a collection bag (via the covered port at the bottom of the bag) or from a disposable diaper. Both urine collection methods yield accurate results.

Evaluation

During this step of the nursing process, evaluate the effectiveness of the care plan by ongoing evaluation of subjective and objective criteria. Evaluation findings should be stated in terms of actions performed or outcomes achieved for each goal. The following examples illustrate appropriate evaluation statements.
- The neonate did not appear cyanotic or dusky.
- The neonate maintained a stable axillary temperature of 97.7° F (36.5° C).
- The neonate voided clear amber urine six times in 24 hours.

Documentation

All steps of the nursing process should be documented as thoroughly and objectively as possible. Thorough documentation not only allows the nurse to evaluate the effectiveness of the care plan, but it also makes the data available to other members of the health care team, helping to ensure consistency of care.

Documentation for the healthy neonate should include:
- vital signs, including temperature, heart rate and rhythm, and respiratory rate and rhythm
- general appearance
- umbilical cord description
- circumcision site description (as appropriate)
- stool and urine passage, including times, amounts, and characteristics

• any abnormal physical or behavioral findings
• parent teaching provided.

STUDY ACTIVITIES   **Short answer**

1. While still in the delivery room, Soledad Verdi, a 21-year-old primipara, has been intently watching as the nurse performs routine care on her daughter, Carolina. As the nurse begins to suction a copious amount of clear mucus from Carolina's nasopharynx with a bulb syringe, Ms. Verdi asks the nurse to explain what she is doing. How might the nurse respond?

_____

2. Ginger Seacrest, a 16-year-old, is about to begin feeding her son, Ian, for the first time. Although Ms. Seacrest has decided on formula feeding, the nurse offers this new mother sterile water. Why is this a common practice, and what would be included in an initial nursing assessment of Ian's first feeding?

_____

3. While conducting the "Preparation for Parenting" class during a childbirth education series, Joyce Gates, the nurse-educator, is asked by one of the fathers about changing diapers. How could Ms. Gates describe the neonate's expected urinary and bowel elimination patterns to the prospective parents who will either breast-feed or formula-feed?

_____

_____

_____

4. What measures must the nurse take to ensure the neonate's environmental safety?

_____

5. Because the neonate does not have localized immune reactions, infection may cause only subtle, nonspecific changes initially. Identify at least five suggestive signs of infection in the neonate.

_____

6. What are the signs of cold stress in the neonate?

_____

7. Briefly discuss the components of a complete teaching plan for new parents prior to discharge.

_____

_____

8. List two nursing prevention measures for each of the four mechanisms of heat loss.

_____

_____

_____

Fill in the blank

9. The most common neonatal complication, respiratory _____,

may be mild (such as _____) or severe (such as _____).

10. Neonatal ophthalmia, an eye infection caused by _____ or

_____, can be prevented if _____ solution, _____

ointment, or _____ ointment is applied to the eyes shortly after delivery.

11. Typically the umbilical cord dries and falls off within _____ after birth.

ANSWERS

Short answer

1. The nurse could explain that at birth, Carolina must begin to breathe through her nose, newly drawing air into her lungs as she adapts to extrauterine life. Increased saliva and mucus production are very common in neonates for the first 2 or 3 days after birth. Suctioning with a bulb syringe prevents aspiration or inhalation of this mucus as well as keeping the nose clear to ensure adequate oxygenation.

2. For the first feeding, the bottle-fed neonate usually is given sterile water because it is less irritating than formula or glucose water if it is aspirated. If Ian tolerates the sterile-water feeding without problems, formula may be given.

During the first feeding the nurse would assess Ian's sucking ability as well as his coordination of sucking, swallowing, and gag reflexes. Immediately after the feeding, his salivation, mucus production, aspiration, and regurgitation would be checked.

3. The neonate's elimination patterns are established within the few days after birth. Voiding should begin by 48 hours after birth, though the majority of neonates start urinating by 24 hours. The urine may appear cloudy and amber; there may be blood in both a girl's diapers (from pseudomenstruation) and in a boy's diapers (from the circumcision site, if present). After the first 24 hours, urine should be clear. As a general rule of thumb, the formula-fed neonate who requires a diaper change every 2 to 4 hours is receiving sufficient fluids. That would be translated into a moderately saturated diaper six to ten times per 24 hours. The breast-fed neonate usually voids slightly less frequently but at least six to eight times a day.

The first stool, usually passed within the first 48 hours, consists of meconium, a thick, dark green, sticky, odorless material. Once feeding patterns have been established, stools change color and consistency. Transitional stools—thinner, lighter green, and seedier than meconium—then appear. After 2 to 3 days, stools change again, taking on distinctive characteristics that vary with the feeding choice. The breast-fed neonate has looser, pale yellow stools and typically passes 2 to 10 stools per day. The formula-fed neonate usually passes 1 stool daily or every other day; the stool is darker, pasty, and somewhat firm.

4. To ensure environmental safety when caring for the neonate, the nurse must consider safety during feeding, bathing, and weighing, never looking away or leaving the neonate unattended. Crib side rails should always be secured in the locked position. Finally, the nurse must ensure that an infant care seat is available for the family's trip home from the health care facility.

5. Signs of infection in the neonate may include a high, low, or unstable body temperature; a weak or high-pitched cry; pallor; cyanosis; feeding problems or fatigue after feedings; diminished peripheral perfusion causing reduced skin temperature; sudden onset of apneic or bradycardic episodes; and jaundice within the first 24 hours.

6. Signs of cold stress include an accelerated respiratory rate, labored respirations, and an increased metabolic rate accompanied by hypoglycemia. Aside from a serum glucose level below 30 mg/dl before the third day after birth or below 40 mg/dl after the third day, other signs of hypoglycemia include tremors, seizures, irritability and lethargy, and apnea or bradycardia.

7. Ongoing parent teaching is an essential part of discharge planning. Such teaching includes bathing, providing cord and diaper rash care, changing diapers, observing stool and voiding patterns, ensuring environmental safety, and integrating the neonate into the family. The nurse also should serve as a caregiver role model for the parents and reinforce their caregiving behaviors. They should be encouraged to ask questions about their child or the required care. They also should be encouraged to interact with their child to enhance bonding. In addition, the nurse explains how to detect early signs of potential problems, such as cold stress, infection, and dehydration to help prevent life-threatening complications.

8. Nursing measures to prevent conductive heat loss include keeping the neonate's bed away from an open window, fan, or air-conditioning vent; covering the neonate with a blanket when moving the neonate; raising the sides of the radiant warmer bed; and avoiding the use of fans in the delivery room or nursery.

Nursing measures to prevent convective heat loss include preheating the radiant warmer bed and linen; warming the stethoscope before use; wrapping the neonate in a warm blanket or allowing the mother to hold the neonate; padding the scale with paper or a preweighed, warmed sheet; and checking the temperature of any surface before placing the neonate on it.

Nursing measures to prevent evaporative heat loss include drying the neonate immediately after delivery; keeping the neonate dry and swaddled in warmed blankets when not in a warming bed; removing wet blankets; delaying the bath until the neonate's temperature is stable; exposing only one body part at a time when bathing the neonate and drying the part immediately; uncovering one area at a time when assessing the neonate; and placing a cap on the neonate's head in the delivery room.

Nursing measures to prevent radiant heat loss include using a radiant heat warmer for initial postdelivery stabilization; placing the neonate in a double-walled incubator; and keeping the neonate away from areas with cold surfaces.

Fill in the blank

9. dysfunction; transient tachypnea; respiratory distress syndrome.

10. *Neisseria gonorrhea*; *chlamydia trachomatis*; 1% silver nitrate; 1% tetracycline; 0.5% erythromycin.

11. the first 2 weeks.

CHAPTER 20

Infant nutrition

OBJECTIVES

After studying this chapter, the reader should be able to:

1. Determine the learning needs of the childbearing family regarding infant nutrition.

2. Teach the patient how breast milk and infant formula differ in composition and nutritional value.

3. Discuss nursing interventions that foster successful feeding outcomes.

4. Describe the nurse's role in identifying and reducing barriers to successful breast-feeding.

OVERVIEW OF CONCEPTS

The rapid physical and developmental growth of the first year necessitates optimal nutrition. Besides playing a crucial part in infant health, nutrition also provides an opportunity for positive feeding experiences and important interactions between infant and caregiver. Teaching about infant nutrition is a major role of the nurse who works with young families. By understanding the nutritional needs of the first year, the nurse can provide the patient with accurate and practical rationales for feeding recommendations.

Infant nutritional needs

The neonate's immature organ systems and the unparalleled growth of the first year impose special requirements for nutrients and fluids. These factors also limit the types and amounts of foods a neonate can ingest and digest. Recommendations for the introduction of solid foods are based on these limitations.

Nutrient and fluid requirements

Like all diets, the neonate's must contain sufficient amounts of carbohydrates, proteins, fats, vitamins, minerals, and fluids.

Energy. Three basic nutrients—carbohydrates, proteins, and fats—supply the body's caloric needs. Carbohydrates should serve as the body's main source of calories. Proteins promote cellular growth and maintenance, aid metabolism, and contribute to many protective substances. Fats provide a concentrated energy storage form, transport essential nutrients (such as fatty acids needed for neurologic growth and development), and insulate vital organs.

Vitamins and minerals. Vitamins regulate metabolic processes and promote growth and maintenance of body tissues. Fat-soluble vitamins (A, D, E, and K) in excess of needs can be stored in the body to some extent and normally are not excreted; therefore, reserves may accumulate. Water-soluble vitamins (C, B_1, B_2, B_6, B_{12}, niacin, folic acid, pantothenic acid, and biotin) are stored only in small amounts. Consequently, if these vitamins are not ingested regularly, deficiencies may develop relatively quickly.

All major minerals and most trace minerals are essential for a wide range of body functions, including regulation of enzyme metabolism, acid-base balance, and nerve and muscle integrity. Calcium and iron are particularly important for growth—calcium for the rapid bone mineralization of the first year and iron for hemoglobin synthesis.

Fluids. The neonate's difficulty concentrating urine plus a high extracellular water content result in a much greater need for fluids (150 ml/kg/day) compared to the adult (20 to 30 ml/kg/day). By age 1, the daily fluid requirement is roughly 700 ml.

Special considerations

The neonate has limited gastric capacity. Also, fat absorption does not reach adult levels until ages 6 to 9 months. For the first 3 months, digestion of complex starches found in solid foods is restricted. Because of the neonate's low glomerular filtration rate (GFR) and difficulty concentrating urine, high renal solute loads may cause fluid imbalance. Some commercial infant formulas have a higher renal solute load than breast milk. Coupled with the neonate's low GFR, solutes such as sodium, potassium, and urea can cause too much fluid to be excreted, increasing the neonate's fluid needs even more.

Although the basic components of the neurologic system are present at birth, myelinization (development of the myelin sheath that protects nerve fibers) is incomplete. Only breast milk, infant formula, and whole milk contain enough linoleic acid to facilitate myelinization and should be used in the first year.

Sleeping through the night, a significant developmental milestone, usually occurs earlier in the formula-fed infant than in the breast-fed infant. Parents may introduce solid foods early, believing this will lengthen the infant's sleep. However, before age 3 months, the infant is ill equipped to ingest solids. The extrusion reflex, in which the tongue pushes out food placed on it, does not diminish until approximately age 4 months. Also, an infant under age 3 months lacks the tongue motion needed to pass solids from the front to the back of the mouth. These limitations indicate unreadiness for solid foods.

Nutritional assessment

Weight, length, and head circumference are the major nutritional assessment indices in the infant. Repeat measurements at various ages show whether the infant is growing at the expected rate. However, current charts are based on formula-fed infants and may be unreliable for exclusively breast-fed infants, who grow rapidly during the first 3 months and more slowly from ages 3 to 6 months.

The neonate typically loses an average of 10% of the birth weight in the first few days. This may alarm parents, who commonly view weight as a reflection of their infant's health status. However, the formula-fed neonate usually returns to birth weight by day 10 and the breast-fed neonate by 3 weeks. Birth weight typically doubles by ages 5 to 6 months and triples by age 1 year. Body length increases by about 50% by age 1; head circumference expands along with the rapidly growing brain.

Infant feeding methods

Choice of an infant feeding method involves more than a comparison of the biophysical properties of breast milk and formula. Cultural, psychosocial, and other factors also come into play. Consequently, the nurse must be familiar with the basic techniques of both breast-feeding and formula-feeding.

Because many patients make infant feeding decisions during pregnancy, the nurse should be prepared to offer guidance at that time to ensure an informed decision. Working with the patient after delivery, the nurse helps her gain skills and confidence in the method she has chosen.

Breast-feeding

Breast-feeding is an evolving, interdependent, and reciprocal relationship between mother and infant. Although the reflexes involved are natural, many of the techniques of breast-feeding must be learned by both mother and infant. The nurse who strives to work successfully with the breast-feeding patient must have a comprehensive understanding of the physiology of lactation and a genuine commitment to facilitating practices that promote breast-feeding.

Physiology of lactation

Lactation operates on a supply-meets-demand basis: The more milk the infant removes, the more milk the breast produces. Hormones control milk production and ejection to make milk available to the infant.

Milk production. Milk is produced in the breast alveoli. The female breast has a rich blood supply from which the alveoli extract nutrients to produce milk. The alveoli are situated in lobules—clusters leading to ductules that merge into lactiferous ducts. These larger ducts widen further into ampullae, or lactiferous sinuses, located behind the nipple and areola.

Lactogenesis—initiation of milk production—begins during the third trimester of pregnancy under the influence of human placental lactogen, a hormone secreted by the placenta. After delivery of the placenta and the resultant decrease in circulating estrogen and progesterone, the anterior pituitary gland releases prolactin. In response, alveolar secretory cells begin extracting nutrients from the blood and converting them to milk. Initial prolactin production also hinges on tactile stimulation of the nipple-areola junction by infant sucking or milk expression. Frequent feeding over the entire 24-hour period enhances prolactin secretion and significantly increases milk production. Prolactin secretion also creates a calm, relaxed feeling in the mother, which may enhance mother-infant bonding.

Milk ejection. The hormone oxytocin makes breast milk available to the infant through the let-down reflex. In this reflex, nipple stimulation or an emotional response to the infant causes the hypothalamus to trigger release of oxytocin by the posterior pituitary gland. Myoepithelial cells surrounding the alveoli then contract and eject milk into the ductules and sinuses, making milk available through nipple openings. A conditioned reflex, let-down occurs after 2 to 3 minutes of sucking during the first days of breast-feeding; several let-downs occur over the course of a feeding.

In the early postpartal period, other let-down symptoms may include uterine cramps (afterpains), caused by the action of oxytocin on the involuting uterus, and a slight increase in lochia (the vaginal discharge emitted after delivery). Also, the breasts may leak. However, let-down may occur even in the absence of milk leakage.

Restricting sucking time can disrupt optimal function of the let-down reflex by preventing the infant from completely emptying the milk ducts. This, in turn, leads to milk buildup and signals the body to stop producing milk. The breasts become engorged and harden; the nipples may become flat, hindering proper infant attachment. The body responds to engorgement by halting milk production. In the early days of breast-feeding, restricted sucking time may establish a negative feedback system that can lead to insufficient milk production. Also, it may force the infant to feed more often to satisfy hunger.

Breast milk composition and digestion

The composition of breast milk undergoes various changes. Initial feedings provide colostrum, a thin, serous fluid. Unlike mature breast milk, which has a bluish cast, colostrum is yellow. However, its color may vary considerably from one woman to the next.

Colostrum contains high concentrations of protein, fat-soluble vitamins, minerals, and immunoglobulins, which function as antibodies. Colostrum's laxative effect promotes early passage of meconium. Also, the low colostrum volumes produced do not tax the neonate's limited gastric capacity or cause fluid overload.

The breasts may contain colostrum for up to 96 hours after delivery. The maturation rate from colostrum to breast milk varies. With increased breast-feeding frequency and duration in the first 48 hours, colostrum matures to milk more rapidly.

Breast milk composition also changes over the course of a feeding. The foremilk—thin, watery milk secreted when a feeding begins—is low in calories but contains abundant water-soluble vitamins. Next, whole milk is released. The hindmilk, available 10 to 15 minutes after the initial let-down, has the highest concentration of calories for satisfying hunger between feedings. The rate of milk transfer to the infant varies among mother-infant couples. Consequently, limiting feeding times or insisting that the woman use both breasts at each feeding may prevent the infant from obtaining the maximum benefit of variable breast milk content.

The whey proteins that predominate in breast milk lead to formation of soft, easily digested curds. The infant typically digests breast milk within 2 to 3 hours after a feeding and thus may become hungry more often than the formula-fed infant, who typically feeds every 4 hours. In the first few weeks after birth, the breast-fed neonate may feed eight to twelve times every 24 hours.

Infant sucking

The dynamics of sucking on a breast involve no frictional movement; therefore, it should be painless, provided the infant is properly attached. Incorrect infant sucking technique, not prolonged feeding, causes nipple soreness. Some infants must be taught to suck correctly.

Intake requirements

A breast-fed infant typically needs to be fed every 2 to 3 hours. During the first 3 to 4 weeks, before the feeding pattern is established fully, parents may wonder if the neonate is receiving adequate nourishment. Signs of adequate intake include 10 to 12 wet diapers in 24 hours, steady weight gain, and contentedness after feeding.

Duration

Lactation insufficiency (lack of milk) is the most common reason for stopping breast-feeding in the early weeks. Lactation insufficiency most commonly stems from mismanagement of lactation. Practices such as glucose and water feedings and arbitrary feeding schedules may strain the adaptability of the mother-infant couple and interrupt the interactions necessary for successful breast-feeding. Also, indiscriminate use of bottles to supplement breast-feeding in the neonate's first days may cause nipple confusion, making the neonate refuse the breast the next time it is offered.

Like the patient's decision to breast-feed initially, her decision to stop involves many factors, including her age, family or social attitudes toward breast-feeding, and her socioeconomic status or educational level. Maternal ambivalence toward breast-feeding also may play a role. However, with proper antepartal teaching, a patient may learn to adjust her expectations about breast-feeding and thus avoid becoming so discouraged that she stops when problems occur.

The nurse can help prevent a poor breast-feeding outcome by teaching the patient about the physiology of lactation, providing anticipatory guidance about the normal course of breast-feeding, and making sure the patient knows how to obtain information and support after discharge. Although the availability of follow-up support varies, some community health nurses make routine home visits after a neonate's birth. Also, the assistance of a lactation nurse has been found to significantly prolong breast-feeding during the first 4 weeks and among women of lower socioeconomic status. Professional and lay breast-feeding support may be available from a lactation consultant or a local LaLeche League group.

Formula-feeding

Because of the current emphasis on breast-feeding, the patient who chooses formula-feeding may feel uncertain about her choice and react defensively if she feels it is being questioned. By recognizing the many factors that go into infant feeding decisions, the nurse can convey respect and offer support to the patient who has made an informed decision to formula-feed. Also, by working with the patient in the antepartal period, the nurse can help ensure that she receives relevant information in a way that would allow her to revise her choice.

Commercial formulas and equipment

Commercial infant formulas fall into three categories: milk-based, soy-based, and casein hydrolysate-based. The American Academy of Pediatrics recommends commercially prepared formulas over other formulas for infants up to age 1 year. Commercial formulas provide all necessary vitamins, so infants receiving them do not require vitamin supplements. However, use of noncommercial formulas necessitates vitamin supplementation.

Product convenience, personal preference, and economic status influence the patient's choice of formula equipment. Commercially available equipment includes glass bottles, boilable plastic bottles, disposable plastic bags (which the preparer places in a hollow plastic holder), and artificial nipples. Because sucking action on the NUK nipple (which is flat and broad) most closely resembles sucking action on the human nipple, some authorities recommend this nipple for breast-fed infants who receive an occasional supplemental bottle.

Intake requirements

The amount and frequency of formula feedings vary with infant size, maturity, and activity level. Daily formula intake averages 180 ml/kg. Like parents of the breast-fed infant, parents of the formula-fed infant may believe all crying signals hunger. The nurse can help them interpret infant behavior more accurately by reviewing guidelines on feeding frequency. (See *Formula guidelines,* for more information.)

Digestion

The casein proteins predominating in formula result in tougher, less digestible curds than does the whey in breast milk. Consequently, infant formula takes more time and energy to digest than breast milk. Homogenization and heat treatment of commercially prepared formulas have improved curd digestibility somewhat.

Formula guidelines

The table below shows recommended formula volume and feeding frequency for infants up to age 1 year who are receiving commercial formula exclusively.

AGE	FORMULA VOLUME PER FEEDING	FEEDINGS PER DAY
1 month	126 ml (4.1 oz)	6
2 months	142 ml (4.6 oz)	5
3 months	161 ml (5.2 oz)	5
4 months	168 ml (5.4 oz)	5
5 months	191 ml (6.2 oz)	4
6 months	179 ml (5.8 oz)	5
7 to 9 months	131 ml (4.2 oz)	5
10 months	136 ml (4.4 oz)	5
11 months	125 ml (4.0 oz)	5
12 months	141 ml (4.5 oz)	4

Adapted from data analysis performed by Ross Laboratories, 1985. Used with permission.

Assessment

The nurse should begin patient assessment by collecting general data and then make specific assessments related to the feeding method.

The breast-feeding patient

Ideally, assessment should begin in the antepartal period with a determination of how much the patient knows about infant nutrition and breast-feeding techniques. Also evaluate nipple graspability and protractility by determining whether the nipples are slightly everted, flat, or inverted.

For the patient in the postpartal period, after breast-feeding has begun, assess:
• consistency of the breasts (softness, mobility, engorgement, and warmth)
• condition of the nipples (tenderness, abrasions, and discoloration)
• sensations experienced during breast-feeding (such as tingling).

For the breast-feeding neonate, assess the sucking reflex before the first feeding because improper sucking will prevent adequate feeding. Also assess for proper patient and infant positioning. The patient may assume a sitting or reclining position, bringing the infant to her. A pillow can be placed under the arms to prevent shoulder elevation, which could cause muscle tension. The patient should hold the infant facing her and level with the breast so that the infant's neck need not twist or flex. Assess the patient and infant during a feeding to determine if the infant is correctly attached on the breast.

Assessment of the patient and infant after discharge can promote breast-feeding success. Many lifestyle adjustments must be made when a neonate joins the family. These adjustments may cause role strain and conflict. Postdischarge nursing assessment may reveal breast-feeding problems caused by such role strain and conflict.

The patient using infant formula
For the patient in the antepartal period, the nurse should assess for:
• knowledge of proper feeding techniques
• understanding of types of formula
• previous experience with infant formula.

Also find out what equipment and facilities the patient will use to prepare formula and determine if the patient will need financial aid to meet the infant's nutritional needs (see *Nutritional aid for mothers and infants*).

For the patient in the postpartal period, assess bottle and infant positioning during feeding and the patient's ability to adjust feeding technique in response to infant cues. Also inspect the patient's breasts for signs of engorgement, such as tenderness, swelling, warmth, hardness, shininess, and redness.

Nursing diagnoses
After gathering all assessment data, review it carefully to identify pertinent nursing diagnoses for the patient or neonate (for a partial list of applicable diagnoses, see Nursing Diagnoses: *Infant nutrition*, page 326).

Planning and implementation
After assessing the patient and formulating nursing diagnoses, develop and implement a plan of care. For example, if the patient lacks knowledge about breast-feeding, plan what and how to teach her. Although the plan will depend on the patient's abilities, it may include written materials, discussion of proper feeding methods and infant positioning, and patient demonstration of breast-feeding.

Care for the breast-feeding patient
The nurse's role in working with the breast-feeding patient includes teaching of proper feeding techniques and intervention to correct any related problems. The nurse also helps the patient deal with physiologic or psychosocial problems related to breast-feeding.

Patient teaching
Ideally, teaching about breast-feeding should begin in the antepartal period and continue postpartum until breast-feeding is well established.
Antepartum. In the antepartal period, teaching should focus on practical knowledge that will help the patient establish and maintain lacta-

Nutritional aid for mothers and infants

In the United States, a government program called the Women, Infants, and Children Nutrition Program (WIC) provides supplemental foods, access to health care, and nutrition education during critical stages of growth and development. Those eligible include pregnant and postpartal women, infants up to age 1 year, and children up to age 5 whom a health care professional has classified as being at nutritional risk. Although federally funded, WIC is administered by states; consequently, eligibility requirements may vary. Further information can be obtained from the Department of Agriculture or from state health departments.

---

tion after delivery. Some general topics that could be incorporated into antepartal teaching include:

- physiologic, emotional, and social factors that influence lactation
- common breast-feeding problems and possible solutions
- the possibility of continuing to breast-feed after the patient returns to work
- the role of support groups or professional services and how to gain access to them.

Postpartum. Encourage the patient to take advantage of the neonate's early responsiveness by breast-feeding as soon as possible. For the healthy full-term neonate, no contraindications exist to feeding immediately after delivery. Many neonates breast-feed shortly after delivery; all at least make licking or nuzzling motions, helping to stimulate the mother's prolactin production. Also, during this time the patient's breasts may be soft and easily manipulated, facilitating proper attachment. Immediate breast-feeding also offers the chance for intimate contact that can enhance mother-infant bonding and have a positive psychological effect on the parents.

Valid reasons for delaying breast-feeding immediately after delivery include such contraindications as the mother or neonate having a life-threatening illness, the mother being heavily sedated or fatigued, or the neonate having a 5-minute Apgar score of 6 or less.

General breast-feeding guidelines

Although lactation is a natural process, breast-feeding skills must be learned and practiced. The nurse can promote breast-feeding success through timely intervention to correct any problems. In addition to helping the patient initiate breast-feeding, the nurse can suggest comfort measures and promote the patient's hygiene; ensure proper position of mother and neonate; ensure correct infant attachment onto the nipple; and assist the patient with establishing an acceptable breast-feeding pattern. Further the nurse can encourage the patient to take advantage of the benefits from night feedings and to cope with the neonate's growth spurts.

NURSING DIAGNOSES

Infant Nutrition

The following are potential nursing diagnoses for problems and etiologies that a nurse may encounter when caring for a patient as she begins to nourish her neonate. Specific nursing interventions for many of these diagnoses are provided in the "Care for the breast-feeding patient" and "Care for the patient using infant formula" sections of this chapter.
- Altered family processes related to infant feeding
- Altered nutrition: potential for more than body requirements, related to breast-feeding
- Altered role performance related to the new task of breast-feeding
- Anxiety related to change in infant feeding pattern secondary to a growth spurt
- Anxiety related to the ability to properly feed the infant
- High risk for fluid volume deficit related to breast-feeding
- High risk for injury related to improper nipple care
- Ineffective breast-feeding related to improper positioning at the breast
- Ineffective infant feeding pattern related to inadequate milk supply
- Knowledge deficit related to breast-feeding
- Knowledge deficit related to formula-feeding
- Pain related to breast engorgement

Throughout the early postpartum period, the nurse can assist the new breast-feeding mother toward understanding the importance of breast care, solutions for commonly encountered problems, such as nipple soreness, breast engorgement, and the issues surrounding supplementary bottle feedings with the breast-feeding neonate.

Ensuring adequate maternal fluid and food intake. Advise the breast-feeding patient to maintain a fluid intake sufficient to keep her urine clear and amber. Provide fluids at each feeding. Also advise the patient to restrict intake of caffeine-containing fluids because caffeine accumulates in the body and transfers to the infant in breast milk, possibly making the infant fussy in the evening.

Although many obstetricians still advise lactating women to consume 500 extra calories daily, the Royal College of Midwives recommends that hunger—rather than a rigid caloric requirement—should guide food intake during breast-feeding. Help the patient establish a well-balanced diet and assure her that she can consume any food in moderation. However, if the infant develops symptoms of food allergy, she may have to restrict some foods. The patient with a family history of food allergy may need to modify her diet.

Advising the patient about drug use. Almost any drug the patient consumes potentially transfers to the infant through breast milk. However, the patient need not necessarily stop breast-feeding during drug therapy. Instead, she should seek her physician's advice. Usually, the breast-feeding woman can safely use therapeutic doses of such drugs as analgesics, antibiotics, stool softeners, and bulk-forming laxatives.

Promoting family support. The breast-feeding patient needs practical and emotional support from those close to her. The patient's partner can play an especially key role. Mothers of neonates have been found to view three types of support from the father as important: physical support (such as helping with housework or other children), verbal reinforcement (such as ensuring the mother that breast-feeding is progressing well), and psychological support or sensitivity to the mother's feelings.

Care for the patient using infant formula

For the patient who plans to formula-feed her infant, teaching on such topics as formula preparation can begin in the antepartal period. As with breast-feeding, initial formula-feeding experiences can prove crucial for both mother and infant. A positive first feeding experience can enhance maternal confidence and set the right tone for subsequent feedings. The nurse who observes early feedings has a unique opportunity to assess patient-infant interaction and, if necessary, provide timely intervention.

Patient teaching

In the antepartal period, develop varied patient teaching methods to present current recommendations about formula-feeding. Usually, antepartal discussion of growth spurts, of alternatives to early introduction of solid foods, and of support systems is more effective than discussion during the postpartal period, when the patient may be fatigued from sleep deprivation and anxiety accompanying new parenthood.

Ensuring proper formula preparation

To teach the patient about formula preparation, find out what preparation facilities and equipment will be available as well as which formula the patient will use. Where water and refrigeration are readily available, rigorous sterilization practices largely have been replaced with an emphasis on cleanliness of the equipment and preparer. However, a patient who lacks easy access to refrigeration and running water may have to modify preparation procedures.

General principles. Some common principles are basic to all formula preparation methods. The preparer must use good hand-washing technique—a point to reinforce frequently. Also, before opening the can, the preparer should wash the can opener and the top of the formula can with soap and water.

Prepared formula should be used within 24 hours (or 30 minutes with the one-bottle method). Opened formula cans should be covered with plastic or foil and refrigerated. Equipment used in formula preparation may be cleaned in an automatic dishwasher (providing the temperature reaches 140° F) or in warm, soapy water. However, latex nipples cleaned in a dishwasher may need to be replaced frequently because repeated exposure to heat weakens them. Instruct the patient to place latex nipples in a covered basket in the dishwasher to prevent their displacement to the heating element, where they could melt. Also instruct the patient to inspect nipples regularly to ensure that no milk particles block the opening, forming a bacterial breeding ground.

Giving the first feeding

No research-based guidelines support delaying formula-feeding. Nonetheless, in many health care facilities, the first feeding is given when the neonate is about 4 hours old. Neonates fed according to readiness cues are less likely to gag during the first feeding because their sucking and rooting responses are active. In some health care facilities, a nurse—rather than the mother—gives the first bottle (usually sterile water).

Helping the patient with early feedings

Help the patient to a comfortable position with good back support and instruct her to hold the infant close to her in a semi-reclining position, with the bottle tilted so that the nipple always is filled with formula. This position minimizes air swallowing and permits air to rise to the top of the infant's stomach.

Instruct the patient to check nipple openings by holding the bottle upside down and noting whether formula drips freely from the nipple. (Formula that runs in a continuous stream is flowing too quickly.) The patient can assume that nipple openings are the correct size if feedings take roughly 15 to 20 minutes, long enough to meet the infant's nutritional needs without causing fatigue. Warn the patient to discard any formula left in the bottle at the end of a feeding because of the risk of bacterial contamination.

Most health care facilities use glass bottles with standard latex nipples; when the infant sucks, air bubbles may appear in these bottles, indicating that the infant is obtaining milk. However, point out that at home, the patient may use a feeding system with a collapsible bag in which she cannot see air bubbles move. Instead, she should watch for the bag to collapse gradually, as a sign that the infant is obtaining formula.

The nurse can assist the formula-feeding patient with the neonate's early feedings by initially assisting the patient to get comfortable and settled, and teaching general information about bottle-feeding equipment, ensuring good burping techniques, and helping the new mother establish an appropriate feeding pattern. Further the nurse can encourage physical contact between mother and neonate as well as encourage family support and participation in the feedings. Information regarding growth spurts, alternatives to early introduction of solid foods, and identification of helpful support systems should also be included.

Evaluation

Evaluation findings should be stated in terms of actions performed or outcomes achieved for each goal. The following examples illustrate appropriate evaluation statements for the breast-feeding patient:

- The patient demonstrated appropriate techniques for attaching the infant to the breast.
- The patient showed no signs of breast problems, such as sore nipples or excessive engorgement.

The following examples illustrate appropriate evaluation statements for the patient who uses infant formula:

- The patient expressed an understanding of formula preparation and feeding techniques.
- The patient maintained close contact with the neonate during feeding.

Documentation

When assisting a patient with infant feeding, include the following points in the documentation:

- maternal vital signs
- maternal fluid intake and output
- maternal position and comfort level during feeding
- choice of feeding method
- maternal understanding of breast-feeding technique
- maternal understanding of proper infant positioning and ability to achieve it
- maternal attitude toward breast-feeding or formula-feeding
- maternal understanding of dietary needs and breast care
- condition of the nipples and breasts
- infant sucking ability.

In addition, when assisting a patient with formula-feeding, include these further points in the documentation:

- maternal understanding of formula preparation
- maternal understanding of normal infant feeding patterns, including amount of formula taken and feeding frequency.

STUDY ACTIVITIES

Short answer

1. During a childbirth education class, Stephanie and Len Childers, first-time prospective parents, ask the nurse-educator about the composition and nutritional value of breast milk. Mr. Childers especially wants to know why his wife thinks breast milk will be so much more beneficial for their new baby. How could the nurse respond?

_____

_____

2. In a postpartum class at the hospital, the nurse-educator determines that the majority of the new mothers are planning to bottle-feed their babies. What infant factors should the nurse be sure to cover in a discussion of formula-feeding?

_____

3. How does breast milk composition change over the course of a feeding session?

_____

4. Why should the nurse discourage parents from introducing solid foods until their baby is at least 4 months old?

_____

5. Briefly describe the typical pattern of weight loss and gain that a neonate experiences in the first year.

_____

6. Identify some of the barriers that the nurse would attempt to overcome in order to facilitate a successful breast-feeding outcome.

_____

_____

Fill in the blank

7. Lactation insufficiency is the most common reason for _____ in the early weeks and most commonly stems from _____ of lactation.

8. _____, _____, and _____ are the major nutritional assessment indices in the infant.

ANSWERS

Short answer

1. Initial breast-feedings provide colostrum, the forerunner of breast milk. Unlike formula, colostrum contains high concentrations of protein, fat-soluble vitamins, minerals, and immunoglobulins, which function as antibodies. Colostrum's laxative effect promotes early passage of meconium. Also, the low colostrum volumes produced do not tax the neonate's limited gastric capacity or cause fluid overload. The whey proteins that predominate in breast milk lead to formation of soft, easily digested curds.

2. The nurse-educator should be sure to include such infant factors as burping techniques as well as feeding pattern recommendations. The nurse should promote physical contact and cuddling between the mothers and their babies and should encourage family support of this method of feeding. Growth spurts, alternatives to early introduction of solid foods, and identifying helpful support systems should also be included.

3. The foremilk—thin, watery milk secreted when a feeding begins—is low in calories but contains abundant water-soluble vitamins. Next, whole milk is released. The hindmilk, available 10 to 15 minutes after the initial let-down, has the highest concentration of calories for satisfying hunger between feedings. The rate of milk transfer to the infant varies among mothers and their infants.

4. The neonate is ill equipped to ingest solids. The extrusion reflex, in which the tongue pushes out food placed on it, does not diminish until approximately age 4 months. In addition, an infant under age 3 months lacks the tongue motion needed to pass solids from the front to the back of the mouth. These limitations indicate unreadiness for solid foods. Also, fat absorption does not reach adult levels until ages 6 to 9 months, and for the first 3 months, the neonate's digestion of complex starches found in solids is restricted.

5. The neonate typically loses an average of 10% of the birth weight in the first few days. Formula-fed neonates usually return to birth weight by day 10 and the breast-fed neonate by 3 weeks. Birth weight typically doubles by ages 5 to 6 months and triples by age 1 year. Body length increases by about 50% by age 1; head circumference expands along with the rapidly growing brain.

6. Like the patient's decision to breast-feed initially, her decision to stop involves many factors, including her age, family or social attitudes toward breast-feeding, and her socioeconomic status or educational level. Maternal ambivalence may also play a role. The nurse can help prevent a poor breast-feeding outcome by teaching the patient about the physiology of lactation, providing anticipatory guidance about the normal course of breast-feeding, and making sure the patient knows how to obtain information and support after discharge.

Fill in the blank
7. Stopping breast-feeding, mismanagement
8. Weight, length, head circumference

CHAPTER 21

Care of high-risk neonates

OBJECTIVES   After studying this chapter, the reader should be able to:

1. Explain the concept of regionalized neonatal care.
2. Identify the goals of neonatal intensive care.
3. Identify the measures used to resuscitate a neonate at delivery.
4. Discuss the concerns of the family of a high-risk neonate.
5. Identify strategies used to encourage parent interaction with a high-risk neonate.
6. Describe interventions that provide support to the family of a neonate who dies.
7. Identify maternal, antepartal, intrapartal, and fetal factors that increase the risk of perinatal problems.
8. Identify perinatal problems commonly seen in preterm neonates.

OVERVIEW OF CONCEPTS   The high-risk neonate is one who has an increased chance of dying during or shortly after delivery or who has a congenital or perinatal problem necessitating prompt intervention. With the birth of any high-risk neonate (one who is preterm or very ill), family members experience a sense of loss. The family of a neonate with a chronic illness or congenital anomaly must find ways to cope with long-term grief and develop strategies to provide the special care the condition will require. If the neonate is stillborn or dies within a few hours or days after birth, family members must complete their bonding with the neonate, then detach themselves gradually so they can focus again on the family's life and needs.

To provide care in the first weeks after the birth of a high-risk neonate, the nurse must:

- assess how family members are responding to and coping with the crisis of the high-risk neonate
- identify and implement strategies to help family members cope
- help family members identify support systems that can provide further help
- teach family members about the condition and care of the high-risk neonate

Neonatal intensive care

Many high-risk neonates require care in a neonatal intensive care unit. Besides a highly skilled, round-the-clock medical and nursing staff, the NICU offers full life-support, resuscitation, and monitoring equipment and extensive ancillary support staff and services.

Regionalization of care

To ensure the highest quality of care for high-risk neonates, the American Academy of Pediatrics has established a system of "leveled" regionalized care in which a neonate is referred to the facility with the most appropriate staff and equipment to manage the neonate's specific problems. Ideally, regionalized care allows the most efficient use of resources by eliminating the need for all facilities to acquire the expensive equipment and staff for an NICU.

Every hospital in the United States is assigned to a region and classified according to the level of neonatal care provided. Level 1 care (as in the normal neonatal nursery) is most appropriate for uncomplicated deliveries; level 2 care, for neonates with mild to moderate problems; level 3 (NICU) care, for more serious problems.

Obstetric facilities also are classified according to the level of care provided; in some cases, this means that a mother may be cared for in a different facility than her neonate. Ideally, when a high-risk delivery is anticipated, however, the mother may be transported before delivery to a facility with level 3 neonatal care so that she and her neonate can be together.

Goals of neonatal intensive care

The goals of neonatal intensive care include averting or minimizing complications, subjecting the neonate to as little stress as possible, and furthering parent-infant bonding. To achieve these goals, the NICU staff:
• anticipates, prevents, and detects potential or actual perinatal problems
• intervenes early for identified problems
• carries out care procedures in a way that minimizes disturbance to the neonate
• uses a family-centered approach.

Nursing care of the high-risk neonate

In many cases, delivery of a high-risk neonate can be predicted from the maternal health history or from antepartal or intrapartal data. Anticipation and preparation can help prevent or minimize perinatal problems. When a patient is due to deliver, check the calculated date of delivery and review the history for factors that help predict neonatal outcome. (For more information, see *Risk factors for perinatal problems,* page 334.)

Although the neonate's condition will dictate the specifics of nursing care, the same nursing goals apply to all high-risk neonates: to ensure oxygenation, ventilation, thermoregulation, nutrition, and fluid

Risk factors for perinatal problems

The health care team can anticipate a neonate's high-risk status from the maternal, antepartal, or intrapartal history or from certain neonatal conditions present at birth.

Maternal risk factors
- Age over 34 or under 19
- Alcohol or drug use during pregnancy
- Chronic illness (including diabetes mellitus, anemia, hypertension, kidney disease, or heart disease)
- Cigarette smoking
- Death of a previous fetus
- Death or illness of a previous neonate
- Exposure to infection during pregnancy
- Exposure to toxic chemicals, radiation, or other hazardous substances or conditions
- Family history of a genetic disease
- Hereditary disease
- Isoimmunization
- Low socioeconomic status
- More than seven previous pregnancies
- Poor prenatal care
- Previous multiple fetuses
- Short interval between pregnancies (less than 12 months)

Antepartal risk factors
- Abruptio placentae
- Accelerated fetal growth
- Fetal surgery
- First-trimester bleeding
- Hydramnios

- Intrauterine growth retardation
- Multiple fetuses
- Placenta previa
- Pregnancy-induced hypertension
- Premature rupture of the membranes

Intrapartal risk factors
- Abnormal fetal presentation
- Cesarean delivery
- Fetal distress
- Maternal anesthetics or analgesics
- Prolonged labor
- Umbilical cord prolapse
- Use of forceps during delivery

Neonatal risk factors
- Abnormal placental weight or appearance
- Cardiorespiratory depression
- Congenital anomaly
- Lack of spontaneous respirations
- Low Apgar score
- Meconium-stained amniotic fluid
- Prematurity or postmaturity
- Small or large size for gestational age
- Unusual number of umbilical vessels

and electrolyte balance; prevent and control infection; and provide developmental care.

Assessment
If a high-risk neonate is expected, a brief assessment immediately after delivery verifies the endangered status, as when the neonate fails to breathe spontaneously or has central cyanosis or an inadequate heart rate. Poor 1-minute and 5-minute Apgar scores also may confirm or suggest high-risk status. In some cases, however, a perinatal problem is not discovered until a complete examination is conducted several hours or days later.

Nursing diagnoses
After gathering all assessment data, review it carefully to identify pertinent nursing diagnoses for the neonate (for a partial list of applicable

diagnoses, see Nursing Diagnoses: *High-risk neonates and their families,* page 336).

Planning and implementation

Once a fetus or neonate is identified as high risk, initial intervention should focus on preventing complications and death. Some high-risk neonates require emergency interventions; others, such as those with relatively minor congenital anomalies, are fairly stable at birth but require prompt treatment to prevent complications.

Performing emergency intervention

In most cases, the need for resuscitation at delivery can be anticipated from maternal, antepartal, or intrapartal factors. Immediately after delivery, the neonate must be evaluated to determine the need for resuscitation. Depending on the neonate's condition and response to each resuscitative measure, neonatal resuscitation typically involves some combination of the following:
- free-flow oxygen
- positive-pressure ventilation (PPV)
- closed-chest cardiac massage
- gastric decompression
- emergency drugs
- endotracheal intubation.

Preparation for resuscitation. Before every delivery, verify that emergency equipment and supplies are present, in working order, and ready to use; ideally, all items should be double-checked. This helps avert problems during resuscitation, when replacement of a missing supply or malfunctioning part could cause a dangerous treatment delay.

Resuscitation personnel. Every delivery should be attended by at least one person skilled in all resuscitation techniques and another person who is an experienced resuscitation assistant. When asphyxia is likely, a third person also should be present in the delivery room to manage the mother so that the resuscitators can attend solely to the neonate.

Resuscitation procedure. Initial neonatal evaluation and subsequent resuscitative measures are based on respirations, heart rate, and skin color—not on the 1-minute Apgar score. Waiting until the end of the first minute to start resuscitation makes the procedure more difficult and increases the chance for brain damage and death. With a severely asphyxiated neonate, a delay is especially dangerous. (However, Apgar scores should be used to help determine whether resuscitative measures are effective.)

As with any resuscitation, the goal of neonatal resuscitation is to ensure the ABCs—airway, breathing, and circulation. Resuscitation follows an orderly sequence; after each intervention, the team quickly evaluates the neonate's condition and response to the intervention, then decides which further measures, if any, are necessary.

NURSING DIAGNOSES

High-risk neonates and their families

The following are potential nursing diagnoses for problems and etiologies that a nurse may encounter when caring for high-risk neonates and their families. Specific nursing interventions for many of these diagnoses are provided in the "Planning and implementation" sections of this chapter.

For the neonate
- Altered growth and development related to functional immaturity, prolonged environmental stress, and lack of stimulation appropriate for gestational age and physical status
- Altered nutrition: less than body requirements, related to increased caloric requirements, respiratory distress, gastrointestinal immaturity, a weak sucking reflex, or metabolic dysfunction
- Fluid volume deficit related to renal immaturity or increased fluid loss
- High risk for aspiration related to meconium in amniotic fluid
- High risk for infection related to immunologic immaturity, altered ventilation, ineffective airway clearance, or frequent invasive procedures
- Hypothermia related to an immature temperature-regulating center, decreased body mass-to-surface ratio, reduced subcutaneous fat, inability to shiver or sweat, and inadequate metabolic reserves
- Ineffective breathing pattern related to respiratory and neurologic immaturity

For the family
- Altered family processes related to the birth of a high-risk neonate and the adjustments necessitated by the neonate's condition and hospitalization
- Anticipatory grieving related to the prospect of the neonate's death
- Anxiety related to the neonate's condition and unknown outcome
- Denial related to immediate and long-term implications of the neonate's condition
- High risk for altered parenting related to the neonate's condition, difficulty coping with a less-than-perfect neonate, and enforced separation
- Ineffective individual coping related to family disorganization secondary to the neonate's condition
- Ineffective individual coping related to the stress of a preterm birth
- Parental role conflict related to limited opportunities to care for the neonate

Respirations. If the neonate lacks spontaneous respirations, PPV with a bag and mask must begin immediately. If the neonate is breathing (as indicated by chest movements), the resuscitation team moves on, evaluating heart rate.

Heart rate. If the heart rate is below 60 beats/minute or between 60 and 80 beats/minute and not increasing, closed-chest cardiac massage (chest compression) typically begins as PPV continues. (PPV should be initiated whenever the heart rate is below 100, even if the neonate has spontaneous respirations.) If the heart rate is above 100 beats/minute, the team evaluates skin color.

Skin color. If the neonate has central cyanosis, reflecting lack of oxygen in the blood, the team administers free-flow oxygen by holding the end of an oxygen tube close to the neonate's nose or by holding an oxygen mask over the neonate's mouth and nose.

Special considerations

Although most neonates respond to PPV and chest compressions, some require other measures.

Gastric decompression. Bag-and-mask ventilation forces air to enter the stomach, which can prevent full lung expansion, cause aspiration of gastric contents, and lead to abdominal distention (which impedes breathing). Consequently, when bag-and-mask ventilation is required for more than 2 minutes, an orogastric tube must be inserted to suction gastric contents; the tube is left in place throughout resuscitation to vent air.

Emergency drugs. Drugs may be administered if the neonate fails to respond to bag-and-mask ventilation and chest compressions. Such drugs typically are administered via the umbilical vein or, in some cases, through a peripheral vein (such as a scalp or extremity vein) or an endotracheal tube.

Endotracheal intubation. This intervention, which should be performed only by an experienced intubator, is indicated when diaphragmatic hernia is suspected, when the neonate requires prolonged ventilation, or when prolonged bag-and-mask ventilation proves ineffective.

Endotracheal intubation also is necessary when meconium aspiration syndrome is suspected. If the amniotic fluid contains thick meconium (a sign of asphyxia experienced in utero), as soon as the neonate's head is delivered, the mouth, oropharynx, and hypopharynx must be suctioned with a flexible suction catheter. Immediately after delivery, an experienced intubator visualizes the larynx with a laryngoscope, then intubates the trachea and suctions any meconium from the lower airway—preferably by applying suction to an endotracheal tube. After the tube has been inserted, continuous suction is applied as the tube is withdrawn. This procedure is repeated until no more meconium is suctioned.

Postresuscitation care. After resuscitation, observe the neonate closely for signs of respiratory distress, including cyanosis, apnea, tachypnea, and inspiratory retractions. Blood pressure and cardiac perfusion are other key indicators; if either is inadequate, expect to administer volume expanders to reverse shock. Ensure thermoregulation by keeping the neonate under a radiant warmer and monitoring skin temperature.

Supporting oxygenation and ventilation

Most neonates who have been successfully resuscitated—as well as many other high-risk neonates—need supplemental oxygen to prevent or correct hypoxia. Supplemental oxygen can be administered by hood, nasal cannula, or continuous positive-airway pressure; it always should be warmed and humidified.

Because oxygen is a drug, the nurse must be familiar with its potential adverse effects and ways to avoid them. For instance, to prevent or minimize the risk of retinopathy of prematurity (ROP), always administer oxygen at the lowest concentration that will correct hypoxia, using an oxygen analyzer to determine the actual concentration of delivered oxygen.

To ensure therapeutic efficacy and avoid oxygen toxicity, monitor the neonate's oxygenation status continuously with a noninvasive technique, such as transcutaneous oxygen pressure ($tcPO_2$) monitoring or pulse oximetry. These measures must be correlated with simultaneously obtained arterial blood gas (ABG) samples in order to be accurate.

Oxygen hood and nasal cannula. An oxygen hood, which fits over the neonate's head, can deliver up to 100% oxygen and allows easy access to the rest of the neonate's body for care procedures. A nasal cannula delivers oxygen concentrations above room air (21%); typically, it is used for a neonate with bronchopulmonary dysplasia or a congenital cardiac defect (the minimal equipment involved allows frequent cuddling and other stimulation).

Continuous positive-airway pressure (CPAP). CPAP delivers air at a constant pressure throughout the respiratory cycle, keeping the lungs expanded at all times to reduce shunting and improve oxygenation. CPAP may be delivered via a nasopharyngeal tube or an endotracheal tube inserted through the mouth or nose. During CPAP therapy, the nurse monitors the neonate's heart rate, blood pressure, and respiratory effort, staying especially alert for tachycardia, tachypnea, and arrhythmias.

Mechanical ventilation. Mechanical ventilation usually is used instead of CPAP if any of the following criteria are present:
- PaO_2 level below 50 mm Hg with administration of 100% oxygen
- $PaCO_2$ level above 60 mm Hg
- arterial pH below 7.2.

During mechanical ventilation, assess the neonate's vital signs, breath sounds, chest movement, respiratory effort, and oxygenation status every hour.

Maintaining thermoregulation

An essential part of care for all neonates, thermoregulation is particularly crucial to the high-risk neonate, whose oxygen and energy reserves may be depleted rapidly by illness. The preterm neonate especially is at risk for cold stress because of limited subcutaneous fat, an extremely high surface-to-mass ratio, inability to shiver, and minimal brown fat (a type of fat that provides body heat).

A neonate who suffers heat loss and progressive cold stress may experience peripheral vasoconstriction, hypoglycemia, reduced cerebral perfusion, metabolic acidosis, exacerbation of respiratory distress syndrome, decreased surfactant production, impaired kidney function, gastrointestinal (GI) disturbances, and, ultimately, death. Thus preventing heat loss is crucial in high-risk neonates (see *Preventing heat loss* in Chapter 19, Care of the healthy neonate).

Neutral thermal environment. Throughout care, aim for a neutral thermal environment (NTE), a narrow range of environmental temperature (89.6° to 93.2° F [32° to 34° C]) that maintains a stable core temperature with minimal caloric and oxygen expenditure.

Thermoregulation during transport. Special measures must be taken if the neonate requires transport to another facility. Causes of heat loss during transport include poor heat retention in the transport bed, radiant heat loss within the transport vehicle, and drafts as the transport bed passes through unheated corridors or as the door or hood to the transport bed is opened to place the neonate inside.

Providing adequate nutrition

The accelerated metabolic rate and energy expenditure of the high-risk neonate demands additional nutrition. The preterm neonate may need 104 to 130 calories/kg/day, compared to the healthy neonate, who requires 100 to 120 calories/kg/day. However, caloric requirements change over time and should be adjusted depending on the neonate's tolerance.

For the high-risk neonate who can take nourishment by mouth, breast milk is the preferred nutritional form. If the neonate cannot receive breast milk, the physician may order a special high-calorie infant formula to provide 24 or 27 calories/oz.

Enteral nutrition (gavage feedings). To avoid aspiration resulting from a weak sucking reflex, uncoordinated sucking and swallowing, or respiratory distress, many high-risk neonates must be fed enterally, typically through a tube passed through the nose or mouth into the stomach. (However, some neonates must be fed through a surgically placed gastrostomy tube.)

Parenteral nutrition. This method, in which nutrients are administered by the I.V. route, may be required by the preterm or postsurgical neonate who cannot tolerate oral or enteral feedings. Parenteral nutrition requirements depend on birth weight and diagnosis. For many high-risk neonates, a solution of dextrose 5% or 10% in water (80 to 100 ml/kg/day) is initiated in the delivery room or soon after transfer to the NICU. Electrolytes typically are added to the solution 24 hours after delivery; the most commonly administered electrolytes are sodium and potassium chloride.

If the neonate will not be fed orally for more than 3 days, the physician will order total parenteral nutrition, which provides adequate carbohydrates, amino acids, lipids, glucose, vitamins, and electrolytes for growth and development.

Maintaining fluid and electrolyte balance

Renal immaturity, small fluid reserves, a high metabolic rate, and pronounced insensible fluid losses make even the healthy neonate susceptible to fluid and electrolyte imbalance. Perinatal problems—especially those causing diarrhea, vomiting, or high fever—and surgery can further upset fluid balance in the high-risk neonate.

Stay alert for signs of fluid deficit and fluid excess; the latter is most likely with a cardiac or renal problem. (For signs of fluid deficit and excess, see *Assessing fluid status,* page 340.)

Preventing and controlling infection

Nearly all high-risk neonates have potential for infection related to immunologic immaturity, altered ventilation, ineffective airway clear-

Assessing fluid status

Various factors place the high-risk neonate in danger of fluid imbalance—particularly fluid volume deficit. To assess for fluid volume deficit or excess, check for the signs listed below.

Signs of fluid volume deficit (dehydration)
- Dry mucous membranes
- Elevated hematocrit, hemoglobin level, and blood urea nitrogen value
- Increasing heart and respiratory rates
- Low-grade fever
- Poor skin turgor
- Slightly decreased blood pressure
- Sunken eyeballs or fontanels
- Urine output less than 1 ml/kg/hour
- Urine specific gravity above 1.013
- Weight loss

Signs of fluid volume excess (overhydration)
- Chronic cough
- Crackles
- Dyspnea
- Edema
- Increasing central venous pressure
- Rhonchi
- Tachypnea
- Urine output exceeding 5 ml/kg/hour

ance, or frequent invasive procedures. Consequently, take the following precautions to help minimize the risk of infection:
- Practice meticulous hand washing. (Scrub for 3 minutes before entering the nursery and wash hands frequently throughout caregiving activities. After providing care, perform a 1-minute scrub after each neonate.)
- Use aseptic technique during all care procedures.
- Make sure all equipment used for neonatal care is sterile or has been cleaned thoroughly.
- Wear gloves and follow other universal precautions during all neonatal care.

To detect infection early, assess the neonate regularly for such systemic signs as hypothermia or hyperthermia, lethargy, jaundice, petechiae, respiratory distress, purulent drainage from the eyes or umbilical site, and subtle behavioral changes. Also check for signs of localized infection from the umbilical and I.V. sites.

If the neonate has potential signs of infection, place in an incubator and, if possible, an isolation room to protect other neonates. The physician would prescribe prophylactic antibiotics (typically ampicillin and gentamicin) and a septic workup, which routinely includes cultures of blood, cerebrospinal fluid (CSF), and urine; a chest X-ray; serum electrolyte analysis; and a complete blood count with differential.

Providing developmental care and environmental support

Research from the past 20 years shows that the neonate is aware of surroundings and responds to sensory stimulation. Within the past decade, health care providers increasingly have aimed to establish a developmentally appropriate environment for the high-risk neonate by reducing detrimental stimulation, providing appropriate stimulation during caregiving activities, and teaching parents how to provide appropriate stimulation.

Carrying out special procedures

Many high-risk neonates require phototherapy or exchange transfusion to treat hyperbilirubinemia; a few require extracorporeal membrane oxygenation (ECMO). General nursing measures during phototherapy and exchange transfusions focus on maintaining body temperature, timing care to avoid unnecessary stress, and assessing oral intake, urine output, and stools. With any of these procedures, observe the neonate closely for respiratory compromise. The neonate with hyperbilirubinemia is at risk for asphyxia and respiratory distress; the neonate who requires ECMO commonly has preexisting respiratory distress.

Supporting the family and promoting parent-infant bonding

The birth of a critically ill neonate creates a crisis for family members. The nurse provides emotional support to the family throughout the neonate's stay but especially during each parent's first visit to the NICU— a potentially overwhelming experience. Explain the use of monitors and other supportive equipment to lessen the intimidating effect these machines can have. To help the parents adjust to their child's appearance, emphasize the neonate's normal features.

Promote communications, paying special attention to the family's needs. Encourage the parents to visit frequently; if this is not possible, they can keep in touch with the NICU staff by telephone. Give them the names and telephone numbers of the physician, primary nurse, social worker, and other contact persons.

To promote parent-infant bonding, allow the parents to touch and hold their child whenever possible and provide simple caregiving tasks, such as diaper changes. Point out how their child responds to their presence, voice, and touch, and show them how to offer appropriate sensory stimulation so that they can take an active role in their child's development—a measure that enhances their self-esteem.

Planning and implementation

The goal of nursing care is to help the family develop the understanding, skills, and confidence to give competent care after the neonate's discharge. Thus the nurse should plan interventions to help them deal with the crisis of a high-risk neonate and to meet the neonate's needs. Such interventions should focus on the neonate's physical and developmental needs and the family's practical and emotional needs.

Whenever possible, involve family members in planning. This not only helps ensure that they can carry out the planned interventions, but it also makes them active participants in their child's care.

Interventions for the family of a high-risk neonate fall into four main categories:
• providing information
• strengthening support systems
• teaching caregiving skills
• enhancing parent-infant bonding.

Depending on the neonate's status, the nurse also may need to help the family plan for their child's discharge or help them cope with their child's death.

Evaluation

During this step of the nursing process, evaluate the effectiveness of the care plan by ongoing evaluation of subjective and objective criteria. Evaluation findings should be stated in terms of actions performed or outcomes achieved for each goal. The following examples illustrate appropriate evaluation statements for the high-risk neonate:
• The neonate maintained an adequate core temperature.
• The neonate's cardiopulmonary status improved or remained within acceptable limits.
• The neonate maintained fluid and electrolyte balance, as evidenced by adequate urine output, no signs of dehydration or fluid overload, and acceptable serum electrolyte levels.

Documentation

All steps of the nursing process should be documented as thoroughly and objectively as possible. Thorough documentation not only allows the nurse to evaluate the effectiveness of the care plan, but it also makes this information available to other members of the health care team, helping to ensure consistency of care.

Documentation for the high-risk neonate should include, as appropriate:
• vital signs and alertness level
• changes in status
• serum bilirubin, calcium, and glucose levels
• fluid intake and output
• stool characteristics
• tolerance for feedings
• location and appearance of any I.V. infusion site
• presence of any gastric distention
• presence of an indwelling nasogastric tube
• amount and appearance of secretions obtained by suctioning

• tolerance for medical and nursing procedures
• parents' level of acceptance of their child's problem.

Perinatal problems

The most common problems seen in NICUs are prematurity and its sequelae, congenital heart defects, and congenital anomalies requiring emergency surgery (such as omphalocele and tracheoesophageal fistula). Other problems involve respiration, maternal diabetes, metabolic disorders, maternal substance abuse, and infection.

Gestational-age and birth-weight abnormalities

Abnormalities in gestational age (prematurity and postmaturity) and birth weight (small or large size for gestational age) predispose the neonate to various problems. (For assessment findings including significant history and physical examination, see *Gestational-age variations,* pages 344 and 345, and *Birth-weight variations,* pages 346 and 347.)

Nursing diagnoses

For a partial list of applicable diagnoses, see Nursing Diagnoses: *High-risk neonates and their families,* page 336.

Planning and implementation

Nursing care of the neonate with gestational-age or birth-weight variations is similar to that for any high-risk neonate. (For more information, see "Nursing care of the high-risk neonate" and "Nursing care of the family" earlier in this chapter.)

Evaluation

During this step of the nursing process, evaluate the effectiveness of the care plan by ongoing evaluation of subjective and objective criteria. Evaluation findings should be stated in terms of actions performed or outcomes achieved for each goal. For examples of appropriate evaluation statements, see the general ones listed in "Nursing care of the high-risk neonate" earlier in this chapter.

Documentation

All steps of the nursing process should be documented as thoroughly and objectively as possible. Thorough documentation not only allows the nurse to evaluate the effectiveness of the care, but it also makes this information available to other members of the health care team, helping ensure consistency of care. (For information about appropriate documentation, see the general points listed in "Nursing care of the high-risk neonate" earlier in this chapter.)

Respiratory problems

Some neonates have trouble initiating respirations or develop respiratory distress after breathing is established. Problems may arise if fluid remains in the lungs or if the blood perfusion of the lungs does not increase; neonates with apnea at birth or a weak respiratory effort (from such conditions as prematurity, asphyxia, or maternal anesthesia) are predisposed to respiratory distress.

Gestational-age variations

Birth before or after full-term gestation markedly increases the risk of perinatal problems. In the past 25 years, advances in research and technology have improved the survival rate dramatically for neonates with gestational-age variations–even extremely preterm neonates.

PRETERM NEONATE

The preterm neonate—the classic high-risk neonate—is one born before completion of week 37 of gestation. Neonatal mortality and morbidity are highest among preterm neonates. Delivery of a preterm neonate is more likely with any of the following maternal conditions:

- Age extreme (under 19 or over 34)
- Antepartal trauma, infection, or pregnancy-induced hypertension
- Chronic disease (such as cardiovascular disease, renal disease, or diabetes mellitus)
- Exposure to known teratogens (including drugs, alcohol, cigarette smoke, and hazardous chemicals)
- History of previous preterm delivery
- Low socioeconomic status
- Poor nutritional status
- Poor prenatal care
- Uterine anomalies or cervical incompetency

Other predisposing factors include more than one fetus, hydramnios (excessive amniotic fluid), fetal infection, premature rupture of the membranes, abruptio placentae, and placenta previa.

Perinatal problems

General immaturity can lead to dysfunction in any organ or body system. Thus, the preterm neonate risks a wide range of problems, including respiratory distress syndrome, apnea, bronchopulmonary dysplasia, patent ductus arteriosus, ineffective thermoregulation, hypoglycemia, intraventricular hemorrhage, gastrointestinal dysfunction, retinopathy, hyperbilirubinemia, and infection. The preterm neonate also may suffer ineffective development from the effects of intensive medical treatment (such as sensory overload and environmental stress); an immature central nervous system compounds this risk. Also, mother-infant bonding may be jeopardized.

POST-TERM NEONATE

The post-term neonate is one whose gestation exceeds 294 days or 42 weeks. Typically, the neonate's weight falls above the 90th percentile on the Colorado Intrauterine Growth Chart (discussed in Chapter 18, Neonatal assessment).

Perinatal problems

Problems associated with postmaturity include fetal dysmaturity syndrome, asphyxia, meconium aspiration, polycythemia, hypothermia, and birth trauma.

Fetal dysmaturity syndrome. Some 20% to 40% of post-term neonates experience placental insufficiency leading to fetal dysmaturity syndrome and a diagnosis of small for gestational age (SGA). After 280 days of gestation, the risk of placental insufficiency, fetal growth retardation, and chronic hypoxia increases. Fetal weight plateaus around the term date until week 42, then drops rapidly. Placental dysfunction after week 42 impairs fetal oxygenation and nutrition and exhausts placental reserves, retarding fetal growth.

Fetal dysmaturity occurs in three forms: chronic, acute, and subacute placental insufficiency. Each form has distinctive manifestations. With chronic placental insufficiency, no meconium staining occurs but the neonate appears malnourished, with skin defects and an apprehensive look reflecting hypoxia. Acute placental insufficiency leads to a malnourished and apprehensive appearance and green meconium staining of the skin, umbilical cord, and placental membranes. With subacute placental insufficiency, the skin and nails are stained bright yellow (from breakdown of green-bile meconium stain), and the umbilical cord, placenta, and placental membranes may be stained greenish brown.

Asphyxia and meconium aspiration. The post-term neonate has a high risk of birth asphyxia and meconium aspiration. Meconium release (defecation) has been found to occur twice as frequently and meconium aspiration syndrome eight times as frequently in post-term neonates as in other neonates.

Oligohydramnios (presence of less than 300 ml of amniotic fluid at term) increases the risk of asphyxia and aspiration by making meconium less diluted and thus unusually thick. Normally, amniotic fluid volume peaks at 1,000 to 1,200 ml at about 38 weeks' gestation, then decreases rapidly. By week 42, it drops to approximately 300 ml; further decreases occur at 43 and 44 weeks. In the neonate with no congenital anomalies, oligohydramnios confirms postmaturity and has been linked to fetal decelerations (as shown on fetal monitoring strips), bradycardia, or both.

Other perinatal problems. Intrauterine hypoxia in the post-term fetus may trigger increased red blood cell production, causing polycythemia; this in turn may lead to sluggish perfusion and complications associated with hyperviscosity. Subcutaneous fat deficiency caused by skin wasting predisposes the post-term neonate to hypothermia, despite a mature thermoregulatory system. Thus, a post-term neonate exposed to cold stress may develop respiratory compromise and hypoglycemia.

Delivery complications
The risk of delivery complications increases after 280 days (40 weeks) of gestation. Excessive size may cause a dysfunctional labor and shoulder dystocia, possibly necessitating cesarean delivery. Because of maternal uterine inefficiency and cephalopelvic disproportion, post-term neonates have a higher-than-average rate of surgical deliveries.

Asphyxia and apnea. Asphyxia may occur late in gestation or during delivery. Chemically, this condition is defined as insufficient oxygen in the blood (hypoxemia), excessive carbon dioxide in the blood, and a decreased blood pH. As carbon dioxide accumulates, respiratory acidosis occurs; poor tissue oxygenation leads to buildup of lactic acid, resulting in metabolic acidosis of the neonate. If hypoxia is prolonged, the foramen ovale and ductus arteriosus—fetal shunts that normally close shortly after delivery—may reopen. This causes a return to fetal circulatory pathways to maintain circulation to the heart and brain, which is referred to as persistent fetal circulation of the neonate.

Without immediate resuscitation, the asphyxiated neonate will die. Complications of prolonged asphyxia include cerebral hypoxia, seizures, intraventricular hemorrhage (IVH), renal failure, necrotizing enterocolitis, and metabolic imbalances.

Several days after delivery, apneic episodes (cessation of breathing for more than 15 seconds) are common among preterm neonates, many of whom have irregular respiratory patterns from neuronal immaturity. Such episodes may result from acidosis, anemia, hypoglycemia, hyperglycemia, hypothermia, hyperthermia, patent ductus arteriosus (PDA), abdominal distention, regurgitation, sepsis, or IVH.

Meconium aspiration syndrome. A lung inflammation, meconium aspiration syndrome (MAS) results from aspiration of meconium-stained amniotic fluid in utero or as the neonate takes the first few breaths after delivery. Meconium staining of amniotic fluid results from fetal asphyxia: In response to asphyxia, the fetus's intestinal peristalsis increases, the anal sphincter relaxes, and meconium enters the amniotic fluid.

As meconium obstructs the bronchi and bronchioles, air can enter but not exit the bronchi and bronchioles because meconium acts as an obstruction, plugging the alveolar sac. Alveoli then become overdistended; pneumothorax, bacterial pneumonia, or pulmonary hypertension may develop secondarily.

Respiratory distress syndrome. Respiratory distress syndrome (RDS, also called hyaline membrane disease) is characterized by respiratory

Birth-weight variations

Like the neonate with a gestational-age variation, one whose weight is inappropriate for the estimated gestational age is at high risk for perinatal problems.

SMALL-FOR-GESTATIONAL-AGE (SGA) NEONATE
The SGA neonate is one whose birth weight falls below the 10th percentile for gestational age. SGA status results from intrauterine growth restriction (IUGR), an abnormal process in which fetal development and maturation are delayed or impeded. After prematurity, IUGR is the leading cause of death during the perinatal period.

Causes of IUGR
IUGR may result from maternal conditions, genetic factors (for example, trisomies), fetal and placental abnormalities, infection, fetal malnutrition caused by placental insufficiency, or exposure to such teratogens as drugs and alcohol.

Maternal conditions. The most common causes of IUGR are maternal conditions that reduce uteroplacental perfusion, such as toxemia, chronic hypertensive vascular disease, and renovascular and cardiac disorders. Maternal hypertension, smoking, renal disease, and diabetes mellitus that progresses to renovascular compromise also can result in IUGR.

Fetal and placental abnormalities. IUGR can result from placental infarction, hemangiomas, aberrant cord insertion, single umbilical artery, and umbilical vascular thrombosis. Premature placental separation and other conditions that diminish placental surface area and thus decrease fetal-placental exchange capability also may cause IUGR.

Placental insufficiency. Placental insufficiency is the inadequate or improper functioning of the placenta, leading to a compromised intrauterine environment. Causes of placental insufficiency include systemic diseases (such as diabetes mellitus and infection) and placental abnormalities that impair fetal circulation and compromise fetal nutrition and oxygenation (such as abnormal placental implantation, abnormal cord attachment, and placental membrane abnormalities). Although placental insufficiency is most common in the post-term period, it may occur at any time during gestation. The severity of IUGR arising from placental insufficiency depends on the duration of fetal distress.

Exposure to cigarettes, drugs, and alcohol. During early pregnancy, smoking is the most important risk factor for IUGR. Maternal use of heroin, cocaine, and methadone significantly reduces the neonate's weight, length, and head circumference at birth. Maternal alcohol consumption may cause fetal alcohol syndrome (FAS). Some neonates show severe manifestations whereas others appear normal. Besides mental retardation—the most serious and common effect—FAS may reduce the neonate's weight and length at birth.

Perinatal problems
Although the SGA neonate may avoid the problems stemming from organ system immaturity seen in the preterm neonate, other perinatal problems may arise.

Asphyxia and meconium aspiration. The SGA neonate who suffered placental insufficiency risks asphyxiation during labor and delivery, as the flow of oxygen and nutrients slows and uterine contractions reduce placental perfusion. Also, the neonate may aspirate meconium that has entered the amniotic fluid. Respiratory distress, cyanosis, pulmonary air trapping, pneumothorax, and pulmonary hypertension may result, along with severe asphyxia and cerebral hypoxia.

Organ size variations. Relative to body weight, the SGA neonate has a larger brain and heart than the preterm neonate but smaller adrenal glands and a smaller liver, spleen, thymus, and placenta.

Hematologic and metabolic problems. The SGA neonate may experience hematologic changes from chronic fetal hypoxia, a condition that triggers compensation through increases in red blood cell volume (polycythemia) and erythropoietin levels. Polycythemia, in turn, may cause hyperviscosity and sluggish microcirculation perfusion.

With increased energy requirements but inadequate glycogen and fat reserves, the SGA neonate is predisposed to hypoglycemia. A stressful labor may further deplete already deficient energy reserves.

Long-term problems
An SGA neonate later may suffer developmental, immunologic, and neurologic problems.

Slowed growth and immunologic deficiencies. Growth rate depends on when IUGR occurred and how long it lasted. Commonly, the child who was SGA at birth remains slimmer and shorter than other children of the same gestational age or birth weight.

Impaired fetal skeletal growth may contribute to delayed tooth eruption and enamel hypoplasia. Severely growth-retarded neonates also have an increased incidence of infection, possibly from immunologic deficiency.

Neurologic impairment. IUGR-induced brain damage and its potential effect on neurologic development remains a major medical concern. Most investigators believe IUGR has more serious neurologic consequences in the preterm than the term SGA neonate. Follow-up evaluations in children who experienced IUGR in utero have revealed defects in speech and language comprehension; outcome studies have described hyperactivity, short attention span, poor fine-motor coordination,

Birth-weight variations *(continued)*

hyperreflexia, and learning problems. Stunted growth and delayed intellectual or neurologic development were found in children who experienced both short and long periods of IUGR. Other factors that worsen the neurologic prognosis include male sex and low socioeconomic status, regardless of the severity of compromise.

LARGE-FOR-GESTATIONAL-AGE (LGA) NEONATE

The LGA neonate is one whose birth weight exceeds the 90th percentile for gestational age. A neonate delivered at term is considered to be LGA if the birth weight exceeds 4,000 g (8 lb, 13 oz). The leading cause of LGA status is maternal diabetes mellitus.

Traditionally, the large neonate was considered a healthy one. However, clinicians now know that the accelerated intrauterine growth of the LGA fetus poses a threat to both mother and neonate during delivery and increases the risk of complications and death in the early neonatal period.

Intrapartal problems

When the membranes rupture, large fetal size and possible high station may result in umbilical cord prolapse. Uterine overdistention from an LGA fetus increases the risk of premature labor. Usually, the physician will initiate labor and delivery before term (once fetal lung maturity has been confirmed) because of the high incidence of unexplained death among term LGA fetuses. If the mother has an adequate pelvis, the physician typically administers oxytocin to induce labor; otherwise, cesarean delivery may be necessary. The risk of shoulder dystocia stemming from cephalopelvic disproportion also may necessitate cesarean delivery, with all its inherent risks.

During vaginal delivery, the neonate's large size may cause birth injury, such as clavicular fracture resulting from shoulder dystocia, skull fracture from increased head size, or other traumatic head injuries (such as cephalhematomas, facial nerve damage, and intracranial bleeding). A difficult delivery also may lead to phrenic nerve damage or brachial plexus palsy.

Perinatal problems

If the mother is diabetic, the neonate may suffer hypocalcemia, hypoglycemia, and polycythemia. Other problems associated with excessive size include congenital anomalies (such as transposition of the great vessels), erythroblastosis fetalis (hemolytic anemia), and Beckwith's syndrome (a hereditary disorder associated with neonatal hypoglycemia and hyperinsulinemia).

If the mother had postconceptional bleeding causing an error in the calculated delivery date, the LGA neonate may be delivered post-term and thus experience respiratory distress from meconium aspiration or intrauterine asphyxiation. The LGA neonate delivered before term to prevent fetal death or intrapartal complications of excessive size may suffer respiratory distress syndrome, hyperbilirubinemia, and other problems linked to prematurity.

---

distress and impaired gas exchange. RDS affects mainly preterm neonates, who have highly pliable and easily overinflated thoracic muscles, weak intercostal muscles, and insufficient surfactant. Surfactant is necessary to keep alveoli expanded, and its production probably becomes sufficient only after about 35 weeks' gestation.

Insufficient surfactant causes alveolar collapse, leading to decreased lung volume and compliance. The resulting atelectasis causes hypoxia and acidosis, which in turn lead to anaerobic metabolism. As lactic acid accumulates in body tissues, myocardial contractility diminishes, impairing cardiac output and arterial blood pressure. Organ perfusion then diminishes; eventually respiratory failure occurs.

Transient tachypnea. This disorder, characterized by transient episodes of tachypnea (accelerated breathing), stems from incomplete removal of fetal lung fluid. Usually accompanied by cyanosis, it affects mainly full-term or nearly full-term neonates born by cesarean delivery.

Bronchopulmonary dysplasia (BPD). In this lung disease, the bronchiolar epithelial lining and alveolar walls become necrotic; in some cases, right-sided heart failure develops as a complication. BPD occurs mainly in preterm neonates as a complication of oxygen therapy or assisted mechanical ventilation—common treatments for RDS. The neonate with BPD typically becomes ventilator-dependent. Low birth weight and overhydration (in a neonate with PDA) may contribute to BPD.

Assessment

Signs of a respiratory problem may be obvious, immediate, and life-threatening, such as with birth asphyxia or apnea, or may arise hours, days, or even weeks later.

The cardinal sign of asphyxia is deep gasping or failure to breathe spontaneously at delivery. Associated signs include a slow heart rate, abnormally low blood pressure, poor muscle tone, and poor reflexes.

Apneic episodes commonly manifest as rapid respirations punctuated by brief pauses. Hypoxemia, cyanosis, and bradycardia may ensue. With central apnea, expect absence of respiratory efforts and muscle flaccidity. With obstructive apnea, expect respiratory motions accompanied by hypoxemia and bradycardia (from inability to draw air into the lungs).

In MAS, signs of respiratory distress may be mild, moderate, or severe. The neonate typically appears barrel-chested because of an increased anteroposterior chest diameter (from bronchial obstruction by meconium or tension pneumothorax). Skin and nails may be meconium-stained.

Signs of RDS may appear at delivery or within a few hours. They include tachypnea (a respiratory rate over 60 breaths/minute), labored respirations, grunting, nasal flaring, cyanosis, and chest retractions. The neonate may become restless and agitated and show fatigue even after simple care procedures. Complex procedures, such as endotracheal suctioning, may thoroughly exhaust the neonate's limited energy reserves, leading to bradycardia and hypoxia.

RDS affects mainly preterm neonates. Other risk factors include maternal diabetes mellitus, infection, or hemorrhage; maternal steroid or analgesic use; more than one fetus; abruptio placentae; umbilical cord prolapse; meconium-stained amniotic fluid; fetal distress; and breech presentation.

Tachypnea—alone or accompanied by hypoxemia, cyanosis, grunting, and chest retractions—is the hallmark of transient tachypnea. Cesarean delivery and term or near-term gestation are common history findings.

Because BPD typically occurs as a complication of treatment for RDS, signs usually arise after supplemental oxygen administration or mechanical ventilation. The severity of these signs reflects the degree of disease progression and pulmonary dysfunction. Expect nasal flaring, retractions, tachypnea, and grunting. However, the first clue to BPD may be difficulty weaning the neonate from a ventilator. As the disease progresses, carbon dioxide retention and pulmonary secretions increase and crackles can be auscultated. Bronchospasm may result from bronchial smooth muscle hypertrophy. Typically, the neonate's condition worsens and oxygen dependency occurs. (Conversely, decreased oxygen dependency may be the earliest sign of recovery.)

Nursing diagnoses

For a partial list of applicable diagnoses, see Nursing Diagnoses: *High-risk neonates and their families,* page 336.

Planning and implementation

Serious respiratory depression at birth calls for immediate resuscitation (as discussed in "Nursing care of the high-risk neonate" earlier in this chapter). After resuscitation, monitor the neonate's cardiopulmonary status and skin temperature. Anticipate collection of blood samples for ABG analysis and samples for serum electrolyte analysis. Monitor arterial blood pressure frequently and observe for subtle changes, which may signal an impending change in respiratory status.

Evaluation

For examples of appropriate evaluation statements, see the general ones listed in "Nursing care of the high-risk neonate" earlier in this chapter. For the neonate with respiratory problems, these additional evaluation statements may be appropriate:
• Signs of increased breathing effort diminished.
• The neonate's ABG and $tcPO_2$ or pulse oximetry values approached normal limits.
• The neonate had no episodes of apnea.

Documentation

For information about appropriate documentation, see the general points listed in "Nursing care of the high-risk neonate" earlier in this chapter. For the neonate with respiratory problems, documentation also should include:
• breathing effort
• any apneic episodes
• administration route and FIO_2 of supplemental oxygen (if given)
• ABG and $tcPO_2$ or pulse oximetry values
• ventilator pressure, rate, and positive end-expiratory pressure settings (if the neonate is on a mechanical ventilator).

Neonate of a diabetic mother

Long-standing maternal diabetes mellitus or gestational diabetes mellitus (diabetes that arises during pregnancy) may cause various fetal and neonatal complications. Exposure to high glucose levels early in gestational development may have a teratogenic effect, causing various congenital anomalies, including heart defects, sacral agenesis, renal vein thrombosis, and small left colon.

The neonate of a woman with diabetes (sometimes called an infant of a diabetic mother, or IDM) also has an increased risk of asphyxia, prematurity, infection, respiratory distress, severe hypoglycemia, hypocalcemia, hyperbilirubinemia, polycythemia, and neonatal death; unexplained fetal death also is higher than normal in IDMs. Typically, the IDM is large for gestational age (with a birth weight exceeding the 90th percentile for gestational age) and thus may suffer birth trauma, such as shoulder dystocia, cephalhematoma, subdural hemorrhage, ocular hemorrhage, or brachial plexus injury.

Previously, large fetal size and the high incidence of fetal death late in gestation led many obstetricians to advise early delivery for pregnant diabetic patients. However, that approach has changed slightly, partly because the fetus affected by maternal diabetes has delayed alveolar maturation and thus cannot synthesize adequate surfactant to establish respirations after delivery. If early delivery is mandatory, however, typically it is scheduled for the 37th week of gestation.

Assessment

Typically, this neonate is macrosomic, with a birth weight in the upper percentile range for gestational age. The face is round with chubby cheeks and the skin is ruddy to bright red. Signs of hypoglycemia and hypocalcemia may be present (see "Metabolic disorders" later in this chapter for details); however, over half of neonates of diabetic mothers have asymptomatic hypoglycemia. Assess for signs of birth trauma, such as bruising, ecchymosis, and shoulder dystocia (sometimes manifested as a flaccid or unusually positioned arm).

For the neonate whose mother had questionably or poorly controlled diabetes during pregnancy, assess for signs of hypoglycemia and check blood glucose levels using a glucose oxidase dipstick at delivery and 30 minutes afterward.

Nursing diagnoses

For a partial list of applicable diagnoses, see Nursing Diagnoses: *High-risk neonates and their families,* page 336.

Planning and implementation

Assess for signs of birth trauma (for example, by evaluating mobility, especially in the upper extremities), correct any fluid or electrolyte imbalances, and evaluate complications stemming from widely fluctuating serum glucose, calcium, and bilirubin levels. Also monitor the neonate's vital signs as well as tcPO2 or pulse oximetry values and ABG values, as ordered. (For specific interventions associated with hypoglycemia, hypocalcemia, and hyperbilirubinemia, see "Metabolic disorders" later in this chapter.)

Evaluation

For examples of appropriate evaluation statements, see the general ones listed in "Nursing care of the high-risk neonate" earlier in this chapter.

Documentation

For information about appropriate documentation, see the general points listed in "Nursing care of the high-risk neonate" earlier in this chapter.

Metabolic disorders

The most common metabolic disorders in high-risk neonates are hypoglycemia, hypocalcemia, and hyperbilirubinemia and jaundice.

Hypoglycemia. This condition is defined as two serum glucose levels below 35 mg/dl in the first 3 hours, less than 40 mg/dl from 4 to 24 hours, or less than 45 mg/dl from 24 hours to 7 days of age in a term neonate. In a preterm neonate, hypoglycemia is diagnosed when two serum glucose values are below 25 mg/dl during the first 72 hours.

Hypoglycemia typically results from prematurity, low birth weight, severe fetal or neonatal stress, or maternal diabetes. Because fetal glycogen is deposited during the last few gestational months, the preterm neonate has deficient glycogen stores; if a stressful event, such as respiratory distress, develops at birth, these stores quickly become depleted. The low-birth-weight neonate has a high metabolic rate and inadequate enzyme supplies to activate glucogenesis—conditions that contribute to hypoglycemia.

Poorly controlled maternal diabetes, on the other hand, triggers increased insulin production by the fetal pancreas. After birth, the neonate continues to produce high levels of insulin; this facilitates the entry of glucose into muscle and fat cells, rapidly depleting serum glucose. Glucose expenditure during the transition to the extrauterine environment and sudden cessation of maternal glucose when the umbilical cord is clamped further tax the neonate's glucose stores.

Hypocalcemia. Defined as a serum calcium level below 7 mg/100 ml, hypocalcemia typically arises within the first 2 days or at 6 to 10 days after birth. It affects about half of neonates born to women with type I (insulin-dependent) diabetes mellitus. Other risk factors include small-for-gestational-age (SGA) status, prematurity, and birth asphyxia.

Hyperbilirubinemia and jaundice. Hyperbilirubinemia—an elevated serum level of unconjugated bilirubin—is common among both low-risk and high-risk neonates. It results from overproduction or underexcretion of bilirubin, as from liver immaturity or increased hemolysis. The disorder sometimes leads to jaundice, a yellow discoloration of the skin and sclerae. (For more information on bilirubin production and excretion and physiologic jaundice, see Chapter 17, Physiology of neonatal adaptation, and Chapter 19, Care of the healthy neonate.)

The risk of hyperbilirubinemia is greatest in preterm neonates, those who are ill, those with isoimmune hemolytic anemia, and those who experienced a traumatic delivery leading to bruising and polycythemia. Such conditions as hypoxia and hypoglycemia (characterized by bilirubin displacement from binding sites) predispose the preterm neonate to hyperbilirubinemia.

Assessment

Signs of metabolic disorders range from extremely mild to severe.

Hypoglycemia. Signs of hypoglycemia include apnea or bradycardia, seizures, irregular respirations, cyanosis, irritability, listlessness, lethargy, tremors, feeding problems, vomiting, hypotonia, and a high-pitched cry. Also, neurologic immaturity may prevent homeostasis in the hypoglycemic neonate, leading to unstable vital signs. However, some hypoglycemic neonates are asymptomatic.

Besides maternal diabetes, risk factors for hypoglycemia include prematurity, SGA status, severe isoimmune hemolytic anemia, and birth asphyxia.

A glucose oxidase dipstick value below 25 mg/100 ml indicates hypoglycemia and warrants a venous blood sample to confirm the diagnosis. Hypoglycemia is confirmed by a blood glucose level below 40 mg/dl before the first day after birth or below 45 mg/dl on or after the third day.

Hypocalcemia. The hypocalcemic neonate may have seizures, irritability, hypotonia, poor feeding, a high-pitched cry, and signs associated with hypoglycemia. Suspect hypocalcemia in the neonate of a diabetic mother. Other at-risk neonates include those who are preterm or SGA and those who experienced birth asphyxia.

To assess for hypocalcemia, attempt to elicit Chvostek's sign by tapping the skin over the sixth cranial nerve (in front of the ear); unilateral contraction of the muscles surrounding the eye, nose, and mouth indicates tetany, a sign of hypocalcemia. A serum calcium level below 7 mg/100 ml confirms the diagnosis.

Hyperbilirubinemia and jaundice. The neonate with hyperbilirubinemia has yellow skin and sclerae. For the most accurate assessment, apply pressure over the tip of the neonate's nose; a yellow tinge appearing as circulation returns indicates jaundice.

With severe hyperbilirubinemia (bilirubin encephalopathy), signs vary with the disease phase. Phase 1 signs include hypotonia, vomiting, lethargy, a high-pitched cry, a poor sucking reflex, a decreased or absent Moro reflex, and diminished flexion. During phase 2, spasticity develops; this may take the form of opisthotonos, a prolonged, severe muscle spasm in which the back arches acutely, the head bends back on the neck, the heels bend back on the leg, and the arms and hands flex rigidly at the joints.

In phase 3, spasticity diminishes, the sclera shows above the iris (a condition called sunset eyes), and seizures may occur. During phase 4, gastric, pulmonary, and CNS hemorrhages may develop (these problems also may occur during phase 2). A neonate who survives phase 4 usually has residual effects, such as mental retardation, cerebral palsy, and such sensory alterations as deafness and poor visual acuity or blindness.

Nursing diagnoses

For a partial list of applicable diagnoses, see Nursing Diagnoses: *High-risk neonates and their families,* page 336.

Planning and implementation

For hypoglycemia, if the neonate has no other problems, early feedings may be initiated to counteract the glucose imbalance. In other cases, expect to give glucose I.V., as 3 ml/kg of dextrose 10% in water.

For hypocalcemia, expect to administer I.V. or oral supplemental calcium. The typical I.V. dosage is 24 mg/kg/day; the typical oral dosage, 75 mg/kg/day. Monitor the serum calcium levels frequently and, once the serum calcium level stabilizes, draw daily blood samples.

For hyperbilirubinemia, the treatment depends on the serum bilirubin level. If the level is elevated only moderately or begins to fall by the fourth or fifth day after birth, the physician may order only early, frequent feedings, which increase intestinal motility and thus speed bilirubin excretion. However, persistent or severe hyperbilirubinemia commonly warrants phototherapy or complete exchange transfusion to prevent bilirubin encephalopathy. The serum bilirubin level at which these treatments are ordered depends on the physician, facility policy, and the neonate's gestational age and condition.

Evaluation

For examples of appropriate evaluation statements, see the general ones listed in "Nursing care of the high-risk neonate" earlier in this chapter. For the neonate with hyperbilirubinemia, these additional evaluation statements may be appropriate:
• The serum bilirubin level decreased to normal or near-normal limits.
• Jaundice diminished, as evidenced by improved skin and sclera color.
• The neonate was free of complications, such as transfusion reaction or infection, after exchange transfusion.

Documentation

For information about appropriate documentation, see the general points listed in "Nursing care of the high-risk neonate" earlier in this chapter.

Effects of maternal substance abuse

Maternal use of alcohol, narcotics, and other chemical substances during pregnancy can have devastating effects on the fetus and neonate.
Fetal alcohol syndrome (FAS). This syndrome involves alterations in intrauterine growth and development. A common finding in the NICU, FAS may lead to growth deficiency, microcephaly, mental retardation, poor coordination, facial abnormalities, behavioral deviations (such as irritability), and cardiac and joint anomalies.
Drug exposure, addiction, and withdrawal. Depending on the stage of fetal development during exposure, maternal narcotic use may cause subtle or profound effects, including congenital anomalies, asphyxia, prematurity, respiratory and cardiac disorders, CNS abnormalities, and

death. Intrauterine growth retardation leading to low birth weight also may occur, possibly from drug-induced slowing of blood flow to the placenta, which reduces nutrient delivery to the fetus. A fetus exposed to such drugs as heroin, methadone, or barbiturates also may become addicted and must go through withdrawal after birth.

A pregnant woman who uses drugs also puts her fetus in jeopardy by increasing her risk of poor nutrition, anemia, systemic or local infection, preeclampsia, and exposure to such diseases as human immunodeficiency virus (HIV), the virus that causes acquired immunodeficiency syndrome. Intrapartal effects of maternal drug use include fetal distress and preterm delivery. After delivery, the neonate who is going through withdrawal may exhibit behavioral deviations that hinder parent-infant bonding, including irritability, continual crying, and poor feeding.

Ironically, the fetal stress caused by maternal heroin use has one positive consequence: It accelerates respiratory maturation. Consequently, the incidence of respiratory infections and RDS is relatively low among neonates of heroin users.

Maternal use of cocaine—a powerful CNS stimulant causing vasoconstriction, hypertension, and tachycardia—may result in various perinatal problems, depending on the gestational period and duration of exposure. These problems include profound congenital anomalies (such as urogenital anomalies in male neonates), abruptio placentae, altered brain-wave activity, cerebral infarcts (which may develop as late as 40 weeks' gestation), and prune-belly syndrome (characterized by a protruding, thin-walled abdomen; bladder and ureter dilation; small, dysplastic kidneys; undescended testes; and absence of a portion of the rectus abdominis muscle). Death also may occur.

Assessment

The neonate with FAS may have cardiac anomalies, decreased joint mobility, behavioral deviations, kidney defects, labial hypoplasia, and distinctive facial features. The last include short palpebral fissures (eye openings); ptosis (drooping eyelids); strabismus (eye muscle deviation); a thin, smooth upper lip with a long philtrum (vertical groove) above it; a short, upturned nose; and a receding jaw. Behavioral deviations include irritability, excessive crying, and poor feeding.

The neonate affected by maternal drug abuse may have muscle tremors, twitching, or rigidity, with inability to extend the muscles; seizures; temperature instability; GI disturbances, including vomiting and diarrhea; tachycardia; tachypnea; diaphoresis with mottling over the extremities; and excessive sneezing and yawning. If the mother used heroin or methadone during pregnancy, the neonate may be SGA or have a low birth weight with cardiorespiratory depression at delivery.

Typically, the behavior pattern of the drug-addicted neonate is disorganized, with marked fussiness and irritability (which may be exacerbated by eye contact), prolonged periods of high-pitched crying, and poor consolability. Normal neonatal reflexes, especially the Moro re-

Assessing for drug withdrawal

The neonate whose mother used such drugs as narcotics, barbiturates, or cocaine during pregnancy may be addicted at birth and go through withdrawal. Classic signs of neonatal drug withdrawal are listed below.

Vital sign deviations
- Profound diaphoresis
- Skin mottling
- Tachycardia or bradycardia (depending on the drug involved)
- Tachypnea
- Temperature instability (fever followed by hypothermia)

Neuromuscular signs
- Absent or strong sucking reflex (may be poorly coordinated with swallowing reflex)
- Difficulty extending muscles
- Exaggeration of other neonatal reflexes
- Jerky movements
- Muscle rigidity with flexion
- Muscle twitching
- Seizures
- Tremors

Behavioral signs
- Decreased sleep periods and lengthened awake periods
- Dislike for cuddling and close body contact
- Frequent or prolonged sneezing or yawning
- High-pitched or weak cry; inconsolability
- Irritability

Gastrointestinal signs
- Frequent vomiting
- Increased gastrointestinal motility, with diarrhea and rapid (possibly visible) peristalsis

---

flex, are highly exaggerated. The sucking reflex is strong and the neonate may suck on the hands and fists frequently. However, sucking may be poorly coordinated with swallowing, impairing feeding. Sleep periods may be abnormally short; unlike the healthy neonate, who spends more time asleep than awake, the addicted neonate may have a sleep-awake ratio of 1 to 3.

Signs of drug withdrawal typically begin about 12 to 48 hours after birth (for a list of these signs, see *Assessing for drug withdrawal*). As withdrawal progresses, these signs worsen. If neonatal drug addiction or withdrawal is suspected, attempt to find out from the mother what drugs she used during pregnancy. However, keep in mind that some women may deny or misrepresent drug use.

If the neonate's mother used I.V. drugs, an HIV test should be done. Maternally conferred IgG may interfere with the accuracy of an

HIV antibody test for the first few months after birth; therefore, an HIV antigen test is preferred. Assess for signs of HIV infection, including facial dysmorphism (malformation), hepatosplenomegaly, interstitial pneumonia, subtle neurologic abnormalities, behavioral changes, and recurrent infection.

Nursing diagnoses

For a partial list of applicable diagnoses, see Nursing Diagnoses: *High-risk neonates and their families,* page 336.

Planning and implementation

For FAS, no treatment exists because the structural damage occurs in utero. Supportive management focuses on developmental care and environmental support. If the neonate has poorly coordinated sucking and swallowing reflexes, expect to give enteral feedings to prevent aspiration; physical therapy also may be implemented to help alleviate this problem.

For the neonate who is addicted to maternal drugs or going through drug withdrawal, nursing goals include:
• ensuring adequate nutritional intake
• improving coordination of the sucking and swallowing reflexes
• reducing irritability by minimizing environmental stimulation
• avoiding abrupt movements near the neonate
• promoting a normal sleep-awake cycle to prolong sleep
• stabilizing body temperature.

To reduce tremors and extraneous movement, swaddle the neonate and touch the tremulous area firmly and calmly. To minimize muscle rigidity or hypertonicity, bathe the neonate in warm water, massage gently, and swaddle in a flexed position.

For the neonate going through withdrawal, treatment varies with the health care facility and the substance involved. Seizures may be controlled with phenobarbital (5 to 8 mg/kg/day).

Evaluation

For examples of appropriate evaluation statements, see the general ones listed in "Nursing care of the high-risk neonate" earlier in this chapter.

Documentation

For information about appropriate documentation, see the general points listed in "Nursing care of the high-risk neonate" earlier in this chapter. For the neonate suffering the effects of maternal substance abuse, documentation also should include:
• vital sign deviations
• reflexes
• muscle twitching or rigidity
• seizures
• behavioral status, including crying, irritability, and sleep and awake periods

- gastrointestinal status, including vomiting, diarrhea, and increased peristalsis.

Infection

An infection can be acquired in utero, during labor and delivery, or after birth. The preterm neonate is especially vulnerable to postnatal infection because of reduced transmission of maternal immunoglobulins, including IgM and IgA.

Agents that can infect the fetus or neonate, causing potentially morbid effects, are referred to as TORCH agents. This acronym stands for toxoplasmosis, others, rubella, cytomegalovirus, and herpes. Most TORCH infections are acquired in utero.

Cytomegalovirus (CMV) is the most common transplacentally acquired infection; it also can be acquired during delivery. CMV may result in CNS damage, although typically it causes no detectable signs at birth. Rubella, another transplacentally acquired infection, also causes serious sequelae. If acquired during the first trimester, it may result in CNS damage and cardiac defects; after the 14th week of gestation, the major sequela is deafness. Other transplacentally acquired infections include measles, chicken pox, smallpox, vaccinia, hepatitis B, HIV, toxoplasmosis, and syphilis.

Bacterial pneumonia, which can lead to intrauterine death, may be acquired by the fetus after prolonged rupture of the membranes (more than 24 hours), in which vaginal organisms may migrate upward. Bacterial organisms that can cause intrauterine bacteria pneumonia include nonhemolytic streptococci, *Escherichia coli* and other gram-negative organisms, *Listeria monocytogenes,* and *Candida.*

HIV can be acquired transplacentally at various times in gestation, intrapartally through contact with maternal blood and secretions, and postnatally through breast milk. The neonate with HIV typically has a distinctive facial dysmorphism and suffers such problems as interstitial pneumonia, hepatosplenomegaly, recurrent infections, behavioral deviations, and neurologic abnormalities. In many cases, the neonate with HIV is SGA and suffers failure to thrive.

Infections that can be acquired as the fetus passes through the birth canal include:

- *Chlamydia trachomatis,* which may lead to conjunctivitis or pneumonia (if secretions pass into the eyes or oropharynx)
- *Neisseria gonorrhoea,* which may cause ophthalmia neonatorum, an acute purulent conjunctivitis
- herpes simplex virus, which may result in skin vesicles, lethargy, respiratory problems, convulsions, disseminated vascular coagulation, hepatitis, keratoconjunctivitis, and death.

A pregnant patient with known herpes simplex virus should be observed closely through frequent cervical cultures to determine whether the virus is active. Active virus at the time of delivery usually warrants cesarean delivery—an approach that has reduced the number of neonatal herpes cases.

Assessment

The neonate with an infection may be SGA at birth, with a nonspecific rash, pallor, hypotonia, jaundice, lethargy, hyperthermia, or hypothermia. Other common signs accompanying infection include apnea or tachypnea, tachycardia or bradycardia, abdominal distention, hepatomegaly, splenomegaly, seizures, diarrhea, occult blood in the stool, and bleeding disorders. The behavior pattern may be abnormal and the reflexes diminished; poor feeding may cause failure to thrive.

With an intrapartally acquired infection, the neonate may not appear ill at birth but will show gradual deterioration in vital signs over the next 6 to 12 hours. In contrast, with group B streptococcal infection—a commonly acquired intrapartal infection—the neonate may have dyspnea and cyanosis and appear quite ill. However, RDS and congenital cardiac anomalies can cause similar signs and must be ruled out.

A neonate who acquired antepartal HIV may be preterm or SGA, with an abnormally small head and distinctive facial features. Disorders seen in neonates with HIV infection include oral candidiasis (thrush) and lymphoid interstitial pneumonitis. Later, such problems as lymphadenopathy, chronic diarrhea, viral and bacterial infections, *Pneumocystis carinii pneumonia,* and parotid gland enlargement may occur.

Because maternal HIV antibodies are transferred to the fetus, a neonate whose mother has the virus may test positive for HIV antibodies even when not infected. Consequently, an HIV culture or antigen test must be used to confirm infection.

Nursing diagnoses

For a partial list of applicable diagnoses, see Nursing Diagnoses: *High-risk neonates and their families,* page 336.

Planning and implementation

When caring for a neonate with an infection, practice meticulous hand washing and asepsis. (For more information, see "Preventing and controlling infection" earlier in this chapter.)

Evaluation

For examples of appropriate evaluation statements, see the general ones listed in "Nursing care of the high-risk neonate" earlier in this chapter. For the neonate with infection, this additional evaluation statement may be appropriate:

The neonate showed a positive response to antibiotic therapy, as evidenced by improved vital signs and reductions in behavioral deviations, high-pitched crying, and temperature instability.

Congenital anomalies

Many congenital anomalies are life-threatening and warrant immediate intervention and referral to a level 3 nursery. Such disorders include tracheoesophageal malformations, diaphragmatic hernia, omphalocele, gastroschisis, meningomyelocele, encephalocele, and imperforate anus. Other anomalies do not require immediate treatment but may lead to chronic disability or deformity.

The exact cause of many congenital anomalies remains unknown. Some have been linked to genetic or chromosomal disorders, congenital rubella, exposure to radiation, maternal diabetes, and maternal drug use. Increased maternal age also has been associated with certain anomalies, including the trisomy disorders.

Central nervous system anomalies

More congenital anomalies involve the CNS than any other body system. Some CNS anomalies result in only minimal dysfunction; others have devastating consequences.

Meningomyelocele ("spina bifida"). Part of the meninges and spinal cord substance protrude through the vertebral column; the defect may be covered by a thin membrane. (When only the meninges protrude, the anomaly is called a meningocele.) Meningomyelocele results from defective neural tube formation during embryonic development. Hydrocephalus (discussed below) commonly accompanies the anomaly. Consequences of meningomyelocele may be severe—for instance, paralysis below the defect. The child's appearance may be noticeably abnormal even after surgical correction. If meningomyelocele is detected, associated anomalies may be present, such as hip dislocation, knee and foot deformities, and hydrocephalus.

If the defect appears above the lumbosacral region, the bladder and bowel may lack innervation, causing impaired bladder and bowel function. This disorder calls for surgery—perhaps within a few hours after birth. The surgeon removes the herniated tissue and covers the defect with surrounding skin. Before surgery, if the defect is open, it is covered immediately with warm saline-solution compresses and plastic wrap. Reduce pressure on the defect and minimize tissue damage by positioning to avoid pressure on the defect; be sure to support the defect when moving the neonate. After surgery, observe the suture line for signs of CSF leakage and infection, indicated by redness or swelling. Closely monitor neurologic status and movement; check head circumference daily for signs of hydrocephalus. Prevent contamination of and trauma to the wound and stay alert for signs of infection (particularly meningitis).

If the neonate's bladder function is disturbed, monitor fluid intake and output and observe for bladder distention. With lack of innervation (neurologic bladder), an indwelling catheter may be necessary both before and after surgery.

Encephalocele. In this defect, the meninges and portions of brain tissue protrude through the cranium, usually in the occipital area. Typically, it occurs at the midline, through a suture line. Like meningomyelocele, encephalocele results from failure of the neural tube to close during embryonic development, may be accompanied by hydrocephalus, and may lead to paralysis. This defect may be accompanied by hydrocephalus, paralysis, and seizures.

The defect must be closed surgically, necessitating removal of external brain tissue. Surgery may cause such problems as paralysis, mental retardation, or even death.

Preoperatively, the neonate is positioned to avoid pressure on the defect. To prevent infection at the defect, administer antibiotics, as prescribed. Postoperatively, monitor neurologic status and vital signs frequently and assess motor function in all extremities.

If the neonate cannot breathe independently, support respirations by maintaining mechanical ventilation. Inspect the dressing for drainage or CSF leakage; to avoid serious neurologic complications, maintain its sterility.

Congenital hydrocephalus. In this anomaly, excessive cerebrospinal fluid (CSF) accumulates within the cranial vault, leading to suture expansion and ventricular dilation. Hydrocephalus may result from obstruction of the foramen of Monro—a passage allowing communication between the lateral and third ventricles. Hydrocephalus sometimes is associated with meningomyelocele and other neural tube defects, intrauterine infection, meningitis, cerebral hemorrhage, head trauma, or Arnold-Chiari malformation (herniation of the brain stem and lower cerebellum through the foramen magnum into the cervical vertebral canal).

The neonate with hydrocephalus has an enlarged head with an excessive diameter. Wide or bulging fontanels, a shiny scalp with prominent veins, and possible separation of the suture lines are common. Downward eye slanting caused by increased intracranial pressure, and sunset eyes (appearance of the sclera above the iris), reflecting upper lid retraction, are also expected findings. Associated findings include an abnormal heart rate (usually bradycardia), apneic episodes, vomiting, irritability, excessive crying, and reduced alertness.

The condition typically warrants surgical placement of a ventriculoperitoneal shunt (or, rarely, a ventriculoatrial shunt). The shunt drains CSF from the dilated ventricle into the peritoneal cavity or atrium for absorption and removal; it must be revised periodically as the child grows.

Preoperatively, place the neonate in the lateral position, to prevent apnea. Postoperatively, maintain suture line integrity and assess for signs of CSF fluid leakage or infection.

Monitor increasing intracranial pressure by measuring and recording head circumference three times a day. As head circumference decreases, discomfort should subside and oral feedings may begin slowly. Also assess for suture line integrity and alertness level, and note how well the neonate tolerates enteral or oral feedings.

Anencephaly and microcephaly. In anencephaly, the cephalic end of the spinal cord fails to close, causing absence of the cerebral hemispheres. Anencephaly commonly causes stillbirth; if not, the neonate typically lives only a few days.

In microcephaly, the head is abnormally small and the brain underdeveloped, usually resulting in severe mental retardation and motor dysfunction. Microcephaly may result from an inborn error of metabolism (such as uncontrolled maternal phenylketonuria), intrauterine infection, or severe prolonged intrauterine hypoxia.

Provide comfort measures and promote hygiene in a neonate with anencephaly who survived the trauma of delivery but who is terminal. Provide sensitivity and privacy to the parents to help them adjust to this neonate's condition and grieve the loss.

Prepare the neonate to look comfortable prior to the family visit. Emphasize the neonate's positive features. Offer anticipatory guidance regarding the grief process.

Cardiac anomalies

Congenital cardiac anomalies—structural defects of the heart and great vessels—can occur during any stage of embryonic development. Cardiac structures are most susceptible to defects from the third to ninth weeks of gestation. In most cases, the cause remains unknown, although researchers believe that these defects probably stem from a combination of genetic or chromosomal disorders and environmental factors. Maternal alcoholism, malnutrition, rubella, or diabetes mellitus may contribute to cardiac anomalies. Defects become noticeable after delivery when fetal circulation normally changes to neonatal circulation. (For more infomation, see *Congenital cardiac anomalies,* pages 362 and 363.)

A heart murmur, which can be assessed on auscultation, is common to most cardiac anomalies. Other general signs of cardiac anomalies include diminished capillary refill time, tachypnea, dyspnea, and tachycardia. Further, signs of CHF, such as increasing respiratory effort, crackles or other moist breath sounds, feeding intolerance, fatigue, and decreasing urine output, may be present.

Nursing goals for the neonate with a congenital cardiac anomaly include maintaining adequate cardiopulmonary function and preventing complications. The neonate will require intensive, expert care and close monitoring. Assess for cyanosis, heart murmurs, arrhythmias, absent or unequal pulses, and respiratory distress, and monitor daily weight fluid intake and output.

Congenital cardiac anomalies are classified as acyanotic or cyanotic.

Congenital cardiac anomalies

Abnormalities during fetal development may cause structural defects of the heart and great vessels. These defects probably stem from a combination of genetic or chromosomal disorders and environmental factors. Maternal alcoholism, malnutrition, rubella, or diabetes mellitus may contribute to cardiac anomalies. In the illustrations, blood flow is indicated by arrows—shaded arrows for oxygenated blood, black arrows for deoxygenated blood, and dotted arrows for mixed blood.

Atrial septal defect

In this defect, an abnormal opening in the atrial septum allows oxygenated blood from the left atrium to shunt to the right atrium where it mixes with deoxygenated blood; thus, blood in the right heart and the pulmonary arteries is mixed. The increased blood flow to the right heart and pulmonary arteries causes the right ventricle and atrium to enlarge. In many cases, this defect results from failure of the foramen ovale to close.

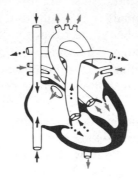

Tetralogy of Fallot

This anomaly consists of four defects—ventricular septal defect, overriding aorta, pulmonic stenosis, and right ventricular hypertrophy. Hemodynamic changes depend on the severity of these defects and typically involve a right-to-left shunt, in which deoxygenated blood from the right ventricle enters the overriding aorta directly. The blood in the aorta is mixed (deoxygenated blood from the right ventricle and oxygenated blood from the left ventricle).

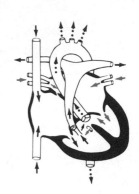

Coarctation of the aorta

This anomaly obstructs preductal or postductal blood flow. The more commonly encountered postductal coarctation illustrated here causes increased pressure in the left ventricle. To compensate, collateral circulation develops, enhancing blood flow from the proximal arteries and bypassing the obstructed area.

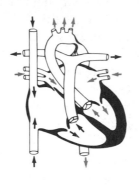

Transposition of the great vessels

In this anomaly, the pulmonary artery arises from the left ventricle and the aorta from the right ventricle, preventing the pulmonary and systemic circulations from mixing. Without associated defects that allow these circulatory systems to mix—such as a patent ductus arteriosus or septal defect—the neonate will die.

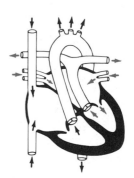

Pulmonic stenosis

This defect may be characterized by poststenotic dilation of the pulmonary trunk and concentric hypertrophy of the right ventricle, which cause a systolic pressure differential between the right ventricular cavity and pulmonary artery.

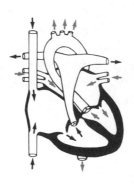

Ventricular septal defect

In this defect, an abnormal opening in the ventricular septum allows oxygenated blood to flow from the left to right ventricle, resulting in recirculation of mixed blood through the lungs and pulmonary artery. If the defect is large, pulmonary vascular resistance increases, causing elevated pulmonary and right ventricular pressures.

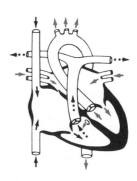

Congenital cardiac anomalies *(continued)*

Patent ductus arteriosus
This anomaly occurs when the ductus arteriosus—a tubular connection that shunts blood away from the fetus's pulmonary circulation—fails to close after birth. Oxygenated blood then shunts from the aorta to the pulmonary artery, resulting in mixed blood distal to the ductus arteriosus.

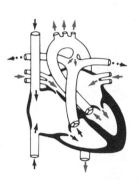

Tricuspid atresia
In this defect, which usually is accompanied by an atrial or ventricular septal defect (both shown), the tricuspid valve is absent or incomplete, preventing the flow of blood from the right atrium to the right ventricle. Right atrial blood then shunts through an atrial septal defect into the left atrium, resulting in mixed blood in the left atrium, left ventricle, and aorta.

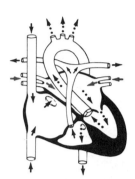

Acyanotic defects. Acyanotic defects do not interfere with shunting of oxygenated blood from the left to the right side of the heart; the left side continues to eject oxygenated blood, preventing cyanosis. However, pulmonary blood flow to the right ventricle increases, placing the neonate at risk for pulmonary edema and congestive heart failure (CHF). With acyanotic defects, cyanosis usually is absent.

With an *atrial septal defect,* an abnormal opening in the atrial septum allows oxygenated blood from the left atrium to shunt to the right atrium where it mixes with deoxygenated blood; thus, blood in the right heart and the pulmonary arteries is mixed. The increased blood flow to the right heart and pulmonary arteries causes the right ventricle and atrium to enlarge. In many cases, this defect results from failure of the foramen ovale to close.

In *ventricular septal defect,* an abnormal opening in the ventricular septum allows oxygenated blood to flow from the left to right ventricle, resulting in recirculation of mixed blood through the lungs and pulmonary artery. If the defect is large, pulmonary vascular resistance increases, causing elevated pulmonary and right ventricular pressures.

Coarctation of the aorta obstructs preductal or postductal blood flow. The more commonly encountered postductal coarctation causes increased pressure in the left ventricle. To compensate, collateral circulation develops, enhancing blood flow from the proximal arteries and bypassing the obstructed area.

Pulmonic stenosis may be characterized by poststenotic dilation of the pulmonary trunk and concentric hypertrophy of the right ventricle, which cause a systolic pressure differential between the right ventricular cavity and pulmonary artery.

Patent ductus arteriosus occurs when the ductus arteriosus—a tubular connection that shunts blood away from the fetus's pulmonary circulation—fails to close after birth. Oxygenated blood then shunts from the aorta to the pulmonary artery, resulting in mixed blood distal to the ductus arteriosus.

For all congenital cardiac anomalies, corrective surgery may be delayed in favor of symptomatic treatment. Surgery may be delayed until the child is a toddler or preschooler.

Cyanotic defects. In cyanotic defects, abnormally high pressure in the right side of the heart permits left-to-right shunting of unoxygenated blood. As this blood mixes with oxygenated blood, arterial blood oxygen becomes desaturated. Peripheral perfusion then decreases and cyanosis develops.

Tetralogy of Fallot consists of four defects—ventricular septal defect, over-riding aorta, pulmonic stenosis, and right ventricular hypertrophy. Hemodynamic changes depend on the severity of these defects and typically involve a right-to-left shunt, in which deoxygenated blood from the right ventricle enters the overriding aorta directly. The blood in the aorta is mixed (deoxygenated blood from the right ventricle and oxygenated blood from the left ventricle).

In *transposition of the great vessels,* the pulmonary artery arises from the left ventricle and the aorta from the right ventricle, preventing the pulmonary and systemic circulations from mixing. Without associated defects that allow these circulatory systems to mix—such as a patent ductus arteriosus or septal defect—the neonate will die.

In *tricuspid atresia,* which usually is accompanied by an atrial or ventricular septal defect, the tricuspid valve is absent or incomplete, preventing the flow of blood from the right atrium to the right ventricle. Right atrial blood then shunts through an atrial septal defect into the left atrium, resulting in mixed blood in the left atrium, left ventricle, and aorta.

With cyanotic cardiac defects, expect cyanosis, especially during hypoxic spells. Palliative surgery typically is performed during the neonatal period. For instance, a temporary shunt may be placed to increase pulmonary blood flow. Palliative medical treatments aim to prevent complications of hypoxemia.

Respiratory tract anomalies

The most common respiratory tract anomaly is diaphragmatic hernia. In this defect, the various segments of the diaphragm fail to fuse during embryonic development, causing the abdominal contents to protrude from the abdominal cavity into the thoracic cavity at birth. Diaphragmatic hernia occurs in 1 of every 2,000 births. In the United States, it is twice as common in males as in females.

The defect may be unilateral or bilateral; most commonly, it occurs on the posterolateral aspect of the diaphragm on the left side. In a left-sided defect, the stomach and intestines typically protrude into the thoracic cavity; protrusion of the liver, spleen, and other abdominal organs is rare.

Most neonates with diaphragmatic hernia have impaired lung development—typically only a lung bud is present (a condition known as hypoplastic lung). This may lead to profound respiratory compromise and death if intervention does not begin immediately after delivery.

Diaphragmatic hernia. Cyanosis and respiratory compromise are the first signs of diaphragmatic hernia; the more severe the defect, the greater the respiratory compromise. The chest typically appears asymmetrical and the abdomen concave (from lack of abdominal contents). Substernal, intercostal, and suprascapular retractions usually occur over the unaffected side. The neonate usually is tachypneic, with a respiratory rate of at least 80 breaths/minute.

Initially, gastric decompression is necessary to relive gastric distention caused by pressure over the stomach and decreased intestinal motility. The sooner the defect is corrected, the better the prognosis.

Surgery for diaphragmatic hernia involves a transthoracic or transabdominal incision to restore the abdominal contents to their proper anatomic position. The surgeon pulls the outer skin layers to cover the abdominal wall defect. Unfortunately, surgical repair does not guarantee survival. If the neonate has respiratory complications or if the unaffected lung is compromised and the affected lung is hypoplastic, the prognosis is guarded at best.

Preoperatively, the main nursing goal is to stabilize and support respiration. Administer prophylactic antibiotics and I.V. fluids. Lab tests would be ordered to monitor signs of hypoxia, infection.

Postoperatively, complications such as right-to-left shunt, pneumothorax, and pulmonary arterial hypertension are possible. Closely monitor airway patency, respiratory support, and fluid and electrolyte balance. Frequently assess signs of infection or leakage.

The neonate probably will require endotracheal intubation. Perform endotracheal suctioning and maintains ventilatory support, as needed. A chest tube also is inserted to help reinflate the lung on the affected side. Maintain and closely evaluate chest tube patency.

GI tract anomalies

These anomalies include tracheoesophageal malformations, abdominal wall defects (omphalocele and gastroschisis), meconium ileus, imperforate anus, and cleft palate and lip.

Tracheoesophageal malformations. Tracheoesophageal malformations, which occur in 1 of every 1,500 live births, result from altered embryonic development of the trachea and esophagus. These anomalies sometimes occur as part of the VACTERL syndrome—vertebral, anal, cardiac, tracheal, esophageal, renal, and limb anomalies. Types of tracheoesophageal anomalies include tracheoesophageal fistula (an abnormal connection between the trachea and esophagus), esophageal atresia (closure of the esophagus at some point), and absence of the esophagus. In almost half of affected neonates, the maternal history includes hydramnios. (See *Tracheoesophageal malformations.*)

Suspect a tracheoesophageal malformation if the neonate has labored breathing, chest retractions, nasal flaring, cyanosis, or frothy secretions. Difficulty inserting a nasogastric tube and choking or aspiration during oral feedings are other suggestive signs.

Surgical intervention is necessary to separate the trachea and esophagus and to maintain the patency of each structure. The surgical procedure used depends on the specific malformation. A gastrostomy tube commonly is inserted during surgery to prevent gastric reflux and aspiration pneumonia.

Nursing goals include maintaining a patent airway and ensuring fluid and electrolyte balance before and after surgery. Oxygen therapy may be required if the neonate's breathing effort increases or if cyanosis develops. Monitor vital signs, respiratory effort, skin color, appearance of the I.V. infusion site, and the amount of secretions suctioned.

Postoperative nursing interventions resemble those used for the neonate with diaphragmatic hernia, except that no chest tube is present. Keep the neonate in an upright position before and after surgery—for instance, by using a cholasia chair, which allows the neonate to remain upright after feeding to prevent reflux of secretions.

When the feedings begin, evaluate how well the neonate tolerates them. A dusky skin color or choking during feedings may indicate fistula leakage; increased mucus may indicate stenosis around the surgical site.

Abdominal wall defects. Omphalocele and gastroschisis occur in approximately 1 of every 7,000 births. In omphalocele, a portion of the intestine protrudes through a defect in the abdominal wall at the umbilicus, in the midline. A thin, transparent membrane composed of amnion and peritoneum typically covers the protruding part. The defect may be quite large—or small enough to elude detection on brief inspection.

Omphalocele arises during embryonic development. Normally, at 9 weeks' gestation, the abdominal contents recede from the umbilical cord, regressing into the abdominal cavity; if the contents fail to recede, omphalocele occurs.

Gastroschisis refers to incomplete abdominal wall closure not involving the site of the umbilical cord insertion. Usually, the small intestine and part of the larger intestine protrude. No membranous sac covers the protrusion.

The neonate with gastroschisis or omphalocele requires immediate intervention in the delivery room—ventilatory support followed by peripheral line placement for I.V. fluid administration. Immediately cover the defect with sterile gauze dressings moistened with warm normal saline solution; place plastic wrap on top of the dressings to help keep tis-

Tracheoesophageal malformations

Tracheoesophageal malformations result from incomplete separation of the trachea and esophagus during the first trimester of pregnancy. Among the most serious surgical emergencies in neonates, they require immediate correction. In many cases, they are accompanied by other congenital anomalies. Common variations of tracheoesophageal malformations are illustrated here.

Esophageal atresia with distal tracheoesophageal fistula is the most common variation.

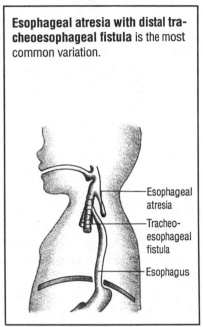

Esophageal atresia

Tracheoesophageal fistula

Esophagus

In **esophageal atresia without tracheoesophageal fistula,** the upper esophageal portion ends in a blind pouch, the upper and lower esophageal portions do not connect, and the trachea and esophagus are not linked by a fistula.

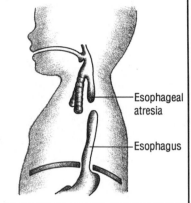

Esophageal atresia

Esophagus

Tracheoesophageal fistula without esophageal atresia (sometimes called an H-type tracheoesophageal fistula) is characterized by an intact esophagus and a connection between the trachea and esophagus.

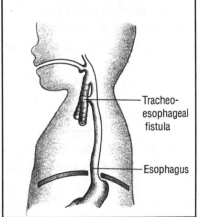

Tracheoesophageal fistula

Esophagus

In some cases, **esophageal atresia** occurs with a **proximal fistula.**

Esophageal atresia

Tracheoesophageal fistula

Esophagus

Esophageal atresia sometimes occurs with a **double** (proximal and distal) **fistula.**

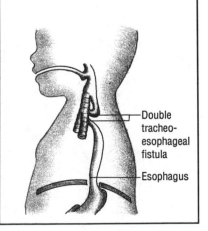

Double tracheoesophageal fistula

Esophagus

sues moist and reduce heat loss. Maintain gastric decompression with a nasogastric tube.

The nursing goal is to minimize the risk of infection and maintain the herniated tissue and organs in optimal condition. Maintain sterile technique throughout caregiving procedures.

Corrective treatment of a small defect involves complete or primary surgical reduction. After the neonate's final surgical closure, feedings are given through a gastrostomy tube.

Cleft lip and palate. These congenital defects, which occur in 1 of every 1,000 live births, sometimes result from chromosomal abnormalities. Cleft palate occurs when the sides of the palate fail to fuse during embryonic development, leading to a fissure in the palatal midline. The fissure may be complete, extending through both the hard and soft palates into the nasal cavities, or incomplete.

In cleft lip (harelip), one or more clefts appear in the upper lip resulting from failure of the maxillary and median nasal processes to close during embryonic development. The defect, which is more common in males than females, may be unilateral or bilateral and sometimes occurs in conjunction with other anomalies. It commonly accompanies cleft palate.

The neonate may have difficulty sucking, with expulsion of milk or formula through the nose. With cleft lip, the neonate may have signs of localized infection in the oral cavity, causing a fever, crying, and irritability.

Surgical repair of these anomalies usually is delayed to prevent disruption of facial growth and tooth-bud formation. However, it must occur early enough so that the defect does not interfere with speech development. Repair of cleft lip (cheilorrhaphy, or Z-plasty) commonly takes place when the child is 3 months old; repair of cleft palate (by joining of the palatal segments) typically is performed when the child is 9 to 15 months old. Ensure adequate nutrition before and after surgery, because air leaks around the cleft and nasal regurgitation typically cause feeding problems.

Many neonates with cleft lip can be breast-fed (except after surgery); the mother may provide breast milk she has pumped. With cleft palate, a feeding neonate requires a syringe or cleft palate feed or a special elongated nipple (such as a Martin's nipple). To prevent aspiration of feeding matter through the palatal opening and the nares, elevate the head of the bed or place the neonate in an infant seat or on the stomach after feedings.

Teach the parents how to provide the special care their child requires. Cleft palate and lip can cause long-term speech, dental, hearing, and other problems, so refer parents to appropriate professionals for follow-up care.

Meconium ileus. This intestinal obstruction results from obstruction of the terminal ileum by viscous meconium. Beyond the ileal obstruction, the colon atrophies and narrows in diameter. In at least 95% of cases, it is a sign of cystic fibrosis, a genetic disease resulting from a pancreatic enzyme deficiency. This disorder manifests as abdominal distention, bilious vomiting, and distended bowel loops in the right lower quadrant (found on palpation).

The initial medical treatment to reduce the obstruction is through a gastrografin or Hypague enema, which is successful 50% of the time. Surgical intervention will be required if the enema was not successful. The neonate may have a temporary ileostomy, which would be closed at a future time.

Nursing goals include postoperative care and prevention of fluid and electrolyte imbalance and nutrition deficit. If the neonate is diagnosed with cystic fibrosis, institute nursing measures to promote parental understanding and adaptation.

Imperforate anus. In this malformation, the anus is closed abnormally. Occurring in 1 of every 20,000 live births, the disorder is more common in males than females. It results from persistence of the membrane that separates the lower rectum from the lower aspect of the large intestine. In many cases, imperforate anus is associated with other defects, such as rectourethral and rectovaginal fistula (both of which permit abnormal evacuation of fecal matter from the rectum).

This anomaly usually is obvious at delivery, although in some cases it is detected only during an attempt to take a rectal temperature. With a complete defect, the anus appears as a dimple in the perineal skin; an incomplete defect may manifest as a narrow opening where the anus should appear. If this anomaly is accompanied by bowel obstruction, the abdomen will be distended. The neonate typically does not pass meconium; however, sometimes meconium passes through a fistula or misplaced anus.

The neonate with this anomaly requires surgical restoration of the anal canal to achieve urinary and bowel continence. For a low defect, a peripheral anoplasty typically is performed during the neonatal period. For an intermediate defect, a colostomy is performed in most cases, with further surgery performed several months later. A high defect always necessitates a colostomy.

Nursing goals include preventing gastric distention and dehydration. Maintain gastric decompression and initiate I.V. therapy. Postoperatively, position the neonate on the stomach or side. Maintain gastric decompression until 24 hours before feedings are to begin. Avoid taking rectal temperatures or examining the rectum. To minimize stool formation until the incision heals, delay feedings at least 24 hours after surgery.

Genitourinary tract anomalies

An anomaly involving the kidneys commonly causes acute renal failure, as reflected by oliguria or anuria. In many cases, the neonate has associated signs, such as hypoplastic lungs or GI defects. Genitourinary tract anomalies include renal agenesis, polycystic kidney disease, and external genital ambiguity.

Renal agenesis. One of the most common congenital anomalies in males, renal agenesis may be unilateral (absence of one kidney) or bilateral (absence of both kidneys). The bilateral form (also called Potter's syndrome) is compatible with life and typically causes stillbirth or death during the neonatal period; autopsies of neonates with bilateral renal agenesis show hypoplastic lung and multiple pneumothoraces. With unilateral agenesis, the single kidney enlarges to maintain normal renal function.

Maternal oligohydramnios during pregnancy is a predictor of renal agenesis; fetal ultrasound examination can confirm it before delivery.

Oliguria or anuria within the first 48 hours after birth is diagnostic of this disorder. Skeletal anomalies that sometimes accompany renal agenesis include bowed legs and flat or broad hands and feet. With bilateral renal agenesis, stillbirth occurs or the neonate dies within a few days after birth.

Nursing goals include anticipatory guidance and support of the grieving process for the family. Possible referral for genetic counseling may be indicated for reassurance regarding future pregnancy outcomes.

Polycystic kidney disease. In this disorder, which occurs as an autosomal recessive disease in the neonate and as an acquired disease in the adult, multiple cysts form within the kidney. As the cysts enlarge, adjacent tissue is destroyed. At birth, the neonate with polycystic kidney disease typically suffers renal failure, respiratory distress, CHF, and hypertension.

A protruding abdomen and greatly enlarged kidneys suggest this disorder; the liver also is enlarged. Fluid buildup may cause signs of acute renal failure, such as oliguria or anuria, edema, and blood pressure fluctuations.

The polycystic kidney is removed surgically. Before surgery, monitor the neonate for infection (especially of the urinary tract).

Nursing goals include maintaining fluid and electrolyte balance and supporting respiration (hypoplastic lungs accompany some renal problems). If surgery is scheduled, preoperative nursing care centers on maintaining fluid and electrolyte balance. Monitor for signs of acute renal failure, such as oliguria or anuria, edema, blood pressure fluctuations, and cardiopulmonary compromise secondary to fluid accumulation. Take postoperative measures to prevent infection. Also assess signs of respiratory compromise, decreased urine output, and drainage from the nephrostomy tube or stent.

External genital ambiguity. This problem may reflect a developmental defect, genetic abnormality, or hormonal influences. In some cases, it complicates determination of the neonate's sex. In males, genital ambiguity typically stems from a developmental abnormality. Genital abnormalities may include abnormally small or undescended testes, hypospadias, and incomplete scrotal fusion.

In females, a common cause is congenital adrenal hyperplasia, a condition stemming from blockage of cortisol precursors (enzymes that convert cholesterol to cortisol). The resulting corticotropin deficiency leads to increased secretion of cortisol precursors and androgens and subsequent masculinization of the female external genitalia. In the affected female, androgen hypersecretion may cause such genital abnormalities as a small penis and the beginning of a scrotal sac.

The nurse who detects ambiguous genitalia should notify the physician immediately so that genetic evaluation can begin. Sex determination not only permits prompt treatment of the underlying adrenal disorder but may help reduce parental anxiety. Definitive sex determination may take up to 2 weeks.

If genital ambiguity stems from congenital adrenal hyperplasia, hydrocortisone is given to arrest the disorder; with severe adrenal hyperplasia, hydrocortisone must be administered immediately to prevent acute adrenocortical failure—a fatal condition. Later, surgical reconstruction of the external genitalia may be attempted.

Anticipate genetic testing and a determination of the neonate's underlying problem if this has not been established. Providing support to the family is a nursing priority.

Musculoskeletal anomalies

The most common congenital musculoskeletal anomaly is clubfoot (talipes). This deformity involves unilateral or bilateral deviation of the metatarsal bones; talus deformation and a shortened Achilles tendon give the foot a clublike appearance. Clubfoot sometimes is associated with other anomalies, such as meningomyelocele. The second most common musculoskeletal disorder is congenital hip dysplasia. This disorder occurs more commonly in females.

Talipes ("clubfoot"). Clubfoot may be mild to severe and occurs in several variations. In equinovarus, the most common form, the heel turns inward from the midline of the leg, the foot is plantarflexed, the inner border of the foot is raised, and the anterior part of the foot is displaced so that it lies medial to the vertical axis of the leg. Other forms of clubfoot include calcaneovalgus, metatarsus adductus, and metatarsus varus.

If the neonate has an obvious foot deformity, first rule out "apparent clubfoot" (caused by fetal positioning) by taking the foot through the full range of motion. If the foot does not revert to a natural position with manipulation, suspect true clubfoot.

Passive stretching exercises and corrective shoes, braces, or splints may be used in treatment. The goals of treatment are to prevent permanent defects and correct the deformity. If these measures fail, surgery may be performed when the child is several years old. Inform the parents of the need for early and continual medical evaluation to avoid problems when the child begins to walk.

Congenital hip dislocation. This abnormality involves the hip joint, with the head of the femur unstable, subluxed, or dislocated from the pelvic joint. It can occur unilaterally or bilaterally. The cause of this condition is not known, although it may occur secondary to a joint, muscular, or neuromuscular irregularity.

Treatment for congenital hip dysplasia involves pressing the femoral head against and into the acetabulum. This pressure allows formation of an adequate socket before ossification is complete. To abduct and externally rotate the leg and flex the hip, apply a triangular pillow over the diaper. At a later date, the neonate typically is placed in a spica cast.

Nursing measures include cast care and parental teaching regarding cast, splint, or brace care. Hygiene is especially important, as is proper positioning.

Inborn errors of metabolism

An inborn error of metabolism is a genetic condition in which a defect of a specific enzyme disrupts metabolism and nutrient use. The involved enzyme may not be produced or its action may be blocked by lack of a precursor necessary for a crucial chemical reaction. The nursing goal for a neonate with an inborn error of metabolism is early detection and prevention of complications.

Congenital hypothyroidism. This condition results from a deficiency of thyroid hormone secretion during fetal development or early infancy. Also known as cretinism, it typically stems from defective embryonic development causing absence or underdevelopment of the thyroid gland or severe maternal iodine deficiency; in some cases, it is inherited as an autosomal recessive disorder involving an enzymatic defect in the synthesis of the thyroid hormone thyroxine. Untreated, congenital hypothyroidism can lead to respiratory compromise and persistent physiologic jaundice. Signs of congenital hypothyroidism in the neonate include inactivity, jaundice, excessive sleep, hoarse cry, constipation, and feeding problems.

Many states require measurement of thyroid hormone levels at birth to detect congenital hypothyroidism early and thus help minimize mental and physical retardation. The disorder is confirmed by an elevated serum level of thyroid-stimulating hormone (TSH) and a low serum thyroxine (T_4) level. (However, test results may be misleading in the preterm neonate—especially one with respiratory distress syndrome, who typically has abnormal TSH and T_4 levels.)

Treatment involves lifelong administration of L-thyroxine, with periodic dosage adjustments to meet the demands of rapid growth periods. During the neonatal period, thyroxine can be given mixed with several milliliters of formula or crushed and mixed with rice cereal or applesauce when the infant begins eating solid foods.

Galactosemia. Galactosemia is a hereditary autosomal recessive disorder in which deficiency of the enzyme galactose-1-phosphate uridyltransferase leads to an inability to convert galactose to glucose and subsequent galactose accumulation in the blood. The disorder can be fatal if not detected and treated within the first few days after birth.

Because the affected neonate cannot tolerate lactose, feeding problems may be the first sign of the disorder. Such problems may include anorexia, diarrhea, vomiting, jaundice, hepatomegaly, growth failure, lack of a red light reflex during eye examination, cataracts, and mental retardation (from elevated fetal galactose levels). Also, birth weight may be somewhat low. With early detection and treatment, these problems may subside.

Diagnosis is confirmed by the galactosemia tolerance test and examination of red blood cells revealing deficient galactose-1-phosphate uridyltransferase activity. In some cases, galactosemia may be detected in utero by amniocentesis. In such cases, the mother should be placed on a galactose-restricted diet to prevent fetal complications and mental retardation.

Treatment involves lifelong avoidance of galactose-containing foods (milk and milk products).

Maple syrup urine disease. This is an autosomal recessive disorder characterized by an enzyme deficiency in the second step of branched-chain amino acid (BCAA) catabolism. BCAAs accumulate in the blood and urine, causing severe ketoacidosis soon after birth. Without intervention, the neonate progresses rapidly to death (usually from pneumonia and respiratory failure).

The neonate typically appears normal at birth but deteriorates within 1 week as respirations become rapid and shallow and the level of consciousness declines. Other signs of the disorder include lethargy, alternating muscle hypotonicity and hypertonicity, brief tonic (rigid) seizures, hypoglycemic manifestations (from altered glucose metabolism), and a maple syrup odor to the urine. Diagnosis is confirmed by a 2,4-dinitrophenylhydrazine test and serum elevation of the essential amino acids leucine, isoleucine, and valine.

Management involves lifelong dietary restriction of BCAAs and close monitoring of serum leucine, isoleucine, and valine levels. An acute episode warrants peritoneal dialysis.

Phenylketonuria (PKU). PKU is an autosomal recessive disorder characterized by the abnormal presence of metabolites of phenylalanine (such as phenylketone) in the urine. It results from deficiency of phenylalanine hydroxylase, the enzyme responsible for converting the amino acid phenylalanine to tyrosine. Phenylalanine is transaminated to phenylpyruvic acid or decarboxylated to phenylthalanine, which then accumulates in the blood. Prolonged exposure to high serum levels of phenylalanine may cause severe brain damage and mental retardation.

Most states require PKU screening at birth. The test usually is done within the first 24 to 48 hours after birth. If results are positive, retesting and referral should take place immediately to ensure early treatment.

Obtain blood for the screening test by heel stick. To prevent a false-negative test result, make sure the neonate has received adequate dietary protein and had no contraindications for oral feedings for 24 to 48 hours before the test.

Dietary restriction of phenylalanine must continue lifelong. Serum phenylalanine blood levels must be monitored closely throughout childhood.

Provide teaching, nutritional counseling, and emotional support to the neonate's family. Emphasize that the neonate cannot be given substitutions for prescribed food products, especially for Lafenalac. Refer the family to any available support groups for help in coping with the disease.

A woman with PKU who contemplates pregnancy should be warned about the possible effects of an elevated maternal phenylalanine level on the developing fetus (including congenital anomalies and mental retardation).

STUDY ACTIVITIES

Short answer

1. After a long and difficult second stage of labor, Laura Phoenix is born at 40 weeks' gestation by vacuum extraction. A tight nuchal cord was clamped and cut prior to her delivery. A neonatal nurse is present at the delivery, in anticipation of the possible need for resuscitation. Emergency equipment and supplies have been verified as ready to use for this delivery. As the nurse receives this neonate, her cyanosis and flaccid tone are apparent. What three parameters are used for the initial neonatal evaluation? What are the goals of neonatal resuscitation?

_____

2. Should the nurse wait until the end of the first minute to start resuscitation on Laura? What is the rationale for this?

_____

3. Positive pressure ventilation (PPV) with a bag and mask was initiated immediately, as Laura was not breathing. Originally, her heart rate was 90 beats/minute, which improved significantly as her oxygenation increased. Her color, dusky and pale at the onset, also recovered dramatically with 1 minute of PPV. After several minutes, Laura cried spontaneously and her vital signs stabilized within normal limits. At 5 minutes, she received an Apgar score of 8, with 1 point off for color and 1 point off for reflexes. Briefly describe the postresuscitation care that would be provided for Laura.

_____

4. Eduardo Peres, a 34-week preterm neonate, was born unexpectedly by precipitous vaginal delivery at home. His mother, Carmella Peres, was unattended and had to deliver the neonate by herself. After Eduardo was transported by ambulance to the hospital soon after the birth, the nursery nurse conducted his initial neonatal evaluation. His rectal, core temperature is noted to be 35.8° C (96.1° F). Why is this preterm neonate at risk for cold stress? What would be the consequences of progressive heat loss for Eduardo?

_____

5. What is the goal of nursing care for the Peres family during this neonatal hospitalization? List the four main categories of nursing interventions that should be provided for the Peres family to help them cope with Eduardo's hospitalization and high-risk, preterm status.

_____

_____

6. Various factors place the high-risk neonate in danger of fluid imbalance. Recognizing signs of either fluid volume excess or deficit is an essential part of neonatal nursing care. Check the clinical findings below and indicate whether they are a fluid volume excess or deficit.

A. _____ Dry mucus membranes
B. _____ Rhonchi
C. _____ Poor skin turgor
D. _____ Edema
E. _____ Tachypnea
F. _____ Sunken fontanels
G. _____ Urine output of 0.5 ml/kg/hr
H. _____ Dyspnea

7. Many congenital anomalies are life-threatening and warrant immediate surgical intervention and referral to a level 3 nursery. Which of the following fall into this category?

A. _____ Diaphragmatic hernia
B. _____ Hydrocephalus
C. _____ Coarctation of the aorta
D. _____ Tracheoesophageal malformations
E. _____ Imperforate anus
F. _____ Tetralogy of Fallot
G. _____ Gastroschisis
H. _____ Transposition of the great vessels
I. _____ Cleft lip and palate
J. _____ Meningomyelocele
K. _____ Ventricular septal defect

8. Distinguish between the preterm and the post-term neonate and between the small-for-gestational-age neonate and large-for-gestational-age neonate. Identify the significance of this status to the neonate's prognosis.

_____

_____

_____

9. Briefly describe the consequences of prolonged neonatal asphyxia would be, especially if the need for resuscitation efforts were delayed or not provided.

_____

True or false

10. Regionalized care permits the most efficient use of health care resources, eliminating the need for every facility to have expensive equipment and staff for an NICU.
☐ True   ☐ False

11. Respiratory distress syndrome (RDS) affects mainly post-term neonates.
☐ True   ☐ False

12. Placental dysfunction after 42 weeks' gestation impairs fetal oxygenation and nutrition and exhausts placental reserves, retarding fetal growth.
☐ True   ☐ False

13. Hyperbilirubinemia and jaundice occur only in high-risk neonates.
☐ True   ☐ False

Fill in the blank

14. The definition of a high-risk neonate is one who has an increased chance of _____ or who has a _____ necessitating prompt intervention.

15. The family of a neonate with a chronic illness or congenital anomaly must find ways to cope with _____ and develop strategies to _____.

16. The goals of neonatal intensive care include _____, _____, and _____.

17. HIV can be acquired transplacentally _____, intrapartally through _____, and postnatally through _____.

18. The most common problems seen in NICUs are _____ and its sequelae, _____, and congenital _____ requiring emergency surgery.

ANSWERS **Short answer**

1. Initial neonatal evaluation and subsequent resuscitative measures are based on respirations, heart rate, and skin color and not on the 1-minute Apgar score. As with any resuscitation, the goal of neonatal resuscitation is to ensure the ABCs: airway, breathing, and circulation. Resuscitation follows an orderly sequence; after each intervention, the team quickly evaluates the neonate's condition and response to the intervention, then decides which further measures, if any, are necessary.

2. Waiting until the end of the first minute to start resuscitation makes the procedure more difficult and increases the chance for brain damage and death. With a severely asphyxiated neonate, a delay is especially dangerous.

3. After resuscitation, the nurse would observe Laura closely for signs of respiratory distress, including cyanosis, apnea, tachypnea, and inspiratory retractions. Blood pressure and cardiac perfusion are other key indicators to be monitored. Thermoregulation would be maintained by keeping Laura under a radiant warmer and monitoring her skin temperature.

4. A preterm neonate such as Eduardo is especially at risk for cold stress because of limited subcutaneous fat, an extremely high surface-to-mass ratio, inability to shiver, and minimal brown fat. A neonate who suffers heat loss and progressive cold stress may experience peripheral vasoconstriction, hypoglycemia, reduced cerebral perfusion, metabolic acidosis, exacerbation of respiratory distress syndrome, decreased surfactant production, impaired kidney function, GI disturbances, and, ultimately, death.

5. The goal of nursing care is to help the Peres family develop the understanding, skills, and confidence to give competent care after Eduardo's discharge. Thus, the nurse should plan interventions to help them deal with the crisis of Eduardo's birth and to meet his needs. Such interventions should focus on the neonate's physical and developmental needs and the family's practical and emotional needs. The four main categories of nursing interventions for the Peres family are providing information, strengthening their support systems, teaching them caregiving skills, and enhancing their parent-infant bonding.

6. Fluid volume deficit (dehydration): A. dry mucus membranes, C. poor skin turgor, F. sunken fontanels, G. urine output less than 1 ml/kg/hour. Fluid volume excess (overhydration): B. rhonchi; D. edema; E. tachypnea; H. dyspnea.

7. Congenital anomalies that are life-threatening include: A. diaphragmatic hernia; D. tracheoesophageal malformations; E. imperforate anus; F. tetralogy of Fallot; G. gastroschisis; H. transposition of the great vessels; J. meningomyelocele.

8. A preterm neonate, the classic high-risk neonate, is one born before completion of the 37th week of gestation; a post-term neonate is one born after the completion of the 42nd week of gestation. Neonatal mortality and morbidity are highest among preterm neonates. Unlike preterm neonates who are generally of low birth weight, the post-term neonate typically weighs above the 90th percentile on the Colorado intrauterine Growth Chart.

A small-for-gestational-age (SGA) neonate is one whose birth weight falls below the 10th percentile for gestational age. SGA status results from intrauterine growth restriction (IUGR), an abnormal process in which fetal development and maturation are delayed or impeded. After prematurity, IUGR is the leading cause of death during the perinatal period. Conversely, a large-for-gestational-age (LGA) neonate is one whose birth weight exceeds the 90th percentile for gestational age. A neonate delivered at term is considered to be LGA if the birth weight exceeds 4,000 g. The leading cause of LGA status is maternal diabetes mellitus.

9. Without immediate resuscitation, the asphyxiated neonate will die. Complications of prolonged asphyxia include cerebral hypoxia, seizures, intraventricular hemorrhage, renal failure, necrotizing enterocolitis, and metabolic imbalances.

True or false
10. True.
11. False. RDS, also called hyaline membrane disease, affects mainly preterm infants who have highly pliable and easily overinflated thoracic muscles, weak intercostal muscles, and insufficient surfactant, the lipoprotein necessary to keep alveoli expanded.
12. True.
13. False. Hyperbilirubinemia—an elevated serum level of unconjugated bilirubin—is common among both low-risk and high-risk neonates.

Fill in the blank
14. Dying during or shortly after delivery, congenital or perinatal problem
15. Long-term grief, provide the special care the condition will require
16. Averting or minimizing complications, subjecting the neonate to as little stress as possible, furthering parent-infant bonding
17. At various times in gestation, contact with maternal blood and secretions, breast milk
18. Prematurity, congenital heart defects, anomalies

Appendix: NANDA taxonomy of nursing diagnoses

The currently accepted classification system for nursing diagnoses is that of the North American Nursing Diagnosis Association (NANDA) as shown in *NANDA nursing diagnoses: Definitions and classifications 1992-1993.* It is organized around nine human response patterns: exchanging, communicating, relating, valuing, choosing, moving, perceiving, knowing, and feeling.

The complete taxonomic structure is listed here. The series of numbers before each diagnosis is its classification number, used to determine the placement of the diagnosis within the taxonomy. The number of digits delineates the level of abstraction of the nursing diagnosis (more specific diagnoses are assigned longer numbers).

Pattern 1. Exchanging

1.1.2.1	Altered nutrition: More than body requirements
1.1.2.2	Altered nutrition: Less than body requirements
1.1.2.3	Altered nutrition: Potential for more than body requirements
1.2.1.1	High risk for infection
1.2.2.1	High risk for altered body temperature
1.2.2.2	Hypothermia
1.2.2.3	Hyperthermia
1.2.2.4	Ineffective thermoregulation
1.2.3.1	Dysreflexia
*1.3.1.1	Constipation
1.3.1.1.1	Perceived constipation
1.3.1.1.2	Colonic constipation
*1.3.1.2	Diarrhea
*1.3.1.3	Bowel incontinence
1.3.2	Altered urinary elimination
1.3.2.1.1	Stress incontinence
1.3.2.1.2	Reflex incontinence
1.3.2.1.3	Urge incontinence
1.3.2.1.4	Functional incontinence
1.3.2.1.5	Total incontinence
1.3.2.2	Urinary retention
*1.4.1.1	Altered (specify type) tissue perfusion (renal, cerebral, cardiopulmonary, gastrointestinal, peripheral)
1.4.1.2.1	Fluid volume excess
1.4.1.2.2.1	Fluid volume deficit
1.4.1.2.2.2	High risk for fluid volume deficit
*1.4.2.1	Decreased cardiac output
1.5.1.1	Impaired gas exchange
1.5.1.2	Ineffective airway clearance
1.5.1.3	Ineffective breathing pattern
#1.5.1.3.1	Inability to sustain spontaneous ventilation
#1.5.1.3.2	Dysfunctional ventilatory weaning response (DVWR)
1.6.1	High risk for injury
1.6.1.1	High risk for suffocation
1.6.1.2	High risk for poisoning
1.6.1.3	High risk for trauma
1.6.1.4	High risk for aspiration
1.6.1.5	High risk for disuse syndrome
1.6.2	Altered protection
1.6.2.1	Impaired tissue integrity
*1.6.2.1.1	Altered oral mucous membrane
1.6.2.1.2.1	Impaired skin integrity
1.6.2.1.2.2	High risk for impaired skin integrity

Pattern 2. Communicating

2.1.1.1	Impaired verbal communication

Pattern 3. Relating

3.1.1	Impaired social interaction
3.1.2	Social isolation
*3.2.1	Altered role performance
3.2.1.1.1	Altered parenting
3.2.1.1.2	High risk for altered parenting

(continued)

Appendix: NANDA taxonomy of nursing diagnoses *(continued)*

Pattern 3. Relating *(continued)*

3.2.1.2.1	Sexual dysfunction
3.2.2	Altered family processes
#3.2.2.1	Caregiver role strain
#3.2.2.2	High risk for caregiver role strain
3.2.3.1	Parental role conflict
3.3	Altered sexuality patterns

Pattern 4. Valuing

4.1.1	Spiritual distress (distress of the human spirit)

Pattern 5. Choosing

5.1.1.1	Ineffective individual coping
5.1.1.1.1	Impaired adjustment
5.1.1.1.2	Defensive coping
5.1.1.1.3	Ineffective denial
5.1.2.1.1	Ineffective family coping: Disabling
5.1.2.1.2	Ineffective family coping: Compromised
5.1.2.2	Family coping: Potential for growth
#5.2.1	Ineffective management of therapeutic regimen (individual)
5.2.1.1	Noncompliance (specify)
5.3.1.1	Decisional conflict (specify)
5.4	Health-seeking behaviors (specify)

Pattern 6. Moving

6.1.1.1	Impaired physical mobility
#6.1.1.1.1	High risk for peripheral neurovascular dysfunction
6.1.1.2	Activity intolerance
6.1.1.2.1	Fatigue
6.1.1.3	High risk for activity intolerance
6.2.1	Sleep pattern disturbance
6.3.1.1	Diversional activity deficit
6.4.1.1	Impaired home maintenance management
6.4.2	Altered health maintenance
*6.5.1	Feeding self-care deficit
6.5.1.1	Impaired swallowing
6.5.1.2	Ineffective breast-feeding
#6.5.1.2.1	Interrupted breast-feeding
6.5.1.3	Effective breast-feeding
#6.5.1.4	Ineffective infant feeding pattern
*6.5.2	Bathing or hygiene self-care deficit
*6.5.3	Dressing or grooming self-care deficit
*6.5.4	Toileting self-care deficit
6.6	Altered growth and development
#6.7	Relocation stress syndrome

Pattern 7. Perceiving

*7.1.1	Body image disturbance
*7.1.2	Self-esteem disturbance
7.1.2.1	Chronic low self-esteem
7.1.2.2	Situational low self-esteem
*7.1.3	Personal identity disturbance
7.2	Sensory or perceptual alterations (specify visual, auditory, kinesthetic, gustatory, tactile, olfactory)
7.2.1.1	Unilateral neglect
7.3.1	Hopelessness
7.3.2	Powerlessness

Pattern 8. Knowing

8.1.1	Knowledge deficit (specify)
8.3	Altered thought processes

Appendix: NANDA taxonomy of nursing diagnoses *(continued)*

Pattern 9. Feeling

*9.1.1	Pain
9.1.1.1	Chronic pain
9.2.1.1	Dysfunctional grieving
9.2.1.2	Anticipatory grieving
9.2.2	High risk for violence: Self-directed or directed at others
#9.2.2.1	High risk for self-mutilation

9.2.3	Post-trauma response
9.2.3.1	Rape-trauma syndrome
9.2.3.1.1	Rape-trauma syndrome: Compound reaction
9.2.3.1.2	Rape-trauma syndrome: Silent reaction
9.3.1	Anxiety
9.3.2	Fear

New diagnostic categorieis in 1992
* Categories with modified label terminology

©North American Nursing Diagnosis Association (1992). *NANDA Nursing Diagnoses: Definitions and Classifications 1992-1993.* Philadelphia: NANDA.

Selected References

Auvenshine, M.S., and Enriquez, M.A. *Comprehensive Maternity Nursing: Perinatal and Women's Health* (2nd ed.). Boston: Jones & Bartlett Wadsworth Publishing Co., 1990.

Bobak, I., and Jensen, M. *Essentials of Maternity Nursing,* (3rd ed.). St. Louis: Mosby Inc., 1991.

Brooten, D., et al. "A survey of nutrition, caffeine, cigarette and alcohol intake in early pregnancy in an urban clinic population." *Journal of Nurse-Midwifery* 32(2):85-90, 1987.

Clinton, J. "Physical and emotional responses of expectant fathers throughout pregnancy and the early postpartum period." *International Journal of Nursing Studies* 24(1):59-68, 1987.

Cohen, S.M., et al. *Maternal, Neonatal, and Women's Health Nursing.* Springhouse, PA: Springhouse Corp., 1991.

Colman, A., and Colman, L. *Pregnancy: The psychological experience.* New York: Bantam, 1977.

Conrad, L.H. *Maternal-Neonatal Nursing* (2nd ed.). Springhouse, PA: Springhouse Corp., 1993.

Cranley, M. "Roots of attachment: The relationship of parents with their unborn." *Birth Defects: Original Article Series* 17(6):59-83, 1981.

Creasy, R.K., and Resnik, R., eds. *Maternal-Fetal Medicine: Principles and Practice* (2nd ed.). Philadelphia: W.B. Saunders Co., 1989.

Cunningham, F.G., et al. *Williams Obstetrics* (18th ed.). Norwalk, CT: Appleton and Lange, 1989.

Doenges, M.E., et al. *Maternal/Newborn Care Plans: Guidelines for Client Care.* Philadelphia: F.A.Davis Co., 1988.

Eden, R.D., and Boehm, F.H., eds. *Assessment and Care of the Fetus: Physiological, Clinical, and Medicolegal Principles,* Norwalk, CT: Appleton and Lange, 1990.

Glazer, G. "Anxiety and stressors of expectant fathers." *Western Journal of Nursing Research* 11(1):47-59, 1989.

Kilpatrick S.J., and Laros, R.K. "Characteristics of Normal Labor," *Obstetrics and Gynceology* 74:85, 1989.

Kintz, D.L. "Nursing Support in Labor," *JOGN* 16:126, March/April 1987.

Kitzinger, S. *The experience of childbirth* (5th ed.). New York: Penguin, 1984.

Klebanoff, M.A., Koslowe, P.A., and Kaslow, R. "Epidemiology of vomiting in early pregnancy." *Obstetrics and Gynecology* 66(5):612, 1985.

Lawrence, R.A. *Breastfeeding: A Guide for the Medical Profession* (3rd ed.). St Louis: Mosby Inc., 1989.

May, K. "A typology of detachment/involvement styles adopted during pregnancy by first-time expectant fathers." *Western Journal of Nursing Research* 2(2):445-453, 1980.

May, K. (1982). "Three phases of father involvement in pregnancy." *Nursing Research* 31(6):337-324, 1982.

Mercer, R., Ferketich, S., DeJoseph, J., May, K., and Sollid, D. "Effect of stress on family functioning during pregnancy." *Nursing Research* 37(5):268-275, 1988.

Miller, M., and Brooten, D. *The Childbearing Family: A Nursing Perspective.* Boston: Little, Brown, (1983).

Muenchow, S., and Bloom-Feshbach, J. "The new fatherhood." *Parents,* pages 64-69, February 1982.

Myles, M.F. *Textbook for Midwives* (11th ed.). New York: Churcill Livingstone, 1990.

Naeye, R. (1981). "Influence of maternal cigarette smoking during pregnancy on fetal and childhood growth." *Obstetrics and Gynecology* 57(1):18-21, 1981.

Nichols, F.H., and Hamenick, S.S. *Childbrith Education: Practice, Research, and Theory.* Philadelphia: W.B. Saunders, 1988.

North American Nursing Diagnosis Association. *NANDA nursing diagnoses: Definitions and classifications 1992-1993.* Philadelphia: NANDA, 1992.

Olds, S., et al. *Maternal-Newborn Nursing: A Family-Centered Approach* (4th ed.). Reading, Mass.: Addison-Wesley Publishing Co., 1992.

Pernoll, M.I., et al. *Diagnosis and Management of the Fetus and Neonate at Risk.* St. Louis, Mosby, 1986.

Poland, M.L., et al. "Quality of Prenatal Care: Selected Social, Behavioral, and Biomedical Factors, and Birth Weight," *AJOG* 75:607, April 1990.

Redder, S.J., and Martin, L.L. *Maternity Nursing: Family, Newborn and Women's Health Care* (16th ed.). Philadelphia: J.B. Lippincott Co., 1987.

Reiber, V. (1976). "Is the nurturing role natural to fathers?" *MCN,* 1:336-371, 1976.

Rolfe, R. *You can postpone anything but love: Expanding our potential as parents.* Edgemont, PA: Ambassador Press, 1985.

Scott, J.R., et al. *Danforth's Obstetrics and Gynecology* (6th ed.). Philadelphia: J.B. Lippincott Co., 1990.

Shapiro, J. *When men are pregnant: Needs and concerns of expectant fathers.* San Luis Obispo, CA: Impact Publishers, 1987.

Varney, H. *Nurse-Midwifery* (2nd ed.). Boston: Blackwell Scientific Publications, 1987.

Index